Second Edition

Interpersonal Psychotherapy

A Clinician's Guide

Scott Stuart MD

Professor of Psychiatry, Psychology and Obstetrics and Gynecology,
University of Iowa, Iowa City, Iowa, USA

Director, IPT Institute

Michael Robertson FRANZCP

Clinical Associate Professor, Centre for Valves, Ethics and Law in
Medicine, University of Sydney, Sydney, Australia

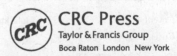

CRC Press
Taylor & Francis Group
Boca Raton London New York

CRC Press is an imprint of the
Taylor & Francis Group, an **informa** business

First published in Great Britain in 2003 by Arnold
This second edition published in 2012 by
Hodder Arnold

Published 2023 by CRC Press
Taylor & Francis Group
6000 Broken Sound Parkway NW, Suite 300
Boca Raton, FL 33487-2742

ISBN 13: 978-1-4441-3754-5 (pbk)

This book contains information obtained from authentic and highly regarded sources. Reasonable efforts have been made to publish reliable data and information, but the author and publisher cannot assume responsibility for the validity of all materials or the consequences of their use. The authors and publishers have attempted to trace the copyright holders of all material reproduced in this publication and apologize to copyright holders if permission to publish in this form has not been obtained. If any copyright material has not been acknowledged please write and let us know so we may rectify in any future reprint.

Visit the Taylor & Francis Web site at
http://www.taylorandfrancis.com

and the CRC Press Web site at
http://www.crcpress.com

Whilst the advice and information in this book are believed to be true and accurate at the date of going to press, neither the author[s] nor the publisher can accept any legal responsibility or liability for any errors or omissions that may be made. In particular (but without limiting the generality of the preceding disclaimer) every effort has been made to check drug dosages; however, it is still possible that errors have been missed. Furthermore, dosage schedules are constantly being revised and new side-effects recognized. For these reasons the reader is strongly urged to consult the drug companies' printed instructions before administering any of the drugs recommended in this book.

British Library Cataloguing in Publication Data
A catalogue record for this book is available from the British Library

Library of Congress Cataloging-in-Publication Data
A catalog record for this book is available from the Library of Congress

Cover Designer: Julie Joubinaux
Cover image © Fotolia

Typeset in MinionPro Disp 10 pts by Datapage (India) Pvt. Ltd.

Contents

Preface

We present herein the second edition of our guide to conducting Interpersonal Psychotherapy (IPT). We are grateful that many clinicians and academicians have used the original edition of this book in their clinical work and teaching over the past decade, as well as in various research projects around the world. Our original intent was (and current intent still is) to publish a text that is useful for clinicians. We seek to encourage clinicians to utilize IPT as a framework in which they can exercise their judgment, recognizing that at least to date, none of the many psychotherapy manuals that have been published (including ours) have been carved in stone and carried down from Mount Horeb.

A flexible approach is needed as manual-based psychotherapies are disseminated from tightly controlled academic settings into the field. Terms such as 'empirically based' or 'empirically supported' treatments are now being used to describe clinical applications, denoting not only that flexibility is important with complex patients,[a] but that rigid adherence to manuals often results in outcomes that are not as good as those obtained when manuals are used as guides and combined with clinical judgment and common sense. Our use of the term 'guide' is intended to convey that IPT is best conceptualized as a treatment which is theoretically grounded, empirical, and clinically validated, and applied with a healthy measure of clinical judgment. We recognize that randomized controlled trials, though critically important, are only one means of obtaining empirical data. The experience of clinicians is also a wealth of qualitative data which should inform clinical practice.

Our primary goal is to assist therapists in their endeavors with the unique individuals with whom they work, with the conviction that IPT is an extremely useful framework for both clinicians and their patients to accomplish the goals that they have mutually set forth. Our objective aim is to provide a guide to the conduct of IPT, but our subjective aim is to help therapists better understand their patients. This mirrors the process of IPT: helping patients alleviate their suffering requires that therapists understand their individual patients, all the while working to help those patients better understand themselves.

Since we last wrote, there have been many changes to IPT which have been disseminated worldwide. Among these are major modifications in the structure of IPT. Acute treatment with IPT is now concluded rather than terminated, with provision made for Maintenance Treatment for most patients. This practice of shifting to maintenance therapy rather than 'terminating' IPT has been the norm in clinical practice for many years. The range of sessions which may be used in IPT has expanded, and is now conceptualized as a flexible dosing range rather than a fixed number. The Problem Areas have been reduced from four to three (eliminating Interpersonal Sensitivity). Each of these changes is grounded in empirical research and clinical experience with IPT.

We have also greatly expanded the application of Attachment and Interpersonal Theory to IPT. A structured IPT Formulation, which has proven to be extremely valuable for clinicians and patients, incorporates this new emphasis. Several specific techniques, such

[a] We have, for convenience sake, chosen to use the term patient throughout the text. In many ways, the term 'patient', which originally meant 'one who suffers', is a very accurate description of the people with whom we work – they are suffering, and are in need of help. In other ways, neither the term 'patient' nor 'client' captures what we would most like to convey; as an alternative, we encourage you to think of the people with whom we work as unique individuals, whose diagnoses, disorders, and distress are but a few of their many human qualities.

as communication analysis, have also been modified. Also new to this edition are some additional clinical tools which have been tested in the field and are now widely disseminated. These include a structured Interpersonal Inventory, a Timeline for Role Transitions, and an Interpersonal Conflict Graph for Interpersonal Disputes. Each is a simple tool designed to help clinicians better understand their patients.

Most importantly, this second edition takes a much broader view of the problems that are amenable to treatment with IPT. Over the past decade there have been a multitude of treatment trials using IPT for many different disorders, and clinical experience has also supported its use transdiagnostically. Given the upcoming shift to *Diagnostic and Statistical Manual of Mental Disorders* (DSM)-V as well as the completely new Research Domain Criteria (RDoC),[1,2] which are under development by the US National Institute of Mental Health, this transdiagnostic approach is both timely and empirically supported. Consequently, we have chosen to use the term 'distress' to encompass these concepts broadly as well as to describe their formulation within IPT.

Since our first edition in 2003, there have been many exemplary studies of IPT for a number of disorders and populations.[b] However, it continues to be the case that, while IPT enjoys even more empirical support for its *efficacy*, there is still limited research evaluating its *effectiveness* in typical clinical settings. As we noted a decade ago, this is the case for all of the empirically validated psychotherapies. In other words, IPT (and other evidence-based practices) have been empirically demonstrated to be of benefit when used:

- In academic settings with therapists specifically devoted to their application
- With subjects (as opposed to patients) who meet carefully selected diagnostic criteria and do not have comorbid diagnoses
- With subjects who agree to be involved in randomized clinical trials
- With subjects who are not required to pay for treatment
- With tightly controlled protocols which dictate strict adherence to a manual.

In contrast, most clinicians work in settings in which it would be nearly inconceivable to meet weekly with a patient for 12, 16, or any arbitrary number of consecutive weeks as research protocols require. Most clinicians are paid for direct patients services rather than being paid by a research grant. Most clinicians do not have the luxury of working with patients with major depression without any comorbid diagnoses – many 'real-life' patients have combinations of depression, anxiety, dysfunctional personality traits, substance abuse, and many other problems. Most patients who seek treatment in community clinics do so with a preconceived idea about the kind of treatment they want, whether it is medication, therapy, or something else. They are different from subjects in research studies who agree to be randomly assigned to treatment. There are no distressed patients who come to community clinics and ask to be treated by being randomized to a placebo.

While empirical research regarding the *efficacy* of a treatment is essential (e.g. its benefit when applied in a strict research setting in a randomized, controlled study), the *effectiveness* of a treatment (e.g. its benefit when applied in clinical settings) is the ultimate measure of its clinical utility.[3,4] Though population-based empirical research regarding the effectiveness of IPT is not well-developed at present, there is a great deal of clinical wisdom and experience which does address its use in the community. This clinical experience is also a form of research: the careful observation of the application of IPT and the responses of patients to adaptations and changes is qualitative data. We believe that the practice of IPT should be

[b] See Chapters 19 and 20.

based on both empirical data gathered from randomized trials and from the qualitative data derived from clinical experience.[c]

This conviction leads to a fundamental conclusion about manualized forms of IPT and manualized treatments in general. Requiring strict adherence to a manual outside of a research protocol is likely to diminish the effectiveness of the treatment because it discourages therapists from utilizing their clinical experience. This assertion is now supported by evidence: experienced therapists have been shown to have better outcomes when they more flexibly deliver empirically validated treatments.[5,6]

The data – observable and inferential data – that a therapist obtains from a patient during therapy, such as the kind of insight the patient is developing, the degree to which she is motivated to change, the effect of the transference on the therapeutic interaction, and the quality of the therapeutic alliance, should assist the therapist to decide whether the patient might benefit from a homework assignment, might develop more insight with a well-timed therapist self-disclosure, or might have greater improvement with 20 as opposed to 16 sessions of therapy. These decisions should be mutually determined within each therapeutic dyad, not dictated 'a priori' by a manual.[7-9] Thus this book is a guide rather than a manual – it provides a set of principles which serve as a framework for the conduct of IPT rather than a set of rules which constrain it.

This is reflected in our description of the structure of IPT in this second edition. For instance, we originally noted that clinical experience had made clear that conducting consecutive weekly sessions of IPT, then terminating treatment abruptly after 12 or 16 sessions, was not the best way to conduct IPT most effectively in a clinical setting. Since then, several well-controlled efficacy trials have been conducted in which Acute Treatment with IPT was concluded, often with sessions tapering in frequency over time, and Maintenance Treatment was then provided.[10-12] Outcomes using this approach have been superior in reducing relapse, as experienced clinicians have known for some time. Since there are data which demonstrate that many disorders such as depression recur,[13,14] and since Maintenance IPT reduces the risk of recurrence,[10,11] it is literally malpractice not to provide it if patients are at high risk.

The provision of Maintenance Treatment means that IPT should not be terminated. It is much more *effective* to negotiate the scheduling of sessions with each patient, to meet for several biweekly or monthly sessions prior to concluding Acute Treatment, and to provide Maintenance Treatment as indicated. Acute Treatment with IPT should be concluded, not terminated. Clinical experience with IPT as well as empirical data also support a Biopsychosocial formulation for IPT. The Biopsychosocial model is used universally in psychiatry, psychology, and medicine.[15-19] More recent clinical experience suggests that expanding this model to include cultural and spiritual factors is likely to be of even more benefit.[d] Human psychological functioning is complex, multifactorial, and far beyond characterization as a simple medical 'disorder'. We are more than the sum of our genes or our 'medical' selves.

It is our belief that strict adherence to a medical model of psychopathology dehumanizes both the therapist and the person with whom she is working. The medical model requires that *patients*, not *people*, must be diagnosed with a specific medical disorder, usually as defined by DSM[20] or the International Classification of Diseases (ICD)[21] criteria. This approach not only categorizes and defines the people with whom we work by their 'symptoms' or 'diagnoses', it limits our ability to understand them as unique individuals, and to work creatively with them to develop solutions to the problems they are experiencing. Since the primary goal of therapy in general, and IPT

[c] This same principle applies to all other empirically validated treatments, whether they are psychotherapeutic or psychopharmacologic.

[d] We are indebted to our colleagues Rob McAlpine and Anthony Hillin for this improvement in IPT.

specifically, is to understand the person seeking treatment, using only strict medical diagnoses to develop that understanding and reflect it to the patient is simply poor clinical practice. IPT should be based on a comprehensive Biopsychosocial/Cultural/Spiritual formulation.

Therefore, although a symptom-based diagnostic system is an important way to understand patients, it should not be used as the primary basis for conceptualizing patients' distress, nor as a requirement for treatment with IPT. IPT can be used clinically with patients who present with interpersonal problems. Some will be depressed, some will be anxious, some will have personality issues, and many will have combinations of these factors. Some will be old, some adolescents; some will be male, some female; some will be from cultural backgrounds different from their therapists'; some will be poor, some wealthy; but all will be individuals who can be understood in part as social beings who are intimately involved in a social network, and are therefore potential candidates for IPT. The question of whether the treatment should be applied in a clinical setting if the patient does not meet strict diagnostic criteria is not relevant; it is the individual's unique problems and distress and social context that should be used to make a determination regarding her suitability for IPT.

In sum, the empirical evidence of efficacy should form the foundation for the clinical delivery of IPT, should be built upon by clinical experience, and should be supplemented by clinical judgment.

The History of IPT

The early developmental trajectory of IPT was different from most of the other 'brands' of empirically supported psychotherapy currently practiced. Most have been derived from clinical observations which gradually coalesced into theories explaining how the treatments 'worked'. In many cases, such as that exemplified by behavioral therapy, these theoretical hypotheses about the mechanisms of change led to specific therapeutic techniques.

Over the past four decades, the movement towards the delivery of evidence-based medicine has required that psychotherapeutic treatments also be empirically validated. Largely influenced by psychopharmacologic trials, randomized and well-controlled efficacy treatment trials have been the 'sine qua non' method for 'proving' that a particular psychotherapy works.[22] Empirically supported treatments (ESTs) are defined as 'clearly specified psychological treatments shown to be efficacious in controlled research with a delineated population',[23] and specific criteria have been established to define what an EST is[24] (Box 0.1). At the time of this writing, the American Psychological Association (APA) Division 12[25] lists 60 psychotherapies that meet these criteria (Box 0.1).

Thus the progression of most recently developed psychotherapies, epitomized by cognitive behavioral therapy (CBT), has moved from clinical observation to theory to randomized treatment trials. Efficacy testing is critical: it is becoming increasingly common around the world that reimbursement and licensure are tied to provision of ESTs. Because of this, there is a lot at stake in ensuring that one's favorite therapy, especially if one is the developer, is on the EST list. This has compounded the rigidity of manualized therapies – once on the list and recognized as empirically validated or supported, there is every reason to insist that one's favored therapy be delivered exactly as described. Manuals become dogma rather than a set of guiding principles.

This same process occurs when pharmaceutical companies market their US Food and Drug Administration (FDA)-approved psychopharmacologic medications. It is in the

Box 0.1 Criteria for well-established empirically validated psychotherapy

I. At least two good between-group design experiments demonstrating efficacy in one or more of the following ways:
   A. Superior (statistically significantly so) to pill or psychological placebo or to another treatment
   B. Equivalent to an already established treatment in experiments with adequate sample sizes
or
II. A large series of single case design experiments (n >9) demonstrating efficacy. These experiments must have:
   A. Used good experimental designs
   B. Compared the intervention to another treatment as in IA

Further criteria for both I and II:
   C. Experiments must be conducted with treatment manuals
   D. Characteristics of the client samples must be clearly specified
   E. Effects must have been demonstrated by at least two different investigators or teams

developer's interest to make every possible distinction between his medication or therapy and all of the others, and to argue for the superiority and universality of his treatment. A treatment that is advertised as better than others increases sales. It is not in the developer's interest to make any adaptations or changes to the treatment because adaptations or changes put the FDA approval or APA approval at risk. This contrasts with the ideal bidirectional collaboration which should occur when empirically validated treatments are disseminated. Ideally, as experience is gained and additional clinical observations accumulate, both theory and techniques should be modified and then tested for efficacy once again. This bidirectional or circular approach to psychotherapy development recognizes that data also come from clinical practice. The best evidence-based practices recognize practice-based evidence (Figure 0.1).

Clinical observations lead to a theoretical understanding of psychopathology and mechanisms of change. These are then translated into clinical strategies and techniques which are refined during pilot testing. A manual or guide is then developed and the treatment empirically tested; those that are efficacious are disseminated clinically. Often, the process stops at this point. Ideally, once the treatment is disseminated, additional clinical observations are collected and used to further refine the theory and improve clinical interventions. These are then pilot tested, added to a revised manual, and empirically tested and disseminated once again. The process is dynamic and evolving, and leads to therapies that are both efficacious and effective.

IPT evolved in a strikingly different fashion than most ESTs. Rather than beginning as a set of clinical observations that were used as the basis for a coherent theory of psychopathology and led to specific techniques to bring about change, IPT began as a manualized treatment developed for a research protocol. In fact, IPT was initially developed not as a clinical treatment, but for the express purpose of serving as a manualized 'placebo condition' for a psychopharmacologic treatment trial for depression.[26-29] It was largely accidental that IPT was discovered to be of benefit.

In order to understand the original IPT model, it is important to note that it was developed in the 1970s,[26] during which time the medical model of psychopathology reigned supreme. At that time, there was an increasing emphasis on medical treatments, particularly psychotropic medications, fueled both by the pharmaceutical industry and the desire of many psychiatrists to be seen as legitimate, empirically based 'medical' specialists.[30,31] It was

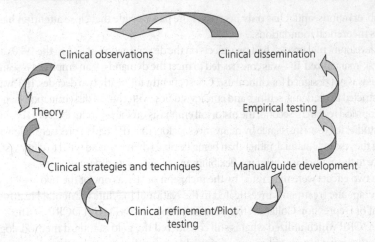

Figure 0.1 Psychotherapy development: an ideal approach

widely held within this model that psychotherapy was not particularly effective, and that it should largely be subsumed by psychopharmacologic treatments.

Nonetheless, some early studies investigating the treatment of depression with medication included psychotherapy as a treatment component, as the trials were designed to mirror the clinical practice of the time, which generally included some form of psychodynamic psychotherapy along with medication.[e] Klerman, Weissman, and their colleagues incorporated a manualized form of psychotherapy in their medication trials for depression for this reason. This manualized treatment, which later became IPT, was initially called a 'high contact' condition,[32] the presumption being that there might be some benefit from the non-specific effects of contact with a therapist, but none that would be attributable to any specific techniques.[29]

Explicitly following the model established by pharmacologic treatment trials, a codified manual describing the procedures and techniques to be used in the psychotherapy condition was developed, so that fidelity to treatment could be preserved. The primary concern of the investigators was that the therapeutic treatment was reproducible – the specific techniques to be used and the theoretical basis for the psychotherapeutic interventions were of secondary importance.[29] In contrast to the investigators' expectations, the early studies of IPT demonstrated that it had a therapeutic effect.[26,28] As IPT was largely conceived of as a 'social work' or 'social support' intervention, it was hypothesized that changes in social circumstances and social relationships were largely the driving force behind improvement. The investigators' enthusiasm to continue to empirically test IPT in rigorously controlled trials led to the use of IPT in many research settings.

In short, IPT was initially constructed in 'retrograde' fashion rather than being derived from clinical observations which were used to develop a theory of psychopathology and to develop specific techniques. IPT began as a manualized therapy which was believed to be an inert treatment, or at most was simply thought to be a codification of 'non-specific' therapeutic factors common to all psychotherapies. The original purpose of IPT was to serve as a credible and reproducible placebo psychotherapy. It was not originally developed from

---

[e] Some have suggested that psychotherapies were included in these medication treatment trials with the intent of demonstrating that they were not effective, thus reinforcing the primacy of biological psychiatry.

clinical observations, and it has only been over the past decade that close attention has been paid to its theoretical foundations.

This developmental process had two effects on the dissemination of IPT in the 1980s and 1990s. First, 'manualized' IPT was constructed to meet the demands of an empirical research protocol; it was not designed for clinical use. Consequently, for nearly two decades, IPT was largely restricted to academic settings and efficacy studies, with clinical dissemination lagging far behind empirical research. Second, the historical emphasis on the reproducibility of IPT in efficacy research studies led to an insistence by many investigators that IPT had to precisely follow the dictates of the research manual, rather than being flexible when it was adapted to clinical settings. Adherence to the manual was primary; flexibility and quality were distant seconds.

These two effects were magnified by the inclusion of IPT as one of the two psychotherapeutic treatments investigated in the National Institute of Mental Health Treatment of Depression Collaborative Research Program (NIMH-TDCRP).[33] The NIMH-TDCRP, which utilized what is still considered the gold-standard methodology for psychotherapy efficacy studies, was designed to definitively answer how efficacious psychotherapy (IPT and CBT specifically) and medication were as acute treatments for depression. The rigorous design dictated that IPT be adapted to the research protocol, rather than adapting the protocol design to reflect good clinical use of IPT.[33] For instance, the description of the NIMH-TDCRP protocol specifically states that the length of the treatments selected for the trial were based on the requirements of the psychopharmacologists, not on the needs of the psychotherapists. To quote Elkin *et al.*:[33]

> All treatment conditions are 16 weeks long. This treatment length was based primarily on pharmacotherapy practice current at the time this program was initiated; the two experimental psychotherapies are frequently only 12 weeks long.

The rigorous NIMH-TDCRP design further entrenched IPT as a 'research' therapy following a medical model. The emphasis on reproducibility and adherence to the IPT manual led to an insistence that it continue to be conducted exactly as specified in the NIMH-TDCRP protocol. Rather than being conceptualized as a dynamically developing treatment which should incorporate new clinical observations and clinical experience, the way IPT was manualized in the NIMH-TDCRP became for many years the singular and 'correct' way to conduct it. For nearly two decades this 16-week protocol was used inflexibly by many IPT clinicians.

Ironically, the flexibility that was included in the NIMH-TDCRP protocol was ignored by those advocating rigid adherence to the manual. In fact, clinical judgment was permitted, and flexibility was explicit. To quote the investigators once again:[33]

> There are, however, some slight differences in the total number and frequency of treatment sessions. These differences are consistent with usual practice for each of the approaches. The patients in CB therapy receive 12 sessions over the course of the first eight weeks, followed by eight sessions once a week, for a total of 20 sessions. The patients in IPT receive 16 weekly sessions with the therapist having the option of scheduling up to four additional sessions, for a total of 16 to 20 sessions.

There was also a wide range of psychotherapy delivery in the NIMH-TDCRP. Though the treatments were planned to be 16 weeks in length, the average number of sessions actually delivered was only 13.0.

The NIMH-TDCRP was structured with the intentional inclusion of therapeutic judgment. Therapists were allowed to schedule up to four additional sessions at their discretion. A reasonable interpretation of the data is that there should be flexibility in the structure of IPT, and that a dosing range should be used for individual patients. This was not the way that IPT was disseminated for nearly two decades. The early manuals became a set of rigid rules rather than clinical guidelines, and dissemination was hindered.

Another ramification of the inclusion of IPT in the NIMH-TDCRP was that some of the components in the original IPT research manual were included (or excluded) primarily as a means of distinguishing it from CBT. By intent, the two psychotherapies to be compared were to be as different as possible in hypothesized effects, therapeutic stance, and specific interventions.[33] Some techniques which are intrinsic to CBT, such as the assignment of homework, were intentionally excluded from IPT. IPT was described as relying largely on 'non-specific' techniques such as non-directive exploration and clarification in order to distinguish it from the behavioral components of CBT. Thus the exclusion of homework specified in the early IPT manuals, for example, was the result of research expedience rather than being supported by a specific theoretical rationale or by clinical experience. The lack of techniques specific to IPT, and the lack of techniques derived from a theoretical base, led some critics to describe IPT as nothing more than a 'time-limited psychodynamic psychotherapy', or a sophisticated means of encouraging social support.[34]

Another major influence of the NIMH-TDCRP on the development of IPT was that the major outcome measures used were focused on symptom reduction. Because medications for depression are targeted specifically at DSM symptoms, the efficacy of IPT as a comparison treatment was measured by the reduction it brought about in depressive symptoms. This reduced IPT (and CBT) to simplistic analogs of antidepressant medication.[35] The implication was that the 'value' of IPT was restricted to the narrow focus of relieving a predefined cluster of symptoms rather than recognizing the benefit of IPT for more broadly defined psychological distress.

While there is no doubt that symptom relief is a highly desirable goal, and no doubt that a multitude of efficacy studies demonstrate that IPT does lead to reduction in symptoms, this narrow focus has displaced attention from the other benefits of IPT. These include potential changes in insight, improvement in social relationships, general life satisfaction and well-being, and an acceptance of life circumstances which is more congruent with the patient's condition. Though these concepts are very difficult to quantify and to measure, neglecting them as changes in IPT, and focusing narrowly on symptomatic outcome alone, runs the risk of missing some of the most powerful and beneficial aspects of the therapy – changes that would be unique to psychotherapy as opposed to the use of medication.

Though the more comprehensive Biopsychosocial/Cultural/Spiritual model is now widely used in IPT, most IPT research still continues to be focused narrowly on symptomatic relief. Most research in IPT continues to examine its application to well-circumscribed DSM psychiatric disorders, rather than examining its impact on interpersonal problems in general. There is a great need for effectiveness studies of IPT in the community with complex patients that focus on presenting problems rather than strict diagnoses, as well as a need for investigation of changes in interpersonal functioning, social functioning, and general distress.

Fortunately, over the past decade, adaptations to IPT have occurred, driven both by clinical experience and research. The application of IPT to more complex populations and to non-affective disorders has led to changes such as the modification of frequency and duration of treatment, development of maintenance treatment, and the combination of IPT with other modalities. These have been implemented in training as well. IPT is now disseminated and practiced as a flexible principle-guided treatment, reflecting what is universally recognized as the most appropriate and effective means of delivering ESTs. To quote the American Psychological Association:[36]

The APA has identified 'best research evidence' as a major component of evidence-based practice. This research evidence for psychological treatments *will necessarily be combined with clinician expertise and patient values and characteristics in determining optimum approaches to treatment.* (emphasis added)

These changes and the flexible approach to IPT that is now used are emphasized in this text. These include a shift to Conclusion of Acute Treatment followed by Maintenance Treatment, a flexible approach to scheduling sessions, and flexibility in utilizing the three Problem Areas. These changes also reflect the further development of the theoretical basis of IPT, from the original description of the use of Attachment and Interpersonal Theory in IPT in our first edition to current data supporting the impact of attachment in the clinical delivery of IPT.[37-39]

These changes are of critical importance in fostering the dissemination of IPT. A new paradigm of clinical practice is emerging. Driven by insurer and governmental demands that therapists deliver evidence-based treatments, IPT and many of the other ESTs are being rolled out across the globe. This trend hearkens a profound change: community-based clinicians will be expected to be trained in IPT and other ESTs in order to be reimbursed or employed in mental health systems. It is our responsibility to ensure that these therapists are well-trained, can utilize a variety of ESTs, and that they can deliver high-quality ESTs *combined with clinician expertise and patient values and characteristics to provide the optimum approach to treatment for the specific individuals with whom they work.*

A Metaphor for IPT and Other Empirically Supported Therapies

Learning psychotherapy is like learning to play chess. If you want to learn how to play chess well, you need to do two things: read books which explain how to play, and play a lot of games against the best competition you can find.

Nearly all chess textbooks divide games into opening, middle, and endgame phases. There are always detailed discussions about how to begin the game, ranging from simple descriptions of the movements of the various pieces to elaborate opening defenses such as the Italian Game or the Vienna Game. Chess manuals also have detailed descriptions of the conclusions of games. As with the opening phases, elaborate descriptions and analyses are offered for the few moves which conclude a game. In contrast, there isn't much information about what happens in the middle of games. This is particularly striking considering how much of the game actually takes place in this 'middle' phase. The middle of the game is shrouded in mystery, a black box which connects the input of the opening phase to the endgame output.

Psychotherapy manuals are like chess textbooks. Most provide detailed information about selecting patients for the specific therapy being described, beginning treatment, and introducing the treatment model to the patient. This is usually followed by a brief review of techniques that might be used (a simple description of how the pieces move outside of the context of an actual game), and then a detailed description of the end of therapy is given. There is good reason to be critical of this approach, which neglects the importance of understanding techniques in the context of the whole treatment. However, much of the reason that disproportionate time is spent on the opening phases of chess games and psychotherapy treatments, and the reason that so much effort is expended on the end of the games/treatments, is that these are the only two times in the process when things can be described with any precision. There are too many permutations and too many possibilities to even begin to describe what happens in the middle of the game or the middle of therapy. In contrast, the limited possibilities of move and countermove, statement and response, during the opening phase make it more amenable to precise description. When only a few pieces are left at the end, or when only a session or two is left, it again becomes possible to offer more precise descriptions – there aren't so many moves that they defy analysis.

Textbooks which give an ordered list of sequential moves to make in a chess game are of little value. Manuals which prescribe what a therapist is to do each and every session are of little value. Patients are different. Some don't want to do homework; some don't want to set an agenda. Some will follow the lead of the therapist; some won't. In each and every case, adaptations have to be made. There are too many ways the middle of the game can be played to script every move.

This is where playing a lot of games with the best competition and working with the most challenging patients comes into the picture. Experience is the best way to learn to conduct the Middle Phase – more so if there is a chess master or psychotherapy supervisor to offer further insights and tips along the way. Experience and skill come from practice. Learning what to do in the Middle Phase, developing a repertoire of moves and strategies and knowing what tactics to use, depends not on rigidly following a manual but on refining intuition and judgment. Master chess players and master therapists develop an intuitive sense of what will work best in a particular session with a particular client, and have the experience to decide when and how to do it. Master chess players and therapists are artisans, not technicians. As one devotes a lifetime to mastering chess, expert clinicians do the same with continual study, self-reflection, and constant practice.

After studying the 'how-to' manuals and getting some experience playing games, chess players move on to the 'case-study' books that describe the great games of the masters. Rather than providing technical information, these case studies are read to hone the chess player's sense of judgment, timing, and intuition – to get inside the mind of the great chess masters. Similarly, at a high level of development, therapists also learn from case studies describing individual cases from which general principles can be gleaned.

Master psychotherapists are those who work to understand the craft of psychotherapy as well as specific techniques. While opening chess defenses and various forms of psychotherapy are important tools to have at one's disposal, they do not constitute the whole of the experience or the process of therapy. Just as chess masters intimately understand a variety of opening strategies, psychotherapy masters should understand and practice a variety of approaches. The art of chess and psychotherapy is making well-informed judgments about when to use which specific strategies and having the ability to carry them out. Master clinicians, like master chess players, recognize that textbooks and manuals are limited. Though helpful in providing a framework for treatment, clinical practice demands that therapists be flexible and that they use clinical judgment in applying the therapy to individual patients. The psychotherapy texts, like the chess books, should be used as guides to treatment. The ability to combine experience and judgment and a willingness to practice diligently is what makes a clinician an expert.

Conclusion

This text is designed to guide clinicians who wish to practice IPT. Our primary goal is to make IPT available and applicable – to encourage the dissemination of what we believe to be an extraordinary treatment for a variety of interpersonal problems and psychiatric syndromes. We offer a paradigm universally accepted by clinicians and researchers alike: IPT is an EST that can be used as a foundation for therapists using their clinical experience within each unique clinical relationship. IPT is grounded in theory, empirical research, and clinical experience, and should always incorporate clinical judgment.

IPT: An Established Paradigm

1. The practice of IPT should be based on theory, empirical data, and clinical experience.
2. Incorporating new empirical data and clinical experience into the IPT model will continue to improve treatment.
3. IPT therapists should utilize IPT as an EST, meaning that adaptations to individual patients and circumstances will enhance outcome.
4. Utilizing clinical judgment within an IPT framework will improve outcome.
5. IPT need not be restricted to specific diagnostic entities, but can be applied to a variety of interpersonal problems.

References

1. Cuthbert BN and Insel TR. Toward new approaches to psychotic disorders: the NIMH Research Domain Criteria project. *Schizophrenia Bulletin*, 2010, **36**(6): 1061–1062.
2. Insel T, *et al*. Research domain criteria (RDoC): toward a new classification framework for research on mental disorders. *American Journal of Psychiatry*, 2010, **167**(7): 748–751.
3. Nathan PE, Stuart S and Dolan S. Research on psychotherapy efficacy and effectiveness: between Scylla and Charybdis? *Psychological Bulletin*, 2000, **126**: 964–981.
4. Barlow DH. Health care policy, psychotherapy research, and the future of psychotherapy. *American Psychologist*, 1996, **51**: 1050–1058.
5. Barber J, *et al*. The role of therapist adherence, therapist competence, and the alliance in predicting outcome of individual drug counseling: results from the NIDA collaborative cocaine treatment study. *Psychotherapy Research*, 2006, **16**: 229–240.
6. Castonguay L, *et al*. Predicting the effect of cognitive therapy for depression: a study of unique and common factors. *Journal of Consulting and Clinical Psychology*, 1996, **64**: 497–504.
7. Edelson M. Can psychotherapy research answer this psychotherapist's questions?, in Talley PF, Strupp HH and Butler SF (eds) *Psychotherapy Research and Practice: Bridging the Gap*. 1994, New York: Basic Books.
8. Garfield SL. Some problems associated with 'validated' forms of psychotherapy. *Clinical Psychology: Science and Practice*, 1996, **3**: 218–229.
9. Strauss BM and Kaechele H. The writing on the wall: comments on the current discussion about empirically validated treatments in Germany. *Psychotherapy Research*, 1998, **8**: 158–170.
10. Frank E, *et al*. Interpersonal psychotherapy and antidepressant medication: evaluation of a sequential treatment strategy in women with recurrent major depression. *Journal of Clinical Psychiatry*, 2000, **61**: 51–57.
11. Frank E, *et al*. randomized trial of weekly, twice-monthly, and monthly interpersonal psychotherapy as maintenance treatment for women with recurrent depression. *American Journal of Psychiatry*, 2007, **164**: 761–767.

12. Talbot N, *et al*. A randomized effectiveness trial of interpersonal psychotherapy for depressed women with sexual abuse histories. *Psychiatric Services*, 2011, **62**: 374–380.

13. Kessler RC, *et al*. The epidemiology of major depressive disorder: results from the National Comorbidity Survey Replication (NCS-R). *Journal of the American Medical Association*, 2003, **289**: 3095–3105.

14. Kessler RC, *et al*. Lifetime prevalence and age-of-onset distributions of DSM-IV disorders in the National Comorbidity Survey Replication. *Archives of General Psychiatry*, 2005, **62**: 593–602.

15. Engel GL. The clinical application of biopsychosocial models. *American Journal of Psychiatry*, 1980, **137**: 535–544.

16. Engel GL. The biopsychosocial model and medical education: who are to be the teachers? *New England Journal of Medicine*, 1982, **306**: 802–805.

17. Sadler JZ and Hulgus YF. Clinical problem solving and the biopsychosocial model. *American Journal of Psychiatry*, 1992, **149**: 1315–1323.

18. Hartmann L. Presidential address: reflections on humane values and biopsychosocial integration. *American Journal of Psychiatry*, 1992, **149**: 1135–1141.

19. Fava G and Sonino N. The biopsychosocial model 30 years later. *Psychotherapy and Psychosomatics*, 2008, **77**: 1–2.

20. American Psychiatric Association. *Diagnostic and Statistical Manual of Mental Disorders*, 4th edn. 1994, Washington, DC: American Psychiatric Association.

21. World Health Organization. *International Statistical Classification of Diseases and Related Health Problems: ICD-10*, 10th edn. 1992, Geneva: World Health Organization.

22. Parloff MB. Placebo controls in psychotherapy research a sine qua non or a placebo for research problems? *Journal of Consulting and Clinical Psychology*, 1986, **54**: 79–87.

23. Chambless DL and Hollon S. Defining empirically supported therapies. *Journal of Consulting and Clinical Psychology*, 1998, **66**: 7–18.

24. Chambless DL, *et al*. Update on empirically validated therapies, II. *Clinical Psychologist*, 1998, **51**(1): 3–16.

25. Society of Clinical Psychology APA Division 12. *Psychological Treatments*. 2011. Available at: www.psychology.sunysb.edu/eklonsky-/division12/treatments.html.

26. Klerman GL, *et al*. Treatment of depression by drugs and psychotherapy. *American Journal of Psychiatry*, 1974, **131**: 186–191.

27. Weissman MM. The psychological treatment of depression. Evidence for the efficacy of psychotherapy alone, in comparison with, and in combination with pharmacotherapy. *Archives of General Psychiatry*, 1979, **36**: 1261–1269.

28. Weissman MM, *et al*. The efficacy of drugs and psychotherapy in the treatment of acute depressive episodes. *American Journal of Psychiatry*, 1979, **136**(4B): 555–558.

29. Weissman MM. A brief history of interpersonal psychotherapy. *Psychiatric Annals*, 2006, **36**(8): 553–557.

30. Detre T. The future of psychiatry. *American Journal of Psychiatry*, 1987, **144**: 621–625.

31. Detre T and McDonald MC. Managed care and the future of psychiatry. *Archives of General Psychiatry*, 1997, **54**: 201–204.

32. DiMascio A, Weissman MM and Prusoff BA. Differential symptom reduction by drugs and psychotherapy in acute depression. *Archives of General Psychiatry*, 1979, **36**: 1450–1456.

33. Elkin I, *et al*. NIMH Treatment of Depression Collaborative Treatment Program: background and research plan. *Archives of General Psychiatry*, 1985, **42**: 305–316.

34. Markowitz JC, Svartberg M and Swartz HA. Is IPT time-limited psychodynamic psychotherapy? *Journal of Psychotherapy Research and Practice*, 1998, **7**: 185–195.

35. Stiles WB and Shapiro DA. Abuse of the drug metaphor in psychotherapy process-outcome research. *Clinical Psychology Review*, 1989, **9**: 521–544.

36. APA Presidential Task Force on Evidence-Based Practice. Evidence-based practice in psychology. *American Psychologist*, 2006, **61**: 271–285.

37. Ravitz P, Maunder R and McBride C. Attachment, contemporary interpersonal theory and IPT: an integration of theoretical, clinical, and empirical perspectives. *Journal of Contemporary Psychotherapy*, 2008, **38**(1): 11–22.

38. McBride C, *et al*. Attachment as a moderator of treatment outcome in major depression: a randomized control trial of interpersonal psychotherapy versus cognitive behavior therapy. *Journal of Consulting and Clinical Psychology*, 2006, **74**: 1041–1054.

39. Stuart S and Noyes R Jr. Attachment and interpersonal communication in somatization. *Psychosomatics*, 1999, **40**(1): 34–43.

Acknowledgments

We are indebted to many for their help with this project. We are particularly grateful to Mike O'Hara and the staff of the Iowa Depression and Research Center, the participants in the IPT Institute, and the many clinicians and colleagues we have had the privilege of working with over the years.

A personal and heartfelt thanks as well to the many patients we have had the privilege of working with. We are grateful for all we have learned from you, and for the graciousness with which you have shared your life stories with us.

Finally we are grateful to our families: Shana, Kaela, Ryson, Darra, and Logan, and to Anna and Lucas.

Scott Stuart – Iowa City, USA
Michael Robertson – Sydney, Australia

Section 1

Introduction

Introduction

Interpersonal Psychotherapy (IPT) is a short-term, attachment-based psychotherapy which aims to alleviate patients' suffering and improve their interpersonal functioning. IPT focuses specifically on interpersonal relationships as a means of bringing about interpersonal change and symptomatic recovery, with the goal of helping patients to improve their interpersonal relationships and to learn to ask more graciously for the emotional and practical support they need. In addition, IPT also aims to assist patients to improve their social support so that they can better manage their current interpersonal distress.

IPT was originally developed in a research context as a treatment for major depression and was codified in a research manual by Klerman *et al.* in 1984.[1] Since that time, as clinical experience and empirical evidence supporting IPT has accumulated, its use has broadened to include not only the treatment of patients with a variety of well-specified diagnoses as described in the *Diagnostic and Statistical Manual of Mental Disorders* (DSM)-IV,[2] but also the treatment of patients presenting with a variety of interpersonal problems and those with psychological 'distress' broadly conceptualized.

IPT reflects the best of both empirical research and clinical experience, incorporating changes as additional data (both quantitative and qualitative) and clinical experience continue to grow. IPT is not static or fixed; clinical experience and research have (and will continue) to inform modifications to IPT. Since the publication of *Interpersonal Psychotherapy: A Clinician's Guide* in 2003, the modified and flexible structure of IPT has fostered its dissemination and utilization in general clinical settings, moving beyond its previously exclusive use in randomized treatment trials in academic research settings. Moreover, this flexible structure, which allows and encourages therapists to apply their clinical judgment when providing IPT, has also increased its effectiveness and allowed it to be applied to a more diverse group of patients.

As was the case with our first edition, this updated guide is written to reflect the current 'state of the art' of IPT, recognizing that future research and clinical experience will lead to further refinements in the treatment, and that IPT will continue to evolve and improve over time. It is our conviction that this should and must be the case in order to maximize its effectiveness. We are grateful to have the opportunity to publish this revision, but our hope is that there will continue to be subsequent revisions as new clinicians and investigators develop even better techniques and tactics within the IPT framework. Both empirical data and clinical experience have contributed, and should continue to contribute, to the IPT model and its clinical application.

Characteristics of IPT

IPT is characterized by four primary elements. First, as is clear from the name, it focuses specifically on interpersonal relationships and social support as points of intervention. Second, IPT is based on a Biopsychosocial/Cultural/Spiritual model of psychological functioning. Third, IPT is short-term in the Acute Phase of Treatment. Fourth, the interventions used in IPT typically do not directly address the patient–therapist relationship as it develops in therapy (Box 1.1).

Box 1.1 Characteristics of IPT

> ○ IPT focuses specifically on **interpersonal relationships and social support** as points of intervention
> ○ IPT is based on a **Biopsychosocial/Cultural/Spiritual model** of psychological functioning
> ○ IPT is **short-term in the Acute Phase of treatment**
> ○ IPT **interventions typically do not directly address the patient–therapist relationship**

IPT Is Interpersonally Oriented

IPT is based on the premise that interpersonal distress is intimately connected with psychiatric symptoms and psychological distress generally. Thus the foci of IPT are twofold. The first is *the conflicts, transitions, and losses in the patient's relationship*: the aim is to help the patient to either improve communication within those relationships, or to develop more realistic expectations about them. The second focus is *helping the patient to build or better utilize her extended social support network* so that she is better able to muster the interpersonal support needed to deal with the crises which precipitated the distress.

This approach is extremely well-suited, for instance, to the treatment of women who may be experiencing postpartum depression.[3] Many women in these circumstances describe that their distress is linked to conflicts in their relationships with their partners. In addition, many also report that they have difficulty making the transition from 'working woman' to 'mother', and that this change in social circumstances and social support contributes to their problems. An IPT therapist would help her to resolve the conflicts with her partner over issues such as division of childcare labor, and would also assist the woman to garner more support from her social network. This might include connecting with and asking for support from other friends who have had children, extended family members, or colleagues at work. It could also include encouraging her to get involved in a new mothers' support group. Resolution of the particular interpersonal conflict, along with improved interpersonal support while the Role Transition is being negotiated, leads to symptomatic improvement and improvement in interpersonal functioning.

This is a clear distinction between IPT and treatments such as Cognitive Behavior Therapy (CBT)[4] and psychoanalytically oriented psychotherapy. In contrast to CBT, in which the primary focus of treatment is the patient's internally based cognitions and schema, IPT focuses first and foremost on the patient's interpersonal communications with others in her interpersonal sphere and on her social support. In contrast to analytically oriented treatments, in which the primary focus of treatment is on understanding the contribution of early life experiences to psychological functioning, IPT focuses primarily on helping the patient to improve her communication and social support in the present. Past experiences, while clearly influencing current functioning, are not a major focus of intervention.

This critical distinction between IPT and other psychotherapies merits further emphasis because it is often missed or glossed over by proponents of other approaches. There is no doubt that all psychotherapies address interpersonal functioning to some degree – it is the bread and butter of the problems that lead people to seek counseling. The difference is in the emphasis. In IPT, these interpersonal issues – Grief and Loss, Interpersonal Disputes, and Role Transitions – are the **primary** foci of treatment. In CBT, psychodynamic psychotherapy, Problem Solving Therapy, Acceptance and Commitment Therapy, Behavioral Activation, and even new-wave 'stand on your head in the corner with crystals' therapies, interpersonal issues are *not* the primary focus. Cognitions, schema, values, or upside-down crystals are. Interpersonal issues are discussed in other treatments, but they are not the primary focus. This is why these therapies are not called 'Interpersonal CBT' or 'Interpersonal Crystal Therapy'.

To be fair and balanced, there is also no doubt that IPT also addresses issues inherent in other therapies. For instance, one could make a compelling Socratic argument that what are called 'expectations' about relationships in IPT are very similar to what are called cognitions in CBT, or that IPT therapists are suppressing the concept that motivations in communication may be driven by psychological factors outside of the patient's awareness. These are valid points. But these issues are not the *primary* foci of IPT, just as interpersonal issues are not the primary foci of these other therapies. While there is overlap between the empirically validated therapies, there are also very clear distinctions.

It is this primary focus on interpersonal issues, however, that is part of the reason why IPT is so effective. IPT directly addresses the here-and-now interpersonal problems that people bring to therapy without having to invoke some kind of sophisticated psychological mechanisms or theories. In IPT, the therapist can state simply and directly that the interpersonal issues which drove the patient to seek help, such as grief, will be talked about in therapy – there's no need to describe hypothetical concepts such as schema or ids or crystalline magnetism.

A corollary of these differences is that by virtue of IPT's primary focus on here-and-now interpersonal functioning, it is designed to resolve psychiatric symptoms and improve interpersonal functioning rather than to change underlying psychodynamic structures. While ego strength, defense mechanisms, and personality characteristics are all important in assessing suitability for treatment, change in these constructs is not presumed to occur in IPT because it is short-term. There's not enough time. Rather, ego strength, personality, and attachment are taken as givens for a particular patient, and the question that drives the IPT therapist's interventions is:

> Given this patient's personality style, ego strength, defense mechanisms, and early life experiences, and the time frame I am working within, how can I help her to improve her here-and-now interpersonal relationships and build a more effective social support network?

IPT Is Based on a Biopsychosocial/Cultural/Spiritual Model

IPT is based on a *Biopsychosocial/Cultural/Spiritual model* of psychological functioning. Rather than viewing psychological distress or psychiatric problems narrowly as medical diseases, the IPT approach is to conceptualize the patient's functioning in broad terms as a product of her temperament, personality, and attachment style, placed upon a foundation of biological factors such as genetics and physiological functioning, in the context of social relationships and general social support. Cultural and spiritual elements are also major factors – this has been increasingly apparent as IPT has been utilized in different settings around the world.

This five-factor model of distress is the most appropriate for IPT for three reasons. First, it is congruent with the theoretical foundation of IPT, in which attachments to others and the individual's ability to communicate effectively are hypothesized to be intimately linked with psychological functioning. Second, the Biopsychosocial/Cultural/Spiritual model leads directly to the specific techniques and interventions that are used in IPT. These include IPT interventions such as the development of Interpersonal Incidents and communication analysis. The acknowledgment of biological factors as one component of distress also makes IPT compatible for use with psychotropic medication when indicated. Third, the Biopsychosocial/Cultural/Spiritual model is strength based – it focuses not only on factors that are diatheses for psychological distress, but also includes factors which are protective. All can be included in the IPT Formulation, which is described in detail in Chapter 6.

The original iteration of IPT over three decades ago was based on a biological model of disease. Given the historical context and the requirements of the research design in which it was developed, this limited perspective is quite understandable. Historically, IPT was developed at a time in which biological mechanisms were primary in medicine; psychiatry was struggling to be taken seriously as a medical discipline, and much of the biological emphasis was an intentional contrast with psychoanalytic psychiatry which had been in the fore for many years. Early research designs, in which IPT (and other psychotherapies) were being compared to medications for specific diagnoses like major depression, also forced IPT into a disease-based biological model.

A consequence of this restrictive medical model was the requirement in the original research manual that patients be given a 'sick role' as they began treatment with IPT. This literally meant instructing the patient that he was medically ill and should be treated as such, i.e. that he should be absolved of life responsibilities for a time, and allowed by others to recover before being asked to take responsibility for change. It didn't matter whether the patient agreed with this idea of the sick role – it was simply imposed upon him rather than developing a collaborative understanding of his experience.

There are several problems inherent in this outmoded biological disease model. First, the field of medicine as a whole has taken a much broader view of illness or dysfunction. No longer is diabetes, for example, seen solely as a 'biological disease'. Instead, the physiologically based disease of diabetes is understood in the context of psychological and social functioning, and cultural and spiritual factors are noted as well. For type 2 diabetes in particular, psychological factors leading to eating behavior, and cultural influences affecting engagement with medical treatment, are seen as critical in the genesis and maintenance of the illness. All physicians now agree that describing diabetes as a simple biological disease, as opposed to a multifaceted illness, is an inappropriate reductionism which compromises treatment and patient care. One simply must pay attention to the whole person, not just his pancreas.

The same is true of psychiatric illnesses. Like diabetes, depression and other psychiatric illnesses have unquestioned biological bases, but they are also embedded within a social and cultural context and infused with psychological and spiritual meaning. Imposing a limited and outdated term such as 'sick role' on the patient does a disservice by discounting his unique individual experience. Moreover, and much more dangerously, it suggests to the patient that he need only 'sit and wait' for a biological change to take effect (i.e. taking medication) rather than taking responsibility for generating change within his social environment and for making changes in his interpersonal relationships. Therapeutically imposing the term 'sick role' also contradicts the evidence that the patient should be active in his own recovery. Behavioral activation[5,6] and motivational interviewing,[7] for example, have provided ample evidence that engagement in treatment is a critical part of recovery. While it is true that the patient is suffering and may be unable to function at full capacity while recovering, it is also true that removing him from normal activities and responsibilities may actually reduce the chances of recovery.

Clinically speaking, it has been often observed that a major problem with 'giving' patients the 'sick role' is that many of them then assume it. The clinician's explicit permission to reduce or avoid activities and to not be held responsible for a 'medical disease' can be used as a bludgeon to get others to take on the patient's responsibilities and as a means of perpetuating the patient's illness behavior. This is an instance in which the term secondary gain has relevance. A far better comparison for understanding the process in IPT is to think about recovery from depression as similar to recovery from an orthopedic injury (or any other physiological dysfunction for that matter). It is acknowledged that the patient has a physiologically based disease, but that there are many other aspects to his illness and recovery. Rather than taking a passive role, the patient should be encouraged to be actively engaged in and committed to rehabilitation, and to recognizing that there may be many difficult and painful exercises that will need to be done as recovery occurs. The degree to which the patient does these things – literally engages in and completes these rehabilitation activities – will play an enormous part in his recovery. The therapist should give no encouragement to the patient to 'sit and wait' – quite the contrary: the patient should be instructed to 'get up and get going' as quickly as possible.

Of course the therapist plays a major role in providing encouragement and expert instruction to the patient as he recovers, and the therapist must take some of the responsibility for motivating him to engage in treatment. Positive reinforcement is critical. The therapist might best be portrayed in the role of a coach in this aspect of IPT. Like a swimming coach, for instance, the therapist should be in the water with the patient, watching carefully to diagnose a problem with arm stroke, kick technique, or timing of breathing. The therapist should, based on this information, help the patient to develop the best possible set of exercises or training regimens to get back into shape and to correct the specific flaw in technique. And the therapist should be a motivator, helping the patient to get back in the water, to start swimming again despite some initial pain, and to be a cheerleader and comforter and taskmaster as needed so that the patient keeps working and progressing. Practice makes perfect.

But no matter how well the therapist does all of these things, *it is the patient who must do the work*. There is no substitute or reframing of this fact, and no 'sick role' to explain it away. The patient has to do the work. He has to swim the long and tedious laps to get back into shape and to rehabilitate the injury. He has to practice, he has to endure, and he has to persist. There is no other road to recovery. The patient is not sick; he is recovering, and he has to work. And he has to work hard. This is not something that you can 'give' to a patient; it is work the patient has to do. It is much more honest, and much more consistent with clinical reality, to tell the patient that he has a lot of hard work to do. But be sure and tell him that, in addition, you will be there to assist and motivate him and to celebrate his accomplishments.

IPT Is Short-term in Its Acute Phase

IPT is characterized by a short-term Acute Treatment Phase. This statement implies two things that we will make explicit: (1) 'short-term' means a dosing range of about 4–20 sessions; and (2) there is a long-term Maintenance Phase of IPT in addition to the Acute

Treatment Phase. There are now IPT studies in which 6,[8] 8,[9,10] 12,[3] 16,[11] and even 24[12] sessions have been used in research paradigms, each of which has demonstrated significant reductions in symptoms. Clinical experience and common sense suggest that these data should be used to inform clinical practice, not to dictate it rigidly. There is no empirically required number of sessions of IPT. Hence the use of the term 'empirically supported psychological treatment' as opposed to 'empirically required psychological treatment'.

Moreover, there is now unequivocal evidence that psychiatric illnesses generally, and depression specifically, are remitting and relapsing illnesses. Since that is the case, patients benefit from Maintenance Treatment which can reduce the risk of relapse. There are a number of studies that suggest that long-term Maintenance IPT in particular is very effective in reducing this relapse risk.[13,14] The obvious data-driven conclusion, supported by clinical experience, is that Maintenance IPT should be provided in some form to most patients.

Finally, despite a great deal of prose devoted to the subject, there is absolutely no evidence whatsoever that terminating therapy after a specified number of sessions is of benefit.[15] The theory that psychotherapy of any sort must have a definitive endpoint that is non-negotiable and that adhering to this rigid endpoint is associated with better outcomes is just that: a theory. And an unsupported one at that. Granted, it is very appealing to hold to this theory with some patients. Those who are more dependent or narcissistic in particular are often deemed by clinicians to be good candidates for termination – the sooner the better. However, though a complete termination may be a relief for clinicians, there is no evidence that it is of benefit to patients.[a]

This 'termination is of benefit' theory is also intuitively appealing to academicians and clinicians of all stripes who know from experience that having a grant deadline, or a deadline for publication, or for completing clinical notes, is a major motivator to getting work accomplished. At first glance, it does make sense. However, a deadline is different than a termination. Consider how you might respond to a deadline-based approach to work if your supervisor, dean, editor, or grant officer made clear that once the grant was submitted or notes were completed your relationship with them would be terminated. No more job, no more submissions, no more grants. Terminated. Your reward for hard work is termination. Most people would find it hard to get motivated.

There is an enormous difference between completing a task by a particular deadline and terminating a relationship – especially an intense clinical relationship – when the task is complete. Setting task deadlines need not require termination of relationship. IPT should not be terminated; IPT should be concluded once Acute Treatment is complete, and Maintenance Treatment provided as necessary.

How should these data and experience be applied clinically? The general answer is obvious: with a good measure of clinical judgment. The data support a dosing range of about 4–20 sessions of IPT for most patients, depending on clinical complexity, followed by longer term Maintenance IPT for most patients, again depending on clinical complexity. Unless the clinician is perfectly prescient in the first session and can predict without fail the exact number of sessions a patient will require for an acute course of IPT, the Treatment Agreement should have some flexibility built into it. Practically speaking this means that a patient with mild depression, good social support, and a secure attachment style who has experienced a recent loss may need only four to six Acute Treatment sessions, while a patient with severe depression complicated by anxiety and personality issues or maladaptive attachment style

---

[a] Of course the idea that termination is complete is also a myth. There is absolutely nothing preventing a patient from walking right back into your office the day after termination, saying he is in distress or is suicidal, and demanding treatment.

may need 16–20 sessions to recover. The first patient may need maintenance contact once every 6 months, while the second would benefit from monthly maintenance sessions to reduce relapse risk. Both are simple examples demonstrating that a combination of data and common sense can lead to efficient and effective clinical care.

Clinical experience is also clear that rather than ending Acute Treatment abruptly, as is required in research settings, IPT is better concluded with a tapering of Acute Treatment sessions. In other words, IPT should be gradually tapered such that the last several sessions are conducted every two to three weeks instead of continuing weekly until the conclusion. In addition to fortifying the gains made in therapy as the patient becomes increasingly autonomous, it greatly eases the pressure on the therapeutic relationship by gradually reducing dependency on the therapist rather than exacerbating it with an abrupt termination. This structure also allows for a smooth transition into maintenance care.

Since there is no evidence that termination – literally complete cessation – is of benefit to patients, an obvious question to ask is why should IPT be time-limited in the Acute Phase. There are at least four different reasons this is the case. The first is that the data support this approach. While the data do not support a specific number of sessions for all patients, all of the studies which have been conducted do support a time limit for Acute Treatment. The 4–20-session dosing range is supported by clinical practice as well. Second, one of the primary targets of IPT is to increase the patient's social support. This means that the therapist, though providing critical support in the early phase of therapy, should gradually move out of a primary support role as the patient increasingly relies on others for practical and emotional support. One way to foster this movement is for the therapist to limit Acute Treatment to the time needed to resolve the interpersonal issues, increase social support, and to transition to attachment relationships outside of therapy. In this sense, the shorter the treatment, the better. Third, the longer the therapy, the more likely that transference will become the focus of treatment. While this is desirable in psychodynamic or psychoanalytic work, it is the opposite of what is desired in IPT. Instead, the goal in IPT is to complete Acute Treatment before transference issues arise. To focus on transference detracts from the IPT focus on interpersonal relationships outside of therapy.

The time frame in IPT is extremely important in helping to prevent the therapy from moving from a treatment focused on symptoms and interpersonal issues to one that focuses on the transference relationship. IPT is focused on the rapid resolution of interpersonal crises, and on the problems that patients are experiencing in their current interpersonal relationships. Shifting this focus to one in which the patient–therapist relationship becomes primary makes it more difficult to generate immediate change in patients' social networks and their relationships outside of therapy. Encouraging the development of transference, which is fostered by increasing the duration and intensity of sessions, is likely to shift the work from relationship change to intrapsychic exploration.[16] Maintaining a time-limited approach helps to keep this from happening.

Finally, clinical utility is a compelling factor in limiting the length of Acute Treatment with IPT. Resources are limited, and though many patients may benefit from long-term therapy, others with more acute needs are waiting for care. The model of providing short-term Acute Treatment with long-term Maintenance is a much better fit given the resources available. In addition, most patients don't stick around for long-term work. Most, when improvement is occurring, are inclined not to come to treatment so often. When IPT is done well – when the therapist listens well and conveys a sense of caring – requests from patients for complete termination will be rare. But many will, as they feel better, begin asking fairly quickly to extend the time between sessions. The cost-benefit of treatment changes as improvement occurs, and expense, travel time, and other logistical issues begin to weigh much more heavily. The Acute Treatment model simply fits clinical reality.

In general, a dosing range of 4–20 acute sessions of IPT is used for the Acute Treatment of interpersonal problems, depression, and other major affective and anxiety disorders. While empirical research regarding Acute Treatment is at present limited to controlled studies in which weekly therapy is provided and then abruptly stopped, clinical experience has been that tapering sessions over time is generally a more effective way of utilizing the treatment. Weekly therapy may be provided for 6–10 weeks, followed by a gradual increase in the time between sessions as the patient improves, such that weekly sessions are followed by biweekly and monthly meetings.

Though Acute Treatment should be short-term, both empirical research and clinical experience with IPT have clearly demonstrated that Maintenance Treatment, particularly for those patients with recurrent disorders such as depression, should be provided for patients who have responded to Acute Treatment in order to reduce relapse risk.[13] This Maintenance Treatment should be distinguished from the Acute Phase of Treatment in IPT, and a specific agreement should be negotiated for the Maintenance Phase as well.[17] There is no need in IPT to 'terminate' at the conclusion of Acute Treatment, especially as it is not in the interest of most patients to do so.

IPT Interventions Do Not Directly Address the Patient–Therapist Relationship

IPT is characterized by a relative absence of interventions which directly address the therapeutic relationship. Though sharing this characteristic with CBT and several other solution-focused therapies, IPT clearly differs in this way from the dynamically oriented therapies. A more thorough explanation of the use of the therapeutic relationship in IPT is necessary to fully appreciate this element of the treatment.

Both Bowlby[18] and Sullivan[19] wrote extensively about the ways an individual's life experiences lead him to interact in subsequent relationships. Sullivan used the term 'parataxic distortion' to describe the way in which individuals impose characteristics of previous relationships upon new relationships.[19] In other words, individuals' experiences in previous relationships inform what they expect in new ones. This expectation then leads them to 'impose' characteristics upon new individuals with whom they come into contact. They expect the new to be like the old. Their expectations are based on the sum of their previous relationship experiences; because of this, the imposition of these expectations are often not accurate in new relationships. New relationships are 'distorted' by these imposed and inaccurate expectations.

For example, if an individual has had previous abusive relationships, she will tend to react to new people as if they too will be abusive. The previous experience is superimposed upon the new. New relationships will be distorted because the expectation is that new significant others will be abusive, even if in reality that is not the case. Similarly, if an individual has had experiences of being deceived, then she will superimpose that lack of trust upon new relationships as well, and will act 'as if' the new person should not be trusted.

Though Sullivan believed that these formative experiences were largely the result of early life experiences, he also believed that parataxic distortions could be modified over time by experiences in adulthood. For instance, a severe trauma, such as an assault, could profoundly change the expectations that an otherwise trusting individual might have about new relationships. Further, Sullivan also argued that the distortions could be modified in both positive and negative ways. While the above examples are indicative of negative modification, the distortions could also be modified positively with the experience of long-term productive, intimate, and trusting relationships.

Bowlby[20] described a similar phenomenon but used the term 'working model' of relationships to describe the ways in which individuals conceptualize new relationships. Their expectations of others in new relationships impact their behavior towards these new people. The purpose of the working model is to organize interpersonal behavior – it allows an individual to predict the behavior of others and to act accordingly. In a fashion similar to Sullivan's concept of parataxic distortion, this working model reflects all of an individual's experiences, with a heavy, but not exclusive, emphasis on early life interactions. The working model of attachment forms the basis for the development of new relationships, as the individual imposes the old working model upon new relationships with the expectation that new acquaintances will behave similarly to people in past relationships.

The problem, according to both Sullivan and Bowlby, is that while parataxic distortions and old working models may be accurate representations of earlier relationships, and may have been adaptive in those previous relationships, they restrict the development of new intimate relationships. New relationships become constrained by the model or the distortion, as opposed to being allowed to develop unfettered. Working models which reflect an accurate view of others as abusive during childhood are no longer accurate in adulthood with all new relationships, yet the imposition of the old model hinders an individual from trusting others or developing any sense of intimacy. It also prevents a realistic appraisal of good and bad relationships. Working models of attachment may reflect a distrust of others which developed honestly as a consequence of real breaches of trust in early relationships, but when they are superimposed upon new relationships in which the development of trust and intimacy would otherwise be possible, they severely limit the individual's ability to function interpersonally.

Because these distortions and working models are imposed upon all relationships, they occur within therapeutic relationships as well. Given enough time, a patient will display behavior towards her therapist which is reflective of her parataxic distortions or working models of attachment. This is the theoretical basis for the occurrence of transference in IPT. The therapist is in a unique position to experience and examine the way in which a patient develops and maintains relationships, because the therapist is in a relationship in which she is the person upon whom the distortions or working models are imposed. Both Sullivan and Bowlby, in the tradition of Freud and other psychoanalysts, believed that one of the most powerful ways to work on correcting these distortions was to examine the relationship between therapist and patient in detail. This was done overtly and explicitly, using techniques such as interpretation in which the transference was directly discussed, and clarifications in which the therapist would directly ask the patient for her reactions to the therapist.

In psychoanalytic treatments in particular, the therapy is structured in such a way that the transference is magnified so that it may be more closely examined. Psychoanalytic therapy is designed to facilitate the patient's projection of her parataxic distortions or working models of relationships onto the 'blank screen' of the therapist. This is enhanced by therapist opacity, by high-frequency sessions (four to five times per week), and by open-ended treatment which may last several years. All serve to intensify the patient–therapist relationship, with the goal of examining the transference as it is displayed in the therapeutic relationship.

Transference, parataxic distortions, and the imposition of working models are universal phenomena in all psychotherapy, including IPT. However, while in IPT the therapist's experience of patient–therapist relationship is used to gather important information about the patient and her interpersonal world, the transference elements of this relationship need not be addressed directly by the therapist as a part of the treatment. Instead, the therapist's experience of the therapeutic relationship in IPT is used as a means of understanding the patient's interpersonal functioning and to assess the patient's attachment style. This information is crucial. The information gleaned from the therapeutic relationship in IPT can then be used to formulate questions about the patient's interpersonal relationships with real people outside of therapy. The use of the transference experience to inform the therapist about potential problems in therapy, and to predict the likely outcome of treatment, and to plan for a good conclusion, is also paramount (Box 1.2).

Box 1.2 Uses of the patient–therapist relationship in IPT

- To assess the patient's attachment style
- To formulate questions about the patient's interpersonal relationships outside of therapy
- To understand the patient's interpersonal functioning outside of the therapeutic relationship
- To inform the therapist about potential difficulties in therapy
- To predict the likely outcome of treatment
- To plan for a good conclusion to therapy

Overt discussion of the patient–therapist relationship is not encouraged in IPT, however, because it switches the focus of treatment from more immediate work on the patient's current social relationships to an intense experience with, and analysis of, the relationship with the therapist. Addressing the patient–therapist relationship directly as a primary technique shifts the therapy from one that is oriented towards improvement in symptoms and immediate interpersonal functioning to a therapy that is oriented towards intrapsychic insight.

While this may be quite helpful for well-selected patients, the majority of patients that are seen in general practice are generally much more concerned with immediate symptom relief than with self-actualization – they are not working at the top of Maslow's hierarchy of needs.[21] Usually, self-actualization isn't even on their radar screens; instead, they come to therapy because they are distressed and lack a sense of intimacy, acceptance, or self-esteem. In other words, they are experiencing interpersonal distress. Their goal is to relieve that distress as quickly as possible. Discussion of transference, an expensive and lengthy course of therapy, and treatment with a therapist who may be perceived as being cold and unsupportive, is neither what they want nor need.

For the reasons described above, the focus of interventions in IPT is not on the therapeutic relationship. To discuss the therapeutic relationship at length shifts away from a more productive focus on social support and interpersonal problems outside of therapy. It is the development and examination of relationships outside of therapy that is the goal of IPT.

IPT is therefore structured in such a way that transference problems are less likely to develop. First and foremost, the patient–therapist relationship is not explicitly discussed. In addition, the IPT therapist generally takes a supportive stance rather than being neutral. The Acute Phase of therapy is time-limited, and the treatment is specifically focused on interpersonal issues in the patient's social relationships. All of these tactical elements in IPT pull the treatment away from a focus on the transference to one which is focused on here-and-now interpersonal relationships in the patient's social environment outside of therapy.

While IPT is specifically designed to delay or diminish the effect of parataxic distortions on the conduct of therapy, it would be a grave mistake to ignore the extraordinary treasure trove of information about the patient which can be gleaned from the therapist's experience of the therapeutic relationship. Though the patient–therapist relationship is not directly addressed in sessions, the clinician can, using her observational skills and finely honed intuitive sense of the relationship that is developing, gather a vast amount of information about the patient. This is because the way in which the patient behaves in therapy is a direct reflection of the way in which she behaves and communicates in relationships outside of therapy. Gathering this information is crucial, as it informs the therapist about the patient's suitability for treatment, her prognosis for therapy, the potential roadblocks that may occur, and about the specific techniques that are likely to be of use during therapy. Understanding the transference, recognizing the distortions that the patient brings to therapy, and developing hypotheses about the patient's interpersonal working model, are all essential to IPT.

As an illustration of this use of information about the parataxic distortions that occur in therapy, consider a patient who forms a relationship with his therapist that is dependent in nature. The patient may manifest this dependency as difficulty in ending sessions, calls to the therapist between sessions, or in more subtle pleas to the therapist for help or reassurance. This transferential relationship should inform the therapist about several aspects of the patient's functioning: (1) the patient is likely to have problems with other people because he relates to them in the same dependent fashion; (2) the patient is likely to have difficulty ending relationships with others; and (3) the patient has likely exhausted others with persistent calls for help. A hypochondriacal patient would be an excellent example of this kind of behavior, manifest in the ways described. This information is then used by the therapist to formulate hypotheses about the patient's difficulties with others, and should lead the therapist to ask questions about how the patient asks others for help, ends relationships, and feels when others aren't responsive to his needs. These questions are directed to relationships outside of the therapy, however – to interpersonal relationships in which the patient is currently engaged, rather than the relationship between therapist and patient.

Further, the information obtained from the transference experience should be used by the therapist to predict potential problems that may arise in treatment, and to modify IPT accordingly. For instance, the therapist might hypothesize that the patient's dependency is likely to cause a problem when concluding therapy, and may begin discussing the Conclusion of Acute Treatment much earlier than with less dependent patients. The therapist might also plan to taper the frequency of sessions later in the course of therapy, moving to sessions once every two weeks as the patient is in recovery. This tapering would allow the patient to depend less on the therapist and increase his sense of independent competence. The principles are the same for all patients: though specific modifications will differ for each, adaptations in structure and tactics in IPT should also be made with those who are avoidant, who manifest other personality characteristics, or have other traits that make treatment more complex. In addition, data gleaned from the therapeutic relationship should provide the therapist with information about the patient's prognosis in therapy. More severe parataxic distortions, and those which become manifest earlier in treatment, suggest a poorer outcome. This information should not be used nihilistically, but rather should lead the therapist to more realistic expectations of outcome.

In sum, the patient–therapist relationship, and particularly the patient-generated distortions in that relationship, are extremely important in IPT, but are not addressed directly in therapy. To do so detracts from the focus on symptom reduction and improvement in interpersonal functioning that is the basis of IPT, and also typically leads to a much longer course of treatment than is required for IPT. The goal in IPT is literally to work with the patient to quickly resolve his interpersonal distress before problematic transference develops and becomes the focus of treatment.

A Metaphor for IPT

The Sydney Harbor Bridge was completed in 1932, and even today is considered an engineering marvel. The single arch, more than 500 meters in length, spans one of the most beautiful harbors in the world, with a magnificent view of the Sydney Opera House, the Rocks, and downtown Sydney. On clear days the view extends to the Pacific Ocean and beyond. It is simply one of the most spectacular sights in the world.

Since 1998, people have been allowed to climb up a very narrow catwalk to the top of the bridge. Not a stairway – the climb is literally on top of the curving superstructure of the bridge, along steel beams at some points only a foot or two across. The top of the arch, which is 134 meters above the harbor, is the highest point on the bridge. It is completely exposed, and on a windy day the whole bridge literally sways back and forth, giving climbers the queasy feeling that they will be pitched over the side and plummet each of those 134 long meters to the water below.

Like most things in life, climbing the bridge requires taking a risk. It requires suspending one's sense of psychological safety. It requires extending oneself. The reward is immense, but it requires physical and psychological effort. For some people who are adventurous or genetically or temperamentally endowed with a predisposition to risk-taking, the bridge climb is an exhilarating experience. No fear, no anxiety, just the thrill and adrenaline rush that comes with being suspended over 120 meters in the air and seeing one of the most breathtaking views in the world. For others, the climb is a bit more anxiety provoking. Some of these mildly anxious people have the psychological resources to literally 'talk themselves' into climbing the bridge. This self-talk might include rationalizations that the climb is really safe (despite appearances to the contrary), or might include continued self-reminders that the effort and risk will be well worth the rewards. Terms such as ego strength and a capacity for delayed gratification might be used when describing these people.

Some people, because of life experience, biological, temperamental, or other factors, need some help to manage the climb. For some, cognitive reassurance is sufficient. A reminder – *from a trusted significant other* – of an accurate cognitive appraisal of the situation is needed. 'After all,' a friend might say, 'the Sydney Harbor Bridge has stood since 1932 without falling down. Hundreds of thousands of people have climbed it without plunging to their deaths.'[b] And in Socratic fashion, a friend serving as amateur clinician might rhetorically ask, 'When was the last time you read in the *Sydney Morning Herald* about someone falling off the bridge? What do you think the realistic chance is that something bad will happen to you if climb?' Thus reassured, these moderately anxious people are able to ascend.

For those who are more anxious, or who are more dependent in personality and attachment, such cognitive reassurance is not sufficient. It is not simply cognitive reappraisal that they require, it is *interpersonal reassurance*. Such people are looking for someone to literally take their hand, to be with them, and to support them psychologically. Such a person, though feeling very anxious about the climb, might be able to say, 'I'll do it if you go with me.'

Some people requiring this kind of reassurance are able to ask for it directly and graciously, and as a result are generally pretty successful in getting the support they need. Their friends can respond to them easily, and are available and willing to provide

---

[b] This is the art of therapy: not only knowing when to reassure, but being aware that words like 'plunging to their deaths' are likely to be less reassuring than noting that hundreds of thousands of people have climbed the bridge safely. As they say, that's what friends are for.

interpersonal and emotional support. In contrast, other people facing the Sydney Harbor Bridge climb have personality or communication styles in which their needs are conveyed either indirectly or in a way that is counterproductive. Whining, complaining, being passive-aggressive, and dependently clinging are not good ways to get someone to hold your hand while climbing the bridge. Finally, there are those that go to Sydney, look at the bridge, and say to themselves, 'I could never do that'. And for a variety of psychological, physical, temperamental, and social reasons, they don't.

The Sydney Harbor Bridge climb is a crisis. It is literally a transcendent experience which requires taking a risk. The approach that people take to this crisis is based largely on their biopsychosocial and cultural and spiritual makeup. Genetics, temperament, early life experience, attachment, personality, social support, and adult experience all play a role in determining who will attempt, and who will succeed, in climbing the bridge. IPT is designed to help those people who need interpersonal support in order to complete the climb. IPT is designed to help people recognize their interpersonal needs for attachment and reassurance, and to express those needs graciously so that others can respond in a helpful way. IPT is not designed for everyone; not everyone needs it. Many people are able to deal with their particular crises without professional help. A few have problems so severe that they need much more extensive help. But there are a significant number of people who need help to resolve a specific crisis, and who need assistance in generating or using their social support system to negotiate it.

IPT is designed to help people to face their bridge climb crises, to reach new heights, and to bring someone along to enjoy the view together.

Conclusion

The defining characteristics of IPT are its four primary elements: an interpersonal orientation; the Biopsychosocial/Cultural/Spiritual model of psychological functioning and distress; a short-term Acute Treatment Phase; and the avoidance of interventions which directly address the patient–therapist relationship. IPT is extremely useful for patients who face acute interpersonal crises that they cannot manage alone.

References

1. Klerman GL, *et al*. *Interpersonal Psychotherapy of Depression*. 1984, New York: Basic Books.

2. American Psychiatric Association. *Diagnostic and Statistical Manual of Mental Disorders*, 4th edn. 1994, Washington, DC: American Psychiatric Association.

3. O'Hara MW, *et al*. Efficacy of interpersonal psychotherapy for postpartum depression. *Archives of General Psychiatry*, 2000, **57**: 1039–1045.

4. Beck AT, *et al*. *Cognitive Therapy of Depression*. 1979, New York: Guilford Press.

5. Jacobson NS, Martell CR and Dimidjian S. Behavioral activation treatment for depression: returning to contextual roots. *Clinical Psychology: Science and Practice*, 2001, **8**: 255–270.

6. Addis ME and Martell CR. *Overcoming Depression One Step at a Time: The New Behavioral Activation Approach to Getting your Life Back*. 2004, Oakland: New Harbinger.

7. Miller WR and Rollnick S. *Motivational Interviewing: Preparing People for Change*, 2nd edn. 2002, New York: Guilford Publications.

8. Schulberg HC, Block MR and Madonia MJ. *Treating Major Depression in Primary Care Practice*. Archives of General Psychiatry, 1996, **53**: 913–919.

9. Swartz HA, *et al*. A pilot study of brief interpersonal psychotherapy for depression among women. *Psychiatric Services*, 2004, **55**(4): 448–450.

10. Grote NK, *et al*. A randomized controlled trial of culturally relevant, brief interpersonal psychotherapy for perinatal depression. *Psychiatric Services*, 2009, **60**(3): 313–321.

11. Elkin I, *et al*. NIMH Treatment of Depression Collaborative Research Program: I. General effectiveness of treatments. *Archives of General Psychiatry*, 1989, **46**: 971–982.

12. Talbot N, *et al*. A randomized effectiveness trial of interpersonal psychotherapy for depressed women with sexual abuse histories. *Psychiatric Services*, 2011, **62**: 374–380.

13. Frank E, *et al*. Three-year outcomes for maintenance therapies in recurrent depression. *Archives of General Psychiatry*, 1990, **47**(12): 1093–1099.

14. Frank E, *et al*. Randomized trial of weekly, twice-monthly, and monthly interpersonal psychotherapy as maintenance treatment for women with recurrent depression. *American Journal of Psychiatry*, 2007, **164**: 761–767.

15. Gelso CJ and Woodhouse SS. The termination of psychotherapy: what research tells us about the process of ending treatment, in Tryon GS (ed.) *Counseling Based on Process Research: Applying What we Know*. 2002, Boston: Allyn and Bacon.

16. Stuart S. Interpersonal psychotherapy, in Dewan M, Steenbarger B and Greenberg R (eds) *The Art and Science of Brief Psychotherapies: A Practitioner's Guide*. 2004, Washington DC: American Psychiatric Press, pp. 119–156.

17. Stuart S. Interpersonal psychotherapy, in Dewan M, Steenbarger B and Greenberg R (eds) *The Art and Science of Brief Psychotherapies: A Practitioner's Guide*, 2nd edn. 2011, Washington DC: American Psychiatric Press.

18. Bowlby J. Developmental psychiatry comes of age. *American Journal of Psychiatry*, 1988, **145**: 1–10.

19. Sullivan HS. *The Interpersonal Theory of Psychiatry*. 1953, New York: Norton.

20. Bowlby J. The making and breaking of affectional bonds: etiology and psychopathology in the light of attachment theory. *British Journal of Psychiatry*, 1977, **130**: 201–210.

21. Maslow A. A theory of human motivation. *Psychological Review*, 1943, **50**: 370–396.

2

Theory and Clinical Applications

Introduction

Interpersonal Psychotherapy (IPT) rests on two primary theoretical foundations. The first and most important is *Attachment Theory*, which forms the basis for understanding patients' relationship difficulties. The second, *Interpersonal Theory*, describes the ways in which patients' maladaptive communication patterns lead to difficulty in their here-and-now interpersonal relationships. Communication is one manifestation of attachment behavior, but it is an extremely important particular in IPT, as it is the point of intervention for many IPT techniques. Social Theory is also a useful way to understand the impact of social support within an IPT framework, but is generally given a lesser theoretical role.[a]

IPT is based on the premise that psychiatric and interpersonal difficulties result from a combination of interpersonal, social, and other factors, following the Biopsychosocial/Cultural/Spiritual model of psychiatric illness and psychological distress. Upon this foundation rests the individual's temperament, personality traits, and early life experiences, which in turn are reflected in a particular attachment style. These factors, as well as cultural and spiritual factors, may be either predisposing or protective. The attachment style may be more or less adaptive, and has effects upon the person's current social support network and her ability to enlist the support of significant others. To put it succinctly, individuals with biological and psychological diatheses will be more likely to become distressed when experiencing interpersonal crises. Interpersonal functioning is determined by the severity of the current stressors in the context of social support. This is depicted in the Interpersonal Triad (Figure 2.1), which is the IPT model that explains why people become distressed.

IPT is therefore designed to treat psychiatric symptoms and improve interpersonal functioning by focusing specifically on patients' primary interpersonal relationships, particularly in the problem areas of *Grief and Loss*, *Interpersonal Disputes*, and *Role Transitions*.[b] Although fundamental change in either personality or attachment style is

---

[a] The de-emphasis of Social Theory is a change from our 2003 guide; however, the emphasis on social support in IPT remains paramount.

[b] Readers of previous IPT manuals, including our first iteration, will note that this list no longer includes interpersonal sensitivity (also called deficits) in the IPT Problem Areas. This former Problem Area is now best understood as an attachment style rather than an acute interpersonal problem. This is addressed at length in subsequent chapters.

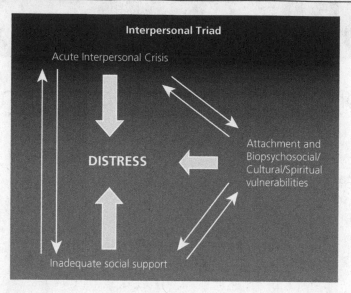

Figure 2.1 Interpersonal Triad

unlikely during short-term treatment, resolution of symptoms and distress is made possible when patients are assisted in repairing their disrupted interpersonal relationships, and when they learn new ways to communicate their needs for emotional and practical support.

A comprehensive and well-articulated theory that supports IPT is necessary for several reasons. *The most important is that it informs the clinician about the nature of the patient's problems and about the kinds of interventions that may be helpful to resolve them.* A comprehensive theory forms the basis for the clinician's formulation of a case, and for determining which specific therapeutic interventions are likely to be most helpful. It also provides guidance in anticipating potential problems with a given individual during the course of therapy (such as problems with forming a therapeutic alliance), and informs the therapist about the ways in which she can prevent or effectively manage these roadblocks.

The theoretical foundation for IPT has the following features:

- It is based on the available empirical evidence.
- It reflects clinical observations and experience as accurately as possible.
- It forms the basis for hypotheses that can be examined clinically.
- It forms the basis for hypotheses that can be tested empirically.
- It is subject to modifications as new empirical and clinical evidence arises.

The theory supporting IPT is, therefore, not a set of static dictums, but is open to investigation and modification as it evolves with clinical experience and as empirical data accumulate (Figure 2.2).

The patient's Biopsychosocial/Cultural/Spiritual diathesis is the template upon which interpersonal crises occur. A sufficiently intense crisis (e.g. Interpersonal Dispute, Role Transition, or Grief and Loss experience) in the context of insufficient social support may lead to interpersonal problems, psychiatric symptoms, and distress. If the crisis is subthreshold, then symptoms and distress are averted. If social support is sufficient, even in the face of a great crisis, symptoms can be averted as well. But if the crisis is great enough, and the social support insufficient, the patient's attachment needs during the crisis go unmet. Maladaptive communication of those needs often follows, and interpersonal distress and psychiatric symptoms are the result.

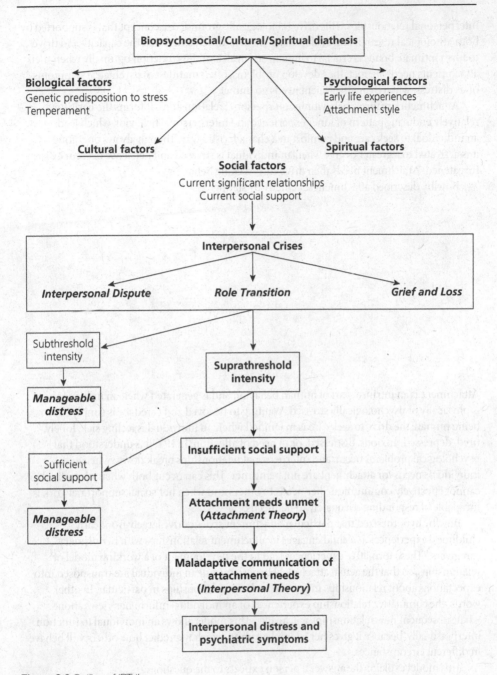

Figure 2.2 Outline of IPT theory

Attachment Theory

Attachment Theory is one of the foundations of IPT. It describes the ways in which individuals form, maintain, and end relationships, as well as the ways they develop problems within them. John Bowlby among others articulated the principles of Attachment Theory,[1-8] which is based on the premise that humans have an intrinsic instinctual drive to form interpersonal relationships. This drive is biologically grounded, a concept that is supported by both ethological research and evolutionary theory,[6] which assert that the capacity and drive to form intimate bonds is crucial to human survival. Humans function optimally when their attachments needs are met; they develop problems, often manifest as psychiatric symptoms or as distress, when their attachment needs go unmet.

Attachment organizes behavior in interpersonal relationships. It forms the basis for a relatively enduring pattern of inner experience and interpersonal behavior, which leads an individual to seek care and comfort in a characteristic way. Though always operating, it is activated to a greater degree when an individual is stressed and her sense of security is threatened. Attachment needs then drive care-seeking behavior.

Bowlby described attachment succinctly by stating:

[A]ttachment behavior is conceived as any form of behavior that results in a person attaining or retaining proximity to some other differentiated and preferred individual. While especially evident during childhood, attachment behavior is held to characterize human beings from the cradle to the grave. In adults it is especially evident when a person is distressed, ill, or afraid. The particular patterns of attachment behavior shown by an individual turn partly on his present age, sex, and circumstances and partly on the experiences he has had with attachment figures earlier in his life.[3] (p. 203)

The desire to be loved and cared for is an integral part of human nature throughout adult life as well as earlier, and the expression of such desires is to be expected in every grown-up, especially in times of sickness or calamity.[4] (p. 428)

Attachment is an intrinsic part of human behavior, and is generated when an individual is physically or psychologically stressed. Wanting to be loved and cared for is simply being human; the drive to seek care is magnified when an individual is feeling sick, lonely, tired, depressed, anxious, distressed, or in need of affection. In IPT, it is understood that psychological problems occur, and interpersonal relationships break down, when an individual's needs for attachment are not being met. This can occur both when the individual cannot effectively communicate her needs to others and when her social support network is incapable of responding adequately to her needs.

Bowlby hypothesized that particular attachment styles derive largely from early childhood experiences as a child engages in attachment relationships with her primary caregivers.[1] These formative experiences lead to the development of a working model of relationships, so that the actual attachment experiences of an individual are transposed into expectations about relationships in general and new relationships in particular. In other words, the cumulative relationship experiences of an individual inform her views about what subsequent new relationships will be like. This model allows an individual to function interpersonally, because it gives her a template upon which to predict how others will behave in different circumstances.

This model explains the answer a person expects to the question:

When I am stressed and in need of care and support, others will typically react towards me by being ...

Different people answer this question in different ways: some expect comfort, some expect rejection, and some expect indifference. But in all cases, the expected answer to this statement forms the basis for the way an individual seeks to meet her attachment needs. If the expectation is that her needs will be met by others, then she will act by directly asking for support. If her expectation, based on her real-life experiences, is that requests for support will be met with rejection, then she is likely to avoid asking for help, or demand it in ways that may be self-defeating. People also develop similar working models about themselves and their ability and competence to deal with stressors. This 'model of self' is also based largely on early life experiences, but can be modified during adulthood. The analogous question here is:

When I am stressed and in need of care and support, I typically react by being …

Different people answer this question in different ways: some feel competent to deal with most stressors; some are anxious about their ability to manage crises. This model of self interacts directly with attachment behavior towards others.

The working models that people develop are based on real-life experiences. No sophisticated intrapsychic mechanisms or abstract constructs are required. An individual who has experienced abuse will understandably and quite reasonably expect the same treatment in new relationships; someone who has experienced rejection will expect more rejection; and someone who has had productive and trusting relationships will anticipate that new relationships will be similar. The attachment effects of these expectations are evident during childhood, but have also been extended to adult behavior as well.[9-14]

Bowlby's concept of a working model of attachment is similar to Sullivan's concept of parataxic distortion,[11] in which the cumulative experiences of an individual inform the way she relates to others. Both Sullivan and Bowlby argued that the working model of relationships, and the subsequent distortions that occurred as a result of the imposition of the model on current and new relationships, are based largely (though not exclusively) on early life relationships with the individual's primary caregiver. Both also hypothesized that an individual experiences interpersonal problems not because her working models are inaccurate reflections of her past experiences, but because the models are imposed inappropriately onto current and new relationships, in which her assumptions about the ways others will behave towards her are not accurate.

For instance, a patient with a history of abuse is quite understandably likely to develop a working model of relationships that people are not to be trusted, or that others will take advantage of her – a model that is imposed consistently upon all relationships. While adaptive and protective when faced with the threat of abuse, this model impairs the ability of the patient to function interpersonally when in situations in which abuse is not likely to occur. She is likely to have difficulty developing intimate relationships because her model of relationships dictates that people can't be trusted – even those who are impeccably trustworthy are pushed away. Therapeutic examples abound: patients with distorted models of relationships frequently impose them upon others in situations in which the models are inaccurate, leading ultimately to self-defeating behavior and distress. This parataxic distortion impairs the ability of the patient to function and feel secure within all relationships, including the therapeutic relationship.

An individual's working model of relationships is generally consistent both within and across relationships, coalescing to form a characteristic attachment style. An individual tends to maintain the same attachment style over time in a given relationship, and also tends to form new relationships with a consistent style of attachment. This phenomena is dramatically illustrated with hypochondriacal patients, for instance, who form dependent relationships with family members, significant others, and healthcare professionals that are all based on a dependent attachment style – they don't suddenly change their way of attaching to others once they are in a relationship, nor do they suddenly change their attachment style when they enter new relationships. Their attachment style is consistent.

This consistency in attachment style forms the theoretical basis in IPT for the development of transference. Given enough time, a patient will manifest the same attachment style with the therapist that she manifests with others outside of therapy. Thus sensitivity to the therapeutic relationship allows the therapist to tap into this extremely important information about the patient's attachment style and model of relationships, and allows the therapist to develop hypotheses about the kinds of interpersonal problems the patient is likely to experience, and the ways others are likely to perceive the patient. Though transference is not addressed directly in IPT, the information obtained from the patient's behavior and communication in the therapeutic relationship is crucial to understanding her attachment and communication problems in her current relationships.

It is absolutely essential for the therapist to keep in mind that the attachment difficulties experienced by the patient and the distortions she imposes upon current and new relationships are all a product of her real experiences. People come by their relationship models honestly. Their models and distortions reflect real attempts to cope with earlier stressors, abuse, or deprivations, and the tragedy is that these past experiences continue to haunt patients through their continuing effect on attachment and interpersonal functioning. Such tragedies call for empathy rather than pathological labels.

Bowlby[1] described three basic styles of attachment: secure, anxious ambivalent, and anxious avoidant.[c] Over the past decade, this model has been replaced in IPT by Bartholomew and Horowitz's[15] four quadrant model of attachment, which has proven to be more useful in clinical work (Figure 2.3). The four quadrants of this model are the result of the intersection of the individual's working model of self (x-axis) and working model of relationships with others (y-axis). Based on real-life experiences, individuals develop a working model of self as either capable of caring for their own needs for the most part, or as needing to rely on others for care because of their belief that they are incapable of caring for themselves. At the same time, based on real-life experience, they also develop a working model of others as either dependable – i.e. willing to provide care if asked – or not dependable. The intersection of the working models of self and others form the four primary attachment styles.

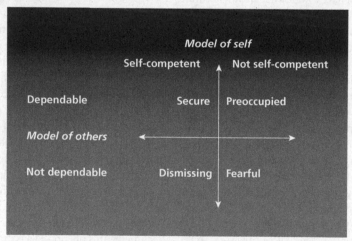

Figure 2.3 The four quadrant model of attachment in IPT

---

[c] Bowlby's model is noted largely for historical reasons; it was first described as the theoretical basis for IPT in our 2003 *Clinician's Guide*. The reader should note that other authors have described additional attachment styles; disorganized attachment has been noted by some and others have described models incorporating different attachment styles. Much work remains to be done to more fully describe the variety of attachment within human relationships throughout the lifespan.

Securely attached individuals base their relationships on working models of self and others which are healthy and flexible – in other words, they generally trust others, believe that their needs will be met, and are able to explore the world and seek out new relationships and experiences with a sense of security. They have a sense of self-competence, and believe that they can manage most crises. They manifest, as Bowlby described, the characteristics of good mental health: they are able to effectively ask for care from others when it is needed, and are also able to provide care to others when asked to do so. Their relationships are generally satisfactory and productive, they have extensive social support networks, and are therefore able to effectively manage most life crises.

Individuals with a *preoccupied* attachment style, in contrast, are constantly anxious that their attachment needs will not be met. Their working model of self develops from the experience of being unable to care for themselves. Their working model of others assumes that others, although they are capable of providing care and support, may choose not to do so. In order to get their attachment needs met, they must constantly seek care and reassurance. These models of self and others often develop from inconsistent or overprotective care during childhood. Hypochondriacal patients are classic examples of this attachment behavior – they constantly seek reassurance, and are so preoccupied with obtaining sufficient care in their attachment relationships that they lack any capacity to provide care for others.[16] Moreover, their constant reassurance seeking behavior eventually wears out their care providers, ultimately resulting in rejection.[17,18] As a result, the intimate relationships they are able to develop are unstable, and they are very vulnerable to conflicts or losses which threaten their attachments. Further, since they are unable to develop mutually supportive relationships, their social support networks are very poor.

Individuals with a *dismissing* attachment style often have early life experiences in which care was never adequately provided. As a result, they develop working models of others based on their belief that care will never be sufficient or will simply not be provided at all, and that their attachment needs will never be met. Narcissistic or antisocial interpersonal behaviors are consistent with this attachment style. The fear of never being cared for sufficiently is covered with a superficial belief that they can meet their own needs and don't need others at all, hence they are quick to dismiss others as incompetent or uncaring. There is little if any capacity for intimate and trusting relationships.

Fearfully attached individuals lack the conviction that they will be cared for in relationships, and therefore form either superficial bonds with others or avoid them altogether. Coupled with a working model of self in which they believe they are unable to meet their own emotional needs, such individuals may manifest avoidance or compulsive self-reliant behavior. Their social support network tends to be very poor as a result. Patients with social phobia or schizoid personality disorders often fit into this category.

Individuals with insecure attachment styles are twice cursed, so to speak. First, their life experiences have led them to develop working models of relationships in which they are convinced that care will not be available to them when needed. Second, because they typically lack the capacity to care for others or to develop intimate relationships, their social support networks are usually very poor. Neither their internal world, nor their external world, is adapted to deal with interpersonal stress.

In sum, Attachment Theory hypothesizes that individuals have difficulty when they experience disruptions in their relationships with other people. This is both because of the loss of or threat to the specific attachment relationship and because their social support network is not able to sustain them during the loss, conflict, or transition. Insecurely attached individuals are much more vulnerable to difficulties with personal conflicts, such as divorce or relationship disruptions, and to transitions such as moving or loss of a job, both because of their tenuous primary relationships and because of their poor social support networks.[19] In addition, they are also more likely to develop problems when faced with a major loss such as the death of a primary attachment.[2,20] These Problem Areas – Interpersonal Disputes, Role Transitions, and Grief and Loss – are specifically addressed in IPT.

The vulnerability of insecurely attached individuals is a result not only of their attachment style, but also the fact that their social support networks are poorly constructed and poorly responsive to their needs. Further, insecurely attached individuals are largely unable to communicate their interpersonal and attachment needs directly[21] or graciously, making it unlikely that others, even if so inclined, will be able to respond to their needs effectively. Even securely attached individuals can become distressed or develop interpersonal problems if faced with a stressor that is great enough, such as the death of a spouse, but their threshold for the development of problems is higher than for those with insecure styles. Both their internal sense of security and their superior social support systems can sustain securely attached individuals in situations in which others might be overwhelmed. Those who are securely attached are also able to ask effectively for support from others when it is needed. Their previous experience and internal working models lead them to expect that support is likely to be provided, and they can communicate more effectively their specific needs for it.

Attachment Theory is consistent with the clearly established biological diatheses for depression and other illnesses. Genetic contributions combine with attachment style to influence the vulnerability of an individual to stress, which, when combined with a sufficient psychosocial crisis, leads to psychiatric symptoms or distress. Given that a maladaptive attachment style often develops because an individual grows up with parents who have psychiatric problems which influence their parenting behavior, and that as a result she has both a heritable biological predisposition to develop psychiatric problems and a maladaptive attachment style, it is not surprising that difficulties develop. In IPT, this is best conceptualized using a Biopsychosocial/Cultural/Spiritual model.

A careful reading of Attachment Theory would likely suggest to the astute clinician that one way to improve a patient's functioning would be to change her basic attachment style. This implies therapeutic goals of helping the patient to recognize her patterns of attachment, to understand how her attachment style developed, and to modify her internal working models of attachment. This reworking of attachment patterns requires the development of insight through the examination of early childhood experiences, as well as an overt discussion of the therapeutic relationship to examine patterns of interaction. The patient's interaction with the therapist would be examined in detail, with the goal of using it as the vehicle for change. A primary technique would be interpretation of the transferential experience. This is essentially an open-ended psychodynamic approach to treatment. In addition to this intensive therapeutic experience, the patient would also have to literally reconstruct her attachment models of self and others. Insight isn't enough to compensate – it is the lived experience of being in long-term trusting relationships and being able to depend on oneself that slowly changes attachment. The time required is great – it may take years of healthy and productive attachment to change the patient's working models at a core level.

While there is utility in a long-term transferential approach with extremely disturbed patients with very maladaptive attachment styles, it takes a great deal of time to bring about a core change in attachment, and the treatment must be quite intensive. Bowlby himself stated that:

> A restructuring of a person's representational models and his re-evaluation of some aspects of human relationships, with a corresponding change in his modes of treating people, is likely to be both slow and patchy.[3] (p. 427)

Long-term therapy which aims to bring about such deep and lasting changes in attachment requires great motivation, insight, time, financial resources, and a patient and therapist who are able to devote themselves to the task without the need for immediate gratification. The key is to determine 'how much therapy' is appropriate for a given patient considering these factors.

In addition, focusing therapy on a patient's internal model of attachment is likely to detract from a focus on the rapid resolution of her current distress. By definition, a therapy that is constructed to look more intensively at the therapeutic relationship will devote less time to resolving the patient's current interpersonal problems outside of therapy. Further, the psychodynamic therapist must always be aware of the fact that, despite her best efforts to support the patient, she will ultimately fail over time to meet the patient's attachment needs as they are manifested in therapy. Thus to continue therapy in an intense and open-ended fashion will eventually require that the therapeutic relationship be discussed as a central feature of the therapy as that disappointment or empathic failure is worked through.

In contrast, rather than attempting to change the patient's fundamental attachment style, *IPT focuses on helping the patient to communicate her attachment needs more directly and graciously, and helping her to construct a more supportive social network.* Taking the patient's attachment style as a constant, IPT works in real-time relationships to help the patient communicate her needs more effectively. It is not designed to change the patient's internal structures, ego functioning, defense mechanisms, or attachment style, but rather to help the patient identify or develop social supports, and to help with the communication of her attachment needs in that context. The experience of having her attachment needs met may help to restructure the patient's internal model in a way that more accurately reflects reality, but this is not the primary goal of treatment. Rather, priority is given to rapid symptom resolution and improvement in interpersonal functioning, and treatment can therefore be short-term (Figure 2.4).

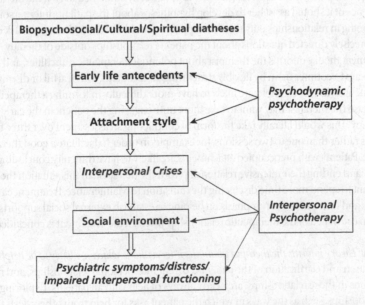

Figure 2.4 IPT and psychodynamic psychotherapy: differing points of intervention. IPT intervenes at the level of the acute interpersonal crises or stressor and the current social environment with the goal of alleviating distress and improving social functioning. Psychodynamic psychotherapy is designed to facilitate fundamental change in attachment style by examining early life experiences and transference within the therapeutic relationship.

The Therapeutic Implications of Attachment Theory

Attachment Theory forms the basis for conceptualizing a patient's distress as attachment needs which are unmet.

This may be because the patient has a maladaptive style of attaching to others which leads her to believe that care from others is insufficient or unavailable. It may also occur when a securely attached individual is faced with an overwhelming interpersonal crisis. In IPT, the emphasis is on quickly assisting the patient to get her needs met more effectively by focusing on communication within the patient's attachment relationships, and on her social support system. Attachment style is not a target of change; communication is. In contrast, in long-term psychodynamic psychotherapy, the emphasis is on modifying the patient's underlying attachment style (Box 2.1).

Box 2.1 Therapeutic implications of Attachment Theory

Attachment Theory forms the basis for:
- Conceptualization of the patient's interpersonal problems and psychological distress
- Understanding the patient–therapist relationship and thereby understanding the patient's relationships outside of therapy
- Anticipating potential problems in therapy and ways to counter them flexibly within the structure of IPT
- Planning interventions that are likely to be of benefit in IPT
- Predicting prognosis.

Attachment Theory connects the way the patient attaches to the therapist to the way the patient attaches to significant others.

Although the patient–therapist relationship is not directly addressed in IPT, the therapist's experience of it should assist her to develop hypotheses about the patient's interpersonal functioning in relationships outside of therapy, and should direct the therapist to ask even more precisely directed questions about the patient's relationships outside of therapy. Attachment theory informs the therapist about potential therapeutic difficulties, and about ways to counter them by flexibly structuring IPT. Patients with fearful or dismissive attachment styles, for example, are likely to have more difficulty in forming a therapeutic alliance, so the therapist may want to take more time engaging the patient in the early sessions of therapy. This would literally take the form of conducting an assessment over three to four sessions rather than one to two sessions, for example, in order to facilitate a good therapeutic alliance. Patients with preoccupied attachments are likely to have difficulty concluding acute therapy and ending their intensive relationship with the therapist; in this situation the therapist may want to spend more time discussing the transition to Maintenance Treatment earlier in therapy, and may put special emphasis on helping to establish external social supports that they can use in lieu of the therapeutic relationship when Acute Treatment is concluded.

Attachment Theory informs the therapist about the interventions which are likely to be helpful in IPT.

Exploration and clarification of the patient's current interpersonal relationships, and recent transitions in those relationships, are nearly always of help with all patients. Exploring patterns of relationships, such as the ways in which the patient asks for help from others, feels that she is understood by others, and the typical ways in which her relationships end, should also be beneficial. However, directive techniques often need to be modified on the basis of attachment style. For example, securely attached patients may benefit from therapist self-disclosure, and are much more likely to be able to constructively use homework assignments or direct advice.

Attachment Theory informs prognosis.

The more securely attached a patient is, the better her prognosis. The prognosis is better not just for IPT, but for all psychotherapies. This is true for a number of reasons. A more securely attached patient generally has better social support, and also has a greater capacity to ask for help when it is needed. A more securely attached patient is also able to form a more productive alliance with the therapist, and enters therapy with the expectation that it will be helpful. Such a patient is also less likely to have difficulty concluding therapy, as her attachments outside of therapy are more satisfying than those of patients who are less securely attached.

Attachment style is a powerful predictor of outcome in all varieties of psychotherapy. The reality is that 'the rich get richer' – those patients with more interpersonal and intrapsychic resources, with better social support networks, and with more adaptive attachment styles, benefit more from therapy. It would be wonderful if there was a therapy that worked better for more severely disturbed patients than it did for securely attached patients – it would get a lot of use – but such an intervention does not exist.

Despite the fact that attachment is intimately related to therapeutic outcome, clinicians should not be nihilistic about their work with patients with more maladaptive attachment styles. There are many patients with varying styles of attachment who do quite well in IPT. Further, there is no evidence that patients with more maladaptive attachment styles do better in other psychotherapies as compared with IPT – in fact, a reasonable argument could be made that for acute problems, IPT is well suited for many insecurely attached patients because the treatment is focal and less intense than more dynamically oriented therapies. The bottom line is that the therapist should recognize that attachment style does influence outcome, and should adjust her expectations about what therapy is likely to achieve on that basis.

Interpersonal Theory

Interpersonal Theory, as articulated by Kiesler,[22-25] Benjamin,[26,27] and Horowitz,[28,29] among others, is intimately connected to Attachment Theory, and can be understood in an IPT framework as describing the way individuals communicate their attachment needs to significant others within specific interpersonal relationships. Attachment Theory describes what happens in the broad, or macro, social context, while Interpersonal Theory describes communication within individual relationships on a micro level. Attachment is the template upon which specific interpersonal communication occurs.

According to Kiesler and Watkins,[30] human personality can be understood as an enduring pattern of recurrent interpersonal interactions. Similarly, attachment can also be understood as an enduring pattern of recurrent interpersonal interactions. These patterns are played out across a wide variety of relationships in the individual's social network. Dysfunctional interpersonal relationships are characterized by disordered interpersonal communications, which in turn are influenced by the individual's expectations about how relationships are formed and maintained. In IPT, this expectation about relationships is based on the working model of attachment described by Bowlby.[6] The distortions imposed upon relationships as a result of these working models, because they are often inaccurate, dramatically influence the interpersonal communication that occurs.

In every interpersonal communication that occurs, individuals negotiate three specific aspects of relationship.[30] Because these aspects are a product of the communication between individuals, they are termed 'metacommunications' – they are communications about the qualities of the relationships itself, and reflect what the relationship is like. The elements are:

- *Affiliation*, i.e. the degree to which individuals have positive (*high affiliation*) or negative (*low affiliation*) feelings about one another
- *Status*, i.e. the degree to which one or the other person is 'in charge' of decisions made within the relationship and the agenda for the relationship (*dominant* versus *submissive*)
- *Inclusion*, i.e. the degree to which the relationship stands as important to each individual (*high* versus *low inclusion*).

The affiliation and status aspects of relationships can be portrayed graphically using two-dimensional axes, and an individuals' communication at any given moment can be graphically displayed on this grid (Figure 2.5). The x-axis denotes affiliation (ranging from low to high) and the y-axis the degree of status (ranging from dominant to submissive). The z-axis (not pictured) could be included in three-dimensional space representing inclusion (ranging from low to high inclusion).

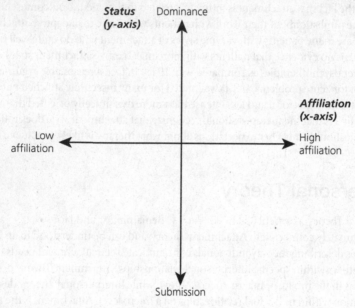

Figure 2.5 Dimensions of interpersonal relationships

The metacommunication of an individual can be plotted on this grid for any specific communication. For instance, the statement 'I love you' spoken to an intimate partner would convey a very high degree of affiliation, a high degree of inclusion reflective of the importance of the relationship, and a neutral degree of dominance. A statement such as 'This project is unacceptable', spoken by a boss to an employee, would convey a high degree of dominance along with low affiliation. Such a statement would also convey a high degree of inclusion if the employee wants to keep her job. A passing comment between strangers, such as 'Nice day today', although fairly high in affiliation, would have a low degree of inclusion as the relationship is not particularly important to either person. On a micro-level, this communication occurs on a moment-by-moment, or statement-by-statement, basis.[31] The cumulative effect of these metacommunications determines the nature of a relationship, and is a manifestation of the attachment styles of both individuals in the relationship.

In addition to the direct communication which occurs in relationships, affiliation, status, and inclusion metacommunications also evoke specific responses from others.[30] These reciprocal responses follow a predictable pattern that has been confirmed by research. The most obvious of these reciprocal responses occurs with affiliative communication: communication which is high in affiliation typically evokes highly affiliative responses (Figure 2.6). This is true both of dominant and submissive communication on the affiliative side of the graph, in which affiliative dominant comments tend to evoke or elicit more submissive affiliative responses and vice versa. For example, a friendly request for advice or assistance (affiliative submissive) usually elicits a pleasant offer of input or help (affiliative dominant); a gracious offer of help (affiliative dominant) is usually gratefully received (affiliative submissive). These interactions are illustrated by the solid arrow on the right side of the graph in Figure 2.6.

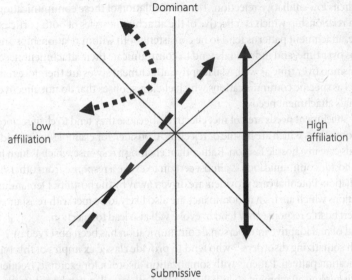

Figure 2.6 Reciprocal interpersonal communication

Reciprocal responses are elicited by specific interpersonal communications. In addition to the responses typically elicited by specific affiliative and status communications, inclusive communications pull for a similar degree of inclusiveness from the other individual.

The dotted curved line in Figure 2.6 represents the elicitations typical for hostile dominant communications. Rather than eliciting a submissive response, hostile dominant comments pull for more of the same – more hostile and more dominant responses. Threats tend to provoke threats, and, unfortunately, the potential for violence tends to escalate quickly as dominant threats are made back and forth.

The one surprising reciprocal communication is the response that is elicited by more submissive hostile communications (the dashes). In contrast to what might be expected (a hostile dominant response), submissive low-affiliation communications tend to initially elicit high-affiliation dominant responses. Significant others (particularly therapists attempting to maintain a positive frame) often attempt to pull the passive-aggressive individual into a more positive relationship by responding positively.[d] This last kind of reciprocal communication occurs frequently in therapeutic encounters. For instance, a low-affiliation submissive

---

[d] An alternative hypothesis would be that the passive-aggressive individual is so good at their communication style that the respondent has no choice but to respond differently – meeting passive-aggressiveness with passive-aggressiveness is a difficult skill to learn!

communication from a patient, such as 'I didn't manage to get my homework done', usually elicits a response from the therapist like, 'That's OK, I'm sure you'll be able to do it next week' or an even more apologetic 'I think I assigned homework that was too difficult for you; we'll try again and I'm sure you'll get it done this time'. The response can be thought of as cheerleading to try to shift the patient out of the passive-aggressive position. It is usually not successful if the patient is skilled at passive-aggressiveness. And it is difficult for the therapist to maintain the cheerleading if the patient continues to be passive-aggressive – eventually, the therapist will respond reciprocally with hostility or rejection.

According to Kiesler, interpersonal problems occur because patients unintentionally elicit negative reciprocal responses from others[31] such as those described above. Hostile aggression, for example, elicits more hostility and rejection. Persistent passive-aggressive communication ultimately elicits low-affiliative rejection. The accumulation of these communications establishes a relationship which is reflective of the attachment styles of both participants. As noted above, attachment patterns tend to be consistent both within relationships and across relationships over time, and individuals tend to communicate their attachment needs in a consistent fashion over time as well. Maladaptive attachment styles are therefore reflected on a micro-level as specific communications which elicit responses that do not effectively meet the individual's attachment needs.

Patients' attachment needs are not met effectively because they tend to elicit reciprocal responses from others which are hostile or rejecting. Consider, for example, an individual who demands care in a hostile fashion. Rather than eliciting a response which is high in affiliation, a hostile communication is almost certain to evoke a response from others which is low in affiliation. Potential care providers are driven away by the hostility. Demanding communications which are high in dominance are also likely to be met with resistance, as the overt or covert hostile response they tend to evoke will also lead to rejection.

This kind of maladaptive interpersonal communication has been observed in patients with somatizing disorders,[16] who tend to provide classic examples of this type of communication pattern. Patients with somatization disorder, for example, frequently manifest a dismissing attachment style, believing that others will never be able to meet their attachment needs. Their communication of this fear and attachment distress, however, comes in the form of statements conveying anger at not being cared for, not being understood, and not being taken seriously. Their demands are usually hostile and aggressive. This ultimately results in the caregiver's rejecting of the somatizer, as well as the somatizing patient's rejection of help from others. Medical professionals are usually quite happy to be rid of such patients, as their persistent hostile communication quashes any desire of the care provider to help. The patient's hostile communications elicit rejection.

Hypochondriacal patients, as another example, often have preoccupied attachment styles which are manifested as persistent help-seeking behavior.[17] Unlike somatizing patients, however, their attachment needs are communicated in a way that is high in affiliation but which is very submissive. Initially, they tend to evoke caring responses from others – many hypochondriacal patients are quite pleasant to work with during the first several sessions. Over time, however, their persistent help-seeking behavior, combined with a very passive and submissive pattern of communication and an inability to be reassured, lead others to become frustrated and ultimately reject the hypochondriac. Again, the patient's communications elicit rejection.

As a final example, consider a patient with schizoid personality traits. Because of his fearful attachment style, such a patient will typically communicate in a fashion which is low in affiliation and inclusion – though not hostile, he may be unable to tolerate a close relationship and will remain distant. This distancing behavior and communication consistently elicits a distancing or low affiliation response from others. A lack of social skills may also inhibit the communication, leading to a frustration of attachment needs when they are communicated ineffectively to others.

In sum, *maladaptive attachment styles lead to inappropriate or inadequate interpersonal communication that prevents the patient's attachment needs from being met.* The continual and rigid verbal and non-verbal pattern of communication elicits a rigidly restricted range of responses from others, usually culminating in rejection. These maladaptive attachment styles and communications are characterized by their rigidity and by the negative responses they evoke.

To make matters worse, patients' maladaptive attachment styles and communication patterns are reinforced by the responses which they provoke. Since those with insecure attachments tend to push others away and elicit rejecting responses as a result of their ineffective communication, their working model of relationships that others will not provide support or will reject them is further reinforced. The very rejection that their behavior and communication evokes becomes further proof that they will never receive adequate care. Since their ability to convey a need for care is greatly restricted, the threat to the minimal care they are able to obtain is met with an even more intense use of the same maladaptive communication, perpetuating and escalating the cycle. For example, angry somatizing patients, upon the elicitation of a rejecting response from a care provider, will communicate even more anger and hostility at being rejected in their next encounter with a medical professional. This makes it even less likely that their attachment needs will be met, and further reinforces their interpersonal working model and their maladaptive attachment style (Figure 2.7).

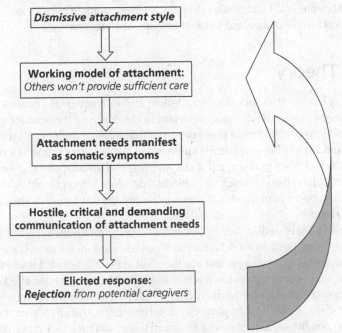

Figure 2.7 The interpersonal communication of somatizing patients. Somatization disorder is characterized by a dismissing attachment style. This reflects a working model of attachment in which the patient is convinced that others won't provide sufficient care. The patient's attachment needs are framed as somatic symptoms for which he needs care, but his requests for care and reassurance are usually hostile, critical, and demanding. This elicits a rejecting and hostile response from potential care providers, further reinforcing the patient's belief that others won't provide sufficient care. The cycle repeats with greater intensity.

Adding insult to injury, patients displaying maladaptive communication patterns typically lack insight into their communication style.[30] In other words, they are at a loss to understand why others are not providing care for them, and do not understand why others ultimately reject them. They are quite aware that they are distressed and that their needs are not being met, but they do not appreciate that this is in large part because the way they are communicating that is leading to their distress. They do not understand that they are not communicating their needs graciously, nor communicating them in a way that others can respond to easily.

This understanding of communication and interpersonal relationships leads to four specific tasks for the IPT therapist.

- First, the therapist should identify the patient's maladaptive communication style and the way her moment-to-moment communication is eliciting rejection or negative responses from others. Interpersonal Incidents (described in Chapter 9) are an excellent way to obtain this information.
- Second, the therapist should help the patient to recognize her ineffective communication, often using communication analysis (another technique described in Chapter 9).
- Third, the therapist should work with the patient to determine ways that she can communicate more effectively.
- Fourth, the therapist should help the patient to put these into practice in her relationships outside of therapy.

Despite the wishes of the therapist and patient that therapy would be easy, it is this last point – working to change communication and practicing, practicing, practicing – that requires the most persistence. There are, in IPT and all other therapies, no magic words or miracle cures that will allow the patient to make changes and sustain them without a lot of practice.

Social Theory

Social Theory has less relevance than Attachment and Interpersonal Theories to the specific interventions in IPT, but it is important in emphasizing the need for general social support in recovering from depression and maintaining wellness. Research in depression and anxiety has consistently emphasized the causative role of interpersonal factors such as loss, poor or disrupted social support, and maladaptive responses to life events.[32] The social milieu in which an individual develops interpersonal relationships, and her social support in particular, strongly influence the way in which she copes with interpersonal stress.

Social Theory has been described by Henderson et al.[33-35] and Brown et al.[36-38] among others. Social Theory posits that a deficiency in social relationships is a causal factor in the genesis of psychological distress, and that the effect of these deficits holds whether an individual is exposed to high or low levels of adversity. Moreover, it is the effect of the individual's *current* environment that is crucial.[34] While past relationships and early life environment may contribute to the picture by distorting the individual's perception of contemporary conditions, it is not invoked in social theory as a necessary causal agent.[34] In sum, stress in current social relationships is an independent causative factor in the genesis of psychological distress.

Social Theory therefore stands in sharp contrast to psychoanalytic theory, and clearly differentiates IPT from more psychoanalytic and psychodynamic approaches. Psychoanalysis rests on two fundamental principles: psychic determinism and the proposition that unconscious mental processes are the foundation for an individual's conscious thoughts and behaviors. According to psychoanalytic theory, individuals are largely unaware of the processes that drive their behavior, and it is these unconscious factors that lead to neurosis and psychopathology.[39] In contrast, Social Theory as it informs IPT invokes neither of these principles. The fundamental basis for Social Theory is that current interpersonal stressors lead to psychopathology – there is no need to rely on either unconscious processes nor psychic determinism as causal factors. The implications of this difference are clear – psychoanalysis is designed to elicit the unconscious determinants of psychopathology, while Social Theory suggests that interventions which affect current social relationships will lead to improved functioning. The latter approach is completely consistent with IPT, and accounts for the emphasis on the development and utilization of social support, a key target in IPT.

Another important concept in Social Theory is that of qualitative responses to social stress. Rather than viewing psychiatric illness as a dichotomous proposition – i.e. one either has an illness or does not have an illness – many social theorists have argued that the distinction between emotional distress and illness is simply one of degree.[40] In other words, there is a spectrum of responses to social stressors which ranges from mild to severe distress; psychiatric illness is simply defined as crossing an arbitrary line of severity. This is the position taken in IPT: distress, whether conceptualized as a formal psychiatric disorder or not, is the appropriate target for therapy. Further, the differences in individuals' experiences of distress, depression, and anxiety are strongly influenced by psychosocial factors.[41] These experiential differences are not reflected in diagnoses, which include only symptoms, but can and should be included in the Interpersonal Formulation. This concept is important in IPT because it is the basis for providing treatment to all individuals who are distressed rather than limiting it only to those who meet a particular set of diagnostic criteria. A number of studies have demonstrated an association between quality of social support and psychological distress, including a series of studies by Henderson et al.,[34,42] who demonstrated that poor social support is associated with depression and other 'neurotic' illnesses.[35,43] Henderson also hypothesized that personality and quality of attachments, among other factors, may be responsible for the difficulties some individuals have in obtaining care and support from others.[33]

The concept of 'social support networks' has been shown to be relevant to interpersonal and psychological distress. Studies confirm that social isolation or limited social interaction places individuals at greater risk for mental illness. The quality of the interaction, however, appears to be more important than the absolute number of relationships. This perceived social support is a function of the individual's subjective evaluation of the dependability of the social network, the ease of interaction within the network, her sense of belonging to the network, and her sense of intimacy with network members.[44] Work by Brown and colleagues has also consistently demonstrated a correlation between adverse social events and the incidence of psychiatric disorders.[45,46] Both current social stressors and childhood experiences of neglect and abuse have been correlated with anxiety and depression.[36]

Marital conflict is one of the most consistent risk factors for depression and is an example of the link between interpersonal problems and distress. Rates of major depressive disorder are highest among separated and divorced individuals and lowest among the single and married. Recent widowhood is associated with higher rates of major depressive disorder across the life cycle,[47] and the absence of a spouse is a risk factor for major depressive disorder.[37] Grief and loss have been associated with depressive symptoms in both men and women, particularly those with poor social supports.[48,49] In contrast, the presence of attachments that can help sustain individuals during a loss appears to be helpful in preventing episodes of depression.[50]

In sum, an individual's social support network greatly influences the likelihood that she will have psychiatric difficulties. This relationship appears to be even stronger when an individual is faced with a significant psychosocial stressor. Those individuals who do not have, or perceive that they have do not have, others they can depend on for support or a good social network, are much more likely to become distressed.

IPT: From Theory to Intervention

The targets of IPT, psychological distress, interpersonal problems, and social support, are all based on Attachment, Interpersonal, and Social Theories. These theories also inform the specific techniques and tactics used in IPT. This theoretical foundation leads to five essential tasks for the IPT therapist (Box 2.2).

Box 2.2 Therapeutic tasks in IPT

> ○ The therapist must create a strong therapeutic alliance (a relationship with a high degree of inclusion and affiliation)
> ○ The therapist must identify the patient's maladaptive communications
> ○ The therapist must help the patient become aware of her maladaptive communications
> ○ The therapist must help the patient modify her communications and practice these changes
> ○ The therapist must assist the patient to build a better social support network, and to utilize the social supports that are currently available

First and foremost, the clinician must create a therapeutic environment in which there is a high degree of inclusion and affiliation: a good therapeutic alliance is absolutely essential in IPT, and the burden to create one is on the therapist! The therapeutic relationship needs to be developed in such a way that it holds importance for both the therapist and patient – both should be actively engaged and attentive to communications from the other. If this does not occur, feedback from the therapist (and from the patient) will be easily dismissed, and the therapy itself will be jeopardized because the patient will simply abandon it. If a productive therapeutic alliance is not established, the patient can easily devalue the therapeutic relationship and consequently ignore any input from the therapist, rendering moot all of the specific techniques the therapist might use.

Creating a meaningful therapeutic relationship is a necessary condition of all psychotherapies. It is of particular importance in IPT, however, as the Acute Phase of Treatment is time-limited. It is incumbent upon the therapist to quickly establish a therapeutic alliance, so that the work of therapy can be accomplished. For this reason, in IPT particular attention must be paid to all of the 'non-specific elements' of therapy: warmth, empathy, affective attunement, positive regard – all of the elements described by Rogers and Truaz[51] as necessary to bring about psychotherapeutic change. It is crucial that IPT therapists be more than technicians – without establishing a productive therapeutic alliance, none of the IPT techniques and strategies will be effective – for that matter, neither will techniques from any other therapeutic approach.

The therapist should also constantly remember that the quality of the alliance is the primary predictor of psychotherapy outcome. Research has consistently demonstrated this in literally every form of therapy in which the alliance has been examined.[52–58] This is not to say that the specific techniques and tactics which characterize different therapies are not important, but rather that they pale in comparison to the effects of the alliance. The therapeutic alliance is even more important with patients who have maladaptive attachment styles,[57] as they will make it difficult for their therapists to consistently respond empathically. Rather than eliciting sympathetic and caregiving responses, such patients will eventually evoke hostility and rejection even from the most gracious therapists. The therapist must be aware of this, and respond by being even more active in conveying empathy and positive regard to those patients who do not naturally evoke such responses.

A patient with a fearful attachment style, for instance, may evoke feelings of boredom or rejection, which will destroy the therapeutic alliance if the therapist responds in kind to this provocation. The therapist must recognize the interpersonal response that is being evoked by the patient, understand the specific communication that is eliciting it, and adapt her responses to create a more productive therapeutic alliance. With such a patient, the therapist may choose to use more empathic statements, or may choose to let the patient set the agenda in early sessions rather than imposing the therapist's agenda too early and risk having the patient feel rejected.

Conversely, a patient with a preoccupied attachment style may 'wear down' the therapist with repeated requests for reassurance, so that over time, the responses that are evoked by the patient are exasperation and rejection. Again, the therapist must recognize the communication pattern, be aware of the responses that the patient evokes, and move to counter the patient's provocation by being consistently caring despite being drawn to do otherwise. Patients with preoccupied attachment are more likely to become dependent on the therapist and therefore have difficulty ending a time-limited therapeutic relationship. The therapist can counter this by placing even greater emphasis on the need for the patient to develop a more supportive social network outside of therapy. Structurally, the therapist can also gradually taper the last several sessions of Acute Treatment over time rather than coming to an abrupt termination, an event which would undoubtedly be very distressing to a preoccupied patient.

Some patients, fortunately, are relatively secure in their attachments, and can communicate their needs effectively, including those in the therapeutic relationship. Such patients require little adjustment on the part of the therapist, are able to receive feedback and use it productively, and are also able to make adjustments within their extended support network. With these patients, the therapist can move to the intermediate phase of IPT and can begin giving feedback to the patient much more quickly, as it will be perceived by the patient as helpful rather than as rejecting.

Herein is a crucial difference between IPT and transference-based psychodynamic psychotherapies. In IPT, the therapist works to recognize the patient's underlying attachment needs and to help the patient meet those needs outside of therapy. In transference-based psychotherapy, the therapist attempts to become a 'blank screen' upon which the patient projects her transference neurosis – this reaction is stimulated with intent as the therapist actively resists meeting the patient's attachment needs in therapy.

The second task of the IPT therapist is to develop an understanding or conceptualization of the patient's communication problems by recognizing the pattern of interpersonal communication as it occurs both in the patient's interpersonal sphere outside of treatment and in the therapeutic relationship. Attachment Theory suggests that attachment styles will be manifest across relationships, including the relationship that develops between therapist and patient. The patient–therapist relationship must be attended to very carefully by the IPT therapist, as it provides extremely valuable information about the way the patient typically attaches to and communicates with others. The difficulties experienced by the patient in communicating within the therapeutic relationship will be manifest in her other relationships. The attachment style which becomes apparent in therapy will be manifest in all of the patient's other relationships, and the ways the therapist is drawn to respond to the patient's communications, particularly those communications involving care-eliciting behavior, will be the ways others outside of therapy are also drawn to respond. Understanding transference in IPT is paramount in developing an accurate formulation of the patient's attachment behavior and interpersonal communication.

In IPT, however, this information is used to ask questions about relationships outside of therapy rather than being used to directly address the relationship between the patient and the therapist. The data gleaned from the therapist's experience of the transference should lead her to ask questions about the way the patient communicates in her relationships outside of therapy; the therapeutic relationship itself need not be addressed as a point of intervention in IPT. When the therapist experiences the patient as passive, for instance, it should lead the therapist to ask questions about the ways the patient may be passive in her extra-therapy relationships. When the therapist feels drawn to respond with hostility, this should lead to queries about incidents when the patient has experienced others outside of therapy reacting with hostility. When the therapist is feeling frustrated, questions which investigate the possibility that others also feel frustrated by the patient should be asked.

While understanding the transference which develops in IPT is crucial to its conduct because it informs the therapist about the ways the patient forms and maintains relationships outside of therapy, IPT, in contrast to psychodynamic psychotherapies, does not focus on transference or the therapeutic relationship as a point of discussion in therapy. The reason for this is that to do so is likely to move the patient away from a here-and-now focus on symptom resolution and into a long-term therapy designed to modify personality or deep-seated attachment problems. While such therapies may be quite helpful for severely disturbed patients, they are outside of the scope of IPT. In IPT, the focus is rapid resolution of symptoms and distress rather than a focus on changing underlying attachment style.

Because the point of IPT is resolution of distress rather than an examination of transference as it develops, the therapist has some latitude in positioning herself in therapy. In transference-based therapies, the therapist ideally is a 'blank screen' upon which the patient has maximum opportunity to project and make clear her transference reactions. Transference-based therapies are designed in such a way that the therapist encourages the development of transference, not only by asking questions about it, but by being non-disclosing and neutral. In contrast, because IPT is designed to focus on relationships outside of therapy and therefore need not encourage the development of transference, the therapist can position herself in the role of a 'coach' or 'mentor'. In attachment terms, the therapist's stance is to be a constant and consistent care-provider, encouraging a positive transferential relationship with the patient in which the therapist is seen as an expert who is willing and able to be of help.

On a practical level, this means that *the IPT therapist has more freedom to use techniques which might otherwise obscure the development of transference*. Self-disclosure, for instance, may be very useful with patients who are more securely attached. The therapist may wish to speak about solutions that other patients with similar problems have found helpful (taking care to maintain confidentiality). The IPT therapist may also be active in helping the patient to extend her social support network, making direct suggestions to attend groups such as Alcoholics Anonymous, religious or spiritual groups, new mothers' support groups, exercise classes and the like, going as far, if needed, as helping the patient find resources for transportation to such groups.

Although the transference experience provides a great deal of information about the patient's style of attachment and communication, it is by no means the only information that the therapist should use. In fact, the primary source of information for understanding the patient's communications should be examples of communication: specific incidents in which the patient has attempted to communicate her needs with significant others. The technique of examining Interpersonal Incidents, described in Chapter 9, is a wonderful method to examine in detail the ways in which the patient is not effectively communicating her needs within relationships. Analyzing these will help the therapist to understand how maladaptive or ineffective communication is occurring.

General patterns in relationships should also be explored, both to help the therapist understand the patient more fully and to assist the patient to see these patterns. The Interpersonal Inventory, in addition to providing information about the patient's social support, should be used as a means of beginning to understand the patient's patterns of relationships. Asking questions about the ways the patient typically forms relationships, ends relationships, or common disappointments that she experiences in relationships can also be extremely helpful.

In essence, the goal of the IPT therapist is to gather information which contributes to an understanding of the patient's attachment style, and then to use specific techniques like Interpersonal Incidents to collect and analyze examples of communication. This provides for a more complete understanding of the patient's difficulties in communication outside of therapy. Within therapy, rather than examining the transference with the patient, the therapist should position herself as an expert help-provider. The idea is literally to have the patient 'get in and get out' of therapy before problematic transference develops. Thus the paramount importance of the time limit in IPT, and the need to focus on here-and-now relationships outside of therapy as the best way to address the primary targets of symptom resolution and relief of distress.

The third task of the IPT therapist is to help the patient become aware of her maladaptive communications: the goal is to help the patient develop insight into her communication style. The therapist needs to understand the ways the patient communicates, the responses that the patient's communication evokes, and the ways the patient's style of communication is perpetuated. In addition, the therapist must assist the patient to appreciate that her communication is not effective – i.e. that it is not achieving the patient's goal of meeting her attachment needs. Communication analysis is a great technique to achieve this. Most patients feel very misunderstood, and once that is acknowledged, the therapist can then work with the patient to communicate differently – to help her to help others understand her more fully.

The goal of treatment with IPT is change in the patient's communication and behavior so that her attachment needs are more fully met. In most cases, this requires at least a limited degree of insight by the patient. This is insight in which the patient recognizes her communication style and the responses it evokes. It does not necessarily require insight into the genesis of the patient's attachment or communication styles. The insight need only be enough that the patient recognize the consequences of her here-and-now communications with others, and in doing so, is motivated to change.

Ideally, the patient would come to recognize something like this:

I have a tendency to communicate in a specific way. My communications tend to draw others to respond in a characteristic way as well. The responses I elicit from others aren't helpful to me, and tend to produce a response which leaves me even more frustrated. I now recognize that I can get my needs met more fully by communicating differently in a way that others respond to more positively.

The fourth task of the IPT therapist is to help the patient modify her communications and practice these changes. The therapist must help the patient to change her communication by developing and practicing new behaviors. IPT techniques such as problem solving can assist the patient both to recognize and to change communications, so that her attachment needs are met more fully. Role playing provides the opportunity to solidify the newly established ways of communicating. Homework can also be used. The goal is to help the patient recognize communication patterns, modify those patterns so that her needs are more effectively met, and maintain the new communication once it is established. It is a simple process, but it takes a great deal of practice.

The fifth task of the IPT therapist is to assist the patient to build a better social support network, and to utilize the social supports that are currently available. The social milieu is intimately connected to the patient's ability to deal with interpersonal crises. The greater the support, the more likely the patient is to weather the interpersonal storm. Thus it is the therapist's task to encourage the patient to identify both existing and potential sources of support, as well as to begin to utilize them constructively.

Conclusion

IPT rests on two primary theoretical foundations: Attachment Theory and Interpersonal Theory. Social Theory provides additional emphasis on the importance of social support. All coalesce within a Biopsychosocial/Cultural/Spiritual model which explains the patient's distress as well as directing the interventions which are used in IPT. The Interpersonal Triad includes an acute psychosocial stressor, coupled with biological and attachment diatheses, in the context of insufficient social support, which lead to the development of symptoms and psychological distress. IPT is specifically designed to help patients by assisting them to improve their interpersonal communication, resolve their interpersonal problems, and more fully develop and utilize their social support systems.

References

1. Bowlby J. *Attachment. Attachment and Loss. Vol. 1.* 1969, New York: Basic Books.

2. Bowlby J. *Separation: Anxiety and Anger. Attachment and Loss. Vol. 2.* 1973, New York: Basic Books.

3. Bowlby J. The making and breaking of affectional bonds: etiology and psychopathology in the light of attachment theory. *British Journal of Psychiatry*, 1977, **130**: 201–210.

4. Bowlby J. The making and breaking of affectional bonds, II: some principles of psychotherapy. *British Journal of Psychiatry*, 1977, **130**: 421–431.

5. Bowlby J. *Loss: Sadness and Depression. Attachment and Loss. Vol. 3.* 1980, New York: Basic Books.

6. Bowlby J. Developmental psychiatry comes of age. *American Journal of Psychiatry*, 1988, **145**: 1–10.

7. Ainsworth MD. Object relations, dependency, and attachment: a theoretical view of the infant-mother relationship. *Child Development*, 1969, **40**: 969–1027.

8. Ainsworth MS, *et al. Patterns of Attachment: A Psychological Study of the Strange Situation.* 1978, MahWah: Erlbaum.

9. George C, Kaplan N and Main M. *Adult Attachment Interview*, 2nd edn. 1985, Berkely: University of California at Berkely Press.

10. Hazan C and Shaver PR. Romantic love conceptualized as an attachment process. *Journal of Personality and Social Psychology*, 1987, **52**: 511–524.

11. Sullivan HS. *The Interpersonal Theory of Psychiatry*. 1953, New York: Norton.

12. Main M and Solomon J. Discovery of an insecure-disorganized/dioriented attachment pattern, in Brazelton TB and Yogman M (eds) *Affective Development in Infancy*. 1986, Norwood: Alblex Publishing, pp. 95–124.

13. Pilkonis PA. Personality prototypes among depressives: themes of dependency and autonomy. *Journal of Personality Disorders*, 1988, **2**: 144–152.

14. Brennan KA, Clark CL and Shaver PR. Self-report measure of adult attachment, in Simpson JA and Rholes WS (eds) *Attachment Theory and Close Relationships*. 1998, New York: Guilford Press, pp. 46–76.

15. Bartholomew K and Horowitz LM. Attachment styles among young adults: a test of a four category model. *Journal of Personality and Social Psychology*, 1991, **61**: 226–244.

16. Stuart S and Noyes R Jr. Attachment and interpersonal communication in somatization. *Psychosomatics*, 1999, **40**(1): 34–43.

17. Stuart S and Noyes R Jr. Treating hypochondriasis with interpersonal psychotherapy. *Journal of Contemporary Psychotherapy*, 2005, **35**: 269–283.

18. Stuart S and Noyes R Jr. Interpersonal psychotherapy for somatizing patients. *Psychotherapy and Psychosomatics*, 2006, **75**: 209–219.

19. Parkes CM. Psycho-social transitions: a field of study. *Social Science and Medicine*, 1971, **5**: 101–115.

20. Parkes CM. Bereavement and mental illness. *British Journal of Medical Psychology*, 1965, **38**: 1–26.

21. Henderson S. Care-eliciting behavior in man. *Journal of Nervous and Mental Disease*, 1974, **159**: 172–181.

22. Kiesler DJ. Interpersonal methods of assessment and diagnosis, in Snyder CR and Forsyth DR (eds) *Handbook of Social and Clinical Psychology: The Health Perspective*. 1991, Elmsford: Pergamon Press, pp. 438–468.

23. Kiesler DJ. Interpersonal circle inventories: pantheoretical applications to psychotherapy research and practice. *Journal of Psychotherapy Integration*, 1992, **2**: 77–99.

24. Kiesler DJ. Standardization of intervention: the tie that binds psychotherapy research and practice, in Talley PF, Strupp HH and Butler SF (eds) *Psychotherapy Research and Practice: Bridging the Gap*.1994, New York: Basic Books.

25. Kiesler DJ. *Contemporary Interpersonal Theory and Research: Personality, Psychopathology, and Psychotherapy*. 1996, New York: John Wiley & Sons.

26. Benjamin LS. *Interpersonal Diagnosis and Treatment of Personality Disorders*. 1996, New York: Guilford Publications.

27. Benjamin LS. Introduction to the special section on structural analysis of social behavior. *Journal of Consulting and Clinical Psychology*, 1996, **64**: 1203–1212.

28. Horowitz LM. *Interpersonal Foundations of Psychopathology*. 2004, Washington DC: American Psychological Association.

29. Horowitz LM, *et al*. How interpersonal motives clarify the meaning of interpersonal behavior: a revised circumplex model. *Personality and Social Psychology Review*, 2006, **10**: 67–86.

30. Kiesler DJ and Watkins LM. Interpersonal complimentarity and the therapeutic alliance: a study of the relationship in psychotherapy. *Psychotherapy*, 1989, **26**: 183–194.

31. Kiesler DJ. An interpersonal communication analysis of relationship in psychotherapy. *Journal for the Study of Interpersonal Processes*, 1979, **42**: 299–311.

32. Weissman MM and Paykel ES. *The Depressed Woman: A Study of Social Relationships*. 1974, Chicago: University of Chicago Press.

33. Henderson S. The social network, support, and neurosis: the function of attachment in adult life. *British Journal of Psychiatry*, 1977, **131**: 185–191.

34. Henderson S, Byrne DG and Duncan-Jones P. *Neurosis and the Social Environment*. 1982, Sydney: Academic Press.

35. Henderson S, *et al*. Social bonds in the epidemiology of neurosis. *British Journal of Psychiatry*, 1978, **132**: 463–466.

36. Brown GW, Harris TO and Eales MJ. Social factors and comorbidity of depressive and anxiety disorders. *British Journal of Psychiatry*, 1996, **168** (suppl 30): 50–57.

37. Brown GW and Harris TO. *Social Origins of Depression: A Study of Psychiatric Disorders in Women*. 1978, London: Tavistock.

38. Brown GW and Harris TO. *Life Events and Illness*. 1989, New York: Guilford Publications.

39. Brenner C. *An Elementary Textbook of Psychoanalysis*. 1973, New York: Anchor Press.

40. Bebbington PE. Inferring causes: some constraints in the social psychiatry of depressive disorders. *Integrative Psychiatry*, 1984, **2**: 69–72.

41. Brown GW. Genetic and population perspectives on life events and depression. *Social Psychiatry and Psychiatric Epidemiology*, 1998, **33**: 363–372.

42. Henderson S, *et al*. Psychiatric disorder in Canberra: a standardized study of prevalence. *Acta Psychiatrica Scandinavica*, 1979, **60**: 355–374.

43. Henderson S, *et al*. Social relationships, adversity and neurosis: a study of associations in a general population sample. *British Journal of Psychiatry*, 1980, **136**: 574–583.

44. Henderson AS. Interpreting the evidence on social support. *Social Psychiatry*, 1984, **19**: 49–52.

45. Brown GW, *et al*. Life stress, chronic subclinical symptoms and vulnerability to clinical depression. *Journal of Affective Disorders*, 1986, **11**: 1–19.

46. Andrews B and Brown GW. Social support, onset of depression and personality: an exploratory analysis. *Social Psychiatry and Psychiatric Epidemiology*, 1988, **23**: 99–108.

47. Paykel ES. Life stress and psychiatric disorder, in Dohrenwend BS and Dohrenwend BP (eds) *Stressful Life Events: Their Naure and Effects*. 1974, New York: Wiley.

48. Walker K, MacBride A and Vachon M. Social support networks and the crisis of bereavement. *Social Sciences in Medicine*, 1977, **11**: 35–41.

49. Maddison D and Walker W. Factors affecting the outcome of conjugal bereavement. *British Journal of Psychiatry*, 1967, **113**: 1057–1067.

50. Parker G. *The Bonds of Depression*. 1978, Sydney: Angus and Robertson.

51. Rogers CR and Truaz CB. *The therapeutic conditions antecedent to change: a theoretical view. The Therapeutic Relationship and its Impact*, ed. C.R. Rogers. 1967, Madison: University of Wisconsin Press.

52. Lambert MJ. Psychotherapy outcome research: implications for integrative and eclectic theories, in Norcross JC and Goldfried MR (eds) *Handbook of Psychotherapy Integration*. 1992, New York: Basic Books.

53. Barber JP, *et al*. Alliance predicts patients' outcome beyond in-treatment change in symptoms. *Journal of Consulting and Clinical Psychology*, 2000, **68**: 1027–1032.

54. Barber J, *et al*. The role of the alliance and techniques in predicting outcome of supportive-expressive dynamic therapy for cocaine dependence. *Psychoanalytic Psychology*, 2008, **25**: 461–482.

55. Martin DJ, Garske JP and Davis MK. Relation of the therapeutic alliance with outcome and other variables: a meta-analytic review. *Journal of Consulting and Clinical Psychology*, 2000, **68**: 438–450.

56. Zuroff DC, *et al*. Relation of therapeutic alliance and perfectionism to outcome in brief outpatient treatment of depression. *Journal of Consulting and Clinical Psychology*, 2000, **68**: 114–124.

57. Diener MJ and Monroe JM. The relationship between adult attachment style and therapeutic alliance in individual psychotherapy: a meta-analytic review. *Psychotherapy*, 2011, **48**(3): 237–248.

58. Horvath AO, *et al*. Alliance in individual psychotherapy. *Psychotherapy*, 2011, **48**(1): 9–16.

Section 2

Assessment/Initial Sessions

3

The Structure of Interpersonal Psychotherapy

Introduction

This chapter is a brief overview of the structure of Interpersonal Psychotherapy (IPT), emphasizing a view of the forest rather than the trees. IPT is divided into four segments: the Assessment/Initial Phase, the Intermediate Phase, the Conclusion of Acute Treatment, and Maintenance Treatment (Figure 3.1).

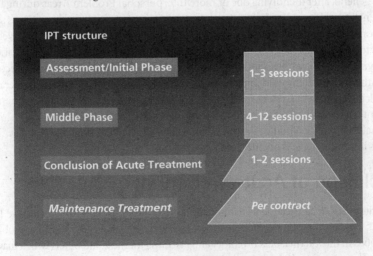

Figure 3.1 The structure of IPT

In the Assessment/Initial Phase, the therapist makes a determination about the patient's suitability for IPT. This assessment includes an Interpersonal Inventory and an Interpersonal Formulation. If the patient is suitable, the therapist then negotiates a Treatment Agreement with the patient. In the Middle Phase, the therapist and patient work at resolving the patient's interpersonal problems (the three IPT Problem Areas) using IPT techniques. When Concluding Acute Treatment, the therapist and patient review progress as well as planning for future problems. Maintenance IPT should be arranged by the patient and therapist depending on the patient's history, severity of distress, and risk for relapse. The Conclusion of Acute Treatment can be tapered so that sessions are less frequent as the conclusion approaches.

Assessment/Initial Phase

The first purpose of the Assessment/Initial Phase is to determine if the patient is a suitable candidate for IPT, and to determine whether IPT is the best treatment. During the assessment the therapist should focus on the patient's presenting problems and attachment style, and should ask about specific instances of interpersonal interaction in order to begin to understand the patient's typical style of communication. Much of this can be accomplished by constructing an Interpersonal Inventory.

The Assessment/Initial Phase of IPT includes a number of specific tasks. The primary goals are to construct an Interpersonal Inventory (Chapter 5) and to develop an Interpersonal Formulation, a detailed hypothesis describing and explaining the patient's interpersonal difficulties (Chapter 6). A Treatment Agreement should be established with the patient to proceed with IPT, and to work on several specific interpersonal problems. Note that the agreement, in contrast to a rigid contract, is flexible, so that a range of acute treatment sessions can be negotiated rather than a fixed number.

Middle Phase

In the Middle Phase of IPT the therapist and patient work together to resolve the patient's Interpersonal Disputes, to adjust to his Role Transitions, or to deal with Grief and Loss issues. In general, after identifying one or more Interpersonal Problem Areas during the Assessment/Initial Phase, the therapist gathers more information about the patient's specific interpersonal problems. Both patient and therapist then work collaboratively to develop solutions to each, usually coming in the form of improving the patient's communication skills or modifying his expectations about a relationship conflict. A suitable option is selected, and then the patient attempts to implement it between sessions. The patient and therapist then work in subsequent sessions to refine the solution and to further assist the patient to implement it if he has had difficulty in carrying it out completely.

The hallmark of the Middle Phase of IPT is a lot of implementation and practice. The key in IPT (as in all therapies) is practice and persistence.

Conclusion of Acute Treatment

The Conclusion of Acute Treatment is a mutually negotiated ending of the intensive time-limited part of IPT. It includes a review of the patient's progress in resolving the interpersonal problems first identified in the Interpersonal Inventory and planning for these and others which may arise in the future. The patient's (and the therapist's) reactions to the conclusion should be acknowledged so that they can be discussed if needed. If IPT is done well, however, the option to taper the frequency of sessions during the Conclusion of Acute Treatment can be utilized so that the transition to Maintenance is seamless and does not cause the patient distress.

Maintenance Treatment

A specific agreement regarding the provision of Maintenance Treatment should always be negotiated with all patients, though this can vary a great deal depending on the patient's risk for relapse and need for ongoing care. In cases where a patient's problems are likely to be recurrent, the patient and therapist should develop an agreement to meet for more frequent maintenance sessions (such as monthly) to monitor ongoing interpersonal problems and to help the patient continue to work on his interpersonal skills. In contrast, if the patient's risk for relapse is low, and his current episode has been mild, the therapist and patient may choose to meet once every 6 months, or even just to have phone or email contact if needed. The scheduling of maintenance IPT sessions requires clinical judgment based on risk and need for longitudinal care. The critical tactic in IPT is simply to have a crystal clear agreement about ongoing contact based on clinical judgment – all patients will benefit from the continuity of care that is provided.

IPT is not a terminable therapy. It does not come to a complete and final end at the Conclusion of Acute Treatment. IPT is structured so that it comes to a conclusion because all of the empirical data point to the need for Maintenance Treatment for most patients. Maintenance Treatment may differ in frequency and intensity based on the individual patient's needs, but it should be provided nonetheless.

The evidence is very clear that affective and anxiety disorders are relapsing and remitting disorders. In addition, IPT has been demonstrated to be a very effective maintenance treatment,[1,2] and it has also been shown that the frequency of Maintenance Treatment can be flexible, as equivalent outcomes resulted when weekly, biweekly, and monthly maintenance sessions were compared.[3] The logical evidence-based conclusion is that Maintenance Treatment should be flexible and based on the needs of the individual patient for whom it is being provided. IPT is much more effective if it is tailored to the individual rather than attempting to use it as a one-size-fits-all approach.

In addition, in contrast to the plethora of theoretical writing on the subject, there is no evidence that terminating psychotherapy leads to better outcomes.[4] Given the well-known risk for relapse, terminating therapy is simply poor clinical practice. Moreover, despite therapists' occasional wishes to the contrary, terminating therapy is in reality nothing more than semantics: there is absolutely nothing to prevent a distressed patient from paying a visit to your office the day immediately following termination, nothing to prevent him from presenting with a new crisis, and nothing to prevent him from suing you if you refuse to treat him again. Clinicians in settings in which the number of sessions are arbitrarily limited by convention are well aware of the many ingenious ways that patients (and therapists) can circumvent the termination rules.

Terminating therapy after a fixed number of sessions is also an affront to the quality of care that virtuoso IPT clinicians should be providing. No ethical or compassionate clinician would terminate IPT after 16 sessions if the patient was still symptomatic and would benefit from a few more sessions. No reasonable clinician would terminate therapy the session after a patient has had a miscarriage or has been diagnosed with cancer or has been assaulted or has experienced any of the innumerable tragic events that randomly occur in life. It would be nice to guarantee that nothing adverse would disrupt the life of a patient as they are coming to the end of treatment, but life happens. And it sometimes happens near the originally agreed upon end of treatment. And if it does happen, then treatment should be extended. Use your common sense and clinical judgment (Box 3.1).

Box 3.1 The structure and components of IPT

Assessment/Initial Phase
- Evaluate the suitability of the patient for IPT
- Evaluate the suitability of IPT for the patient
- Assess psychiatric and interpersonal problems
- Construct an Interpersonal Inventory
- Develop an Interpersonal Formulation
- Identify specific IPT Problem Areas: Disputes, Role Transitions, Grief and Loss
- Explain the rationale for IPT
- Collaboratively establish a Treatment Agreement

Middle Phase
- Attend to the therapeutic relationship
- Maintain the focus of discussion on the specific IPT Problem Area(s)
- Explore the patient's expectations and perceptions of the specific interpersonal problem(s)
- Help the patient to develop solutions to the interpersonal crises
- Help the patient to implement the proposed solutions
- Practice, practice, practice

Conclusion of Acute Treatment
- Review the patient's progress
- Anticipate future problems
- Positively reinforce the patient's gains
- Establish a specific agreement for Maintenance Treatment

Maintenance Treatment
- Focus on Problem Areas
- Monitor progress

IPT and the Biopsychosocial/Cultural/Spiritual Model

IPT is based on the Biopsychosocial/Cultural/Spiritual model of psychological functioning, expanding beyond the Biopsychosocial model described in the first iteration of this book[5] and the long discarded and antiquated medical model. Biological diatheses in conjunction with early life experiences and attachment style lead to vulnerabilities in individual patients. Cultural and spiritual factors may also be vulnerabilities or strengths. Coupled with a sufficiently intense interpersonal stressor, individuals without adequate social support are likely to develop interpersonal difficulties. This explanatory model of distress is depicted in the Interpersonal Triad in Figure 3.2.

The structure used in IPT is directly linked to Attachment and Interpersonal Theory. The IPT therapist focuses on the patient's interpersonal relationships, particularly the way in which the patient's attachment is manifest in them. The therapist also examines the communication style that the patient uses in initiating, maintaining, and disengaging from relationships. This occurs within the time-limited Acute Treatment format of IPT, and focuses on here-and-now resolution of symptoms and distress rather than on the patient–therapist relationship.

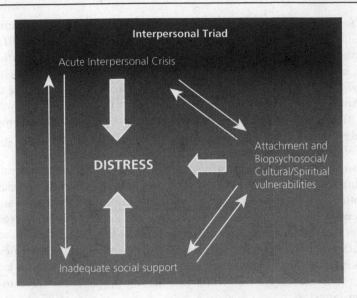

Figure 3.2 Interpersonal Triad

IPT Problem Areas

IPT focuses on three specific Problem Areas which reflect the interpersonal nature of the treatment. These are: *Grief and Loss*, *Interpersonal Disputes*, and *Role Transitions*. Psychosocial stressors from any of the Problem Areas, when combined with an attachment disruption in the context of poor social support, can lead to interpersonal problems, psychiatric syndromes, or distress. The Problem Areas should be used as guidelines, not rigid categories. They are simply a way of focusing treatment as it proceeds.

- Though often understood as a reaction to the literal death of a significant other, the Grief and Loss Problem Area in IPT can best be conceptualized as any loss experienced by the patient. *That loss, whatever it may be, should be defined by the patient, not the therapist.* It is the therapist's job to understand the patient and his perspective, not to force it into a particular category. Thus if the patient conceptualizes his experience as a Grief and Loss issue, then it is. Common sense and therapeutic graciousness should prevail in a therapist who wishes to do IPT well. In addition to loss through death, losses such as divorce may be seen by the patient as Grief and Loss issues. Loss of physical functioning, such as that following a heart attack or traumatic injury, may also be considered in the Grief and Loss Problem Area.[6] Anticipatory grief in the setting of a terminal illness, or the anticipation of the death of a loved one, such as with caregivers of patients with Alzheimer's disease, are additional examples. There is no 'right' or 'wrong' way to use the Grief and Loss category – it is simply a way to focus treatment on the specific interpersonal problem.
- Interpersonal Disputes involve a conflict between the patient and another person, and may result from either the communication problems or the unrealistic expectations of either person. Like Grief and Loss, disputes should be patient defined.
- Role Transitions, as the name suggests, involve changes in a patient's social role and the changes in social support which may accompany such transitions. These include not only life-phase transitions, such as adolescence, childbirth, and aging, but also include many social changes such as leaving home, getting married, or changes in school or job status.

Therapists familiar with previous work in IPT will note that the Problem Area formerly known as interpersonal sensitivity or interpersonal deficits is no longer used in IPT. The reason is that these concepts describe a long-standing attachment style in the fearful range of attachment rather than an Acute Interpersonal Crisis. There are patients with this style, and without doubt, they are more difficult to treat. They are difficult because they have a paucity of interpersonal support, and because it is difficult to form a therapeutic alliance with them. All of the IPT literature notes that these individuals are more complex, and that prognosis is not as good.[5,7-9] It is their fearful attachment style that leads to this complexity.

Therefore interpersonal sensitivities or deficits are best understood as a characteristic style of attachment in which the patient has difficulty forming satisfying interpersonal relationships. The poor social support network which is a consequence of this style often leads the patient to be more likely to become distressed when an acute interpersonal problem occurs. The acute problem – the Role Transition, Interpersonal Dispute, or Grief and Loss issue – should be the primary focus of IPT rather than the fearful attachment style. The fearful attachment style, manifested as sensitivities or difficulties in establishing relationships, is an additional psychological factor just like all of the other attachment styles, and it influences the way the patient will react to an acute interpersonal stressor.

There is *always* an acute crisis that leads a patient to seek treatment. Even if there have been long-standing attachment problems or a paucity of social relationships, something acute happens which finally leads a patient to make the decision to seek help – to seek therapy. It may be the death of a family member, it may be the loss of a job, it may be a perceived personal rejection, but something acute tips the balance just enough for the patient to make the decision to go to treatment. It is this crisis that should be the focus of treatment.

While the Problem Areas are very helpful as a means of focusing the patient on specific interpersonal problems, it is important for the therapist to be flexible when using them. Rather than providing the patient with the proper Problem Area 'diagnosis', the Problem Areas should be used primarily as tools to maintain focus upon one or two interpersonal problems, particularly as the time available in IPT for Acute Treatment is limited. The patient's view of the nature of the problem should be used – for example, if the patient feels that his recent divorce is a Grief issue rather than a Role Transition, then the Grief and Loss Problem Area should be used. The therapeutic alliance should not be sacrificed in order to impose the 'correct' Problem Area 'diagnosis' upon the patient.

The therapist should also be mindful that the interpersonal problems experienced by patients are similar in that they are all derived from the combination of an acute interpersonal stressor combined with a social network that does not sufficiently support them. In addition to addressing the specific problem, effort should always be directed towards improving patients' social support.

The Benefits and Limitations of Structured Psychotherapies

One of the more useful ways to describe psychotherapeutic approaches is to draw a distinction between 'structured' and 'unstructured' psychotherapies. Psychotherapeutic interventions can be placed on a spectrum on this dimension, with most of the short-term treatments at the more structured end of the scale, and most of the analytically oriented therapies at the other. There are obvious benefits and limitations to both structured and unstructured approaches – the point is to consider how specific treatments best meet the needs of a given patient. Table 3.1 compares the 'structured' and 'unstructured' psychotherapies.

Table 3.1 Characteristics of structured and unstructured therapies

	Structured	Unstructured
Examples	IPT, cognitive behavioral therapy (CBT)	Psychoanalysis, self-psychology
Time frame	Time-limited	Open-ended
Focus	Improved functioning	Psychodynamic change and insight
Therapeutic		
Relationship	Supportive, active	Non-transparent, passive
Discussions	Directed primarily by therapist	Directed primarily by patient
Transference	Not a point of intervention	Primary point of intervention

A helpful way of conceptualizing the place of IPT and other more structured psychotherapies in clinical practice is to compare them with pharmacologic treatments for physical problems such as diabetes or hypertension. From this point of view, IPT can literally be 'prescribed' as an appropriate and indicated treatment for the patient's specific problem. For example, the structure of IPT lends itself to a prescriptive treatment in a fashion analogous to the use of antibiotic therapy for pneumonia. Most patients with pneumonia require a structured course of antibiotics that is time-limited and specific to one bacterial pathogen; this treatment is usually highly effective in resolving the illness. There are, however, a few patients who are prone to recurrent infections or who are immunosuppressed. These patients require longer term use of multiple agents, with marked variations in dosing and time course.

To carry the analogy further, all patients who are treated for acute pneumonia – literally all of them – receive maintenance care as well. A primary care physician would never 'terminate' treatment; instead, he would schedule the patient for a follow-up visit a week or two later, invite the patient to call him if the problem recurred, and would ensure that the patient was scheduled for a routine physical exam at some point in the future depending on the patient's age, health profile, and risk for additional problems. A primary care physician uses his clinical judgment and continues to care for his patient.

Similarly, many patients who present for mental healthcare tend to have acute and specific problems, and will benefit from an acute intervention. In these cases, a structured intervention like IPT is likely to offer the greatest benefit in a limited time frame. As in primary care, the IPT therapist should ensure that appropriate maintenance treatment is provided to all patients. In contrast, those patients who require ongoing and less structured interventions, such as those with severe and complex trauma experiences, profound disturbance in personality functioning, or severely debilitating mood or psychotic disorders, will likely require longer term and more transference-based psychological treatments. Borrowing further from this analogy, the concept of 'dose–response' can also be applied to the more structured psychotherapies. There is evidence that benefits to the patient accrue exponentially during the first 5–10 sessions of psychological interventions, with an attenuation of improvement thereafter.[10] Though there continue to be benefits with more sessions, the amount of additional improvement appears to diminish with each additional session. Thus the benefit or 'response' to treatment must be considered in light of the 'dose' or number of sessions that are provided.

Research also suggests that there is a rapid decline in clinic attendance and continuation in psychotherapeutic treatments after 5–10 sessions.[11,12] One study found that 40 percent of appointments with psychiatrists are 'one-off' (i.e. only one session), and that the average number of visits to a psychiatrist for a given patient is approximately seven.[13] There seems to be a brief window of opportunity for most patients, and that window opens when they experience an acute crisis that leads them to seek treatment. This window of opportunity is often best entered with a structured and time-limited treatment like IPT that focuses on the acute crisis.

Research aside, it is an unfortunate fact that the current climate of rationed healthcare and the emphasis on cost-effective treatments has had a profound effect on the healthcare system. If anything, this situation has gotten worse since the original iteration of our book in 2003; no doubt it will continue to be an issue for the foreseeable future. While there are many advantages to more open-ended treatments, IPT and other more structured interventions can often be provided within the constraints of managed care systems. IPT is also well-suited to this environment because there is evidence supporting its efficacy, a point of emphasis for managed care.

Conclusion

The structure of IPT is one of its key virtues. However, maintaining structure should not supersede the fact that the patient's unique needs are of primary concern. A course of IPT that adheres concretely to a manual at the expense of the patient's needs is almost certain to be a less effective treatment than that provided by a flexible therapist who follows the principles of IPT using clinical judgment.

References

1. Frank E. Interpersonal psychotherapy as a maintenance treatment for patients with recurrent depression. *Psychotherapy*, 1991, **28**: 259–266.

2. Frank E, *et al.* Three-year outcomes for maintenance therapies in recurrent depression. *Archives of General Psychiatry*, 1990, **47**(12): 1093–1099.

3. Frank E, *et al.* Randomized trial of weekly, twice-monthly, and monthly interpersonal psychotherapy as maintenance treatment for women with recurrent depression. *American Journal of Psychiatry*, 2007, **164**: 761–767.

4. Gelso CJ and Woodhouse SS. The termination of psychotherapy: what research tells us about the process of ending treatment, in Tryon GS (ed.) *Counseling Based on Process Research: Applying What We Know*. 2002, Boston: Allyn and Bacon.

5. Stuart S and Robertson M. *Interpersonal Psychotherapy: A Clinician's Guide*. 2003, London: Edward Arnold Ltd.

6. Stuart S and Cole V. Treatment of depression following myocardial infarction with interpersonal psychotherapy. *Annals of Clinical Psychiatry*, 1996, **8**: 203–206.

7. Klerman GL, *et al. Interpersonal Psychotherapy of Depression*. 1984, New York: Basic Books.

8. Klerman GL and Weissman MM. *New Applications of Interpersonal Psychotherapy*. 1993, Washington DC: American Psychiatric Press.

9. Weissman MM, Markowitz JW and Klerman GL. *Comprehensive Guide to Interpersonal Psychotherapy*. 2000, New York: Basic Books.

10. Howard KI, *et al.* The dose-effect relationship in psychotherapy. *American Psychologist*, 1986, **41**: 159–164.

11. Howard KI, *et al.* Patterns of psychotherapy utilization. *American Journal of Psychiatry*, 1989, **146**: 775–778.

12. Howard KI, *et al.* The psychotherapeutic service delivery system. *Psychotherapy Research*, 1992, **2**: 164–180.

13. Goldberg D. Impressions of psychiatry in Australia. *Australasian Psychiatry*, 2000, **8**: 307.

4

Assessment and Patient Selection

Introduction

The primary purpose of conducting an assessment is simply to determine if the patient is a good candidate for Interpersonal Psychotherapy (IPT), and if so, to make a judgment about how to modify the therapeutic structure. Though it is obvious, it is worth emphasizing that the treatment and patient must be compatible to ensure the greatest likelihood of resolving the patient's interpersonal problems. When making this determination, the therapist should be guided by several factors including the patient's attachment style, her communication style, her motivation and insight, and the empirical evidence regarding IPT. All of these factors should be integrated using a good measure of clinical judgment.

A thorough evaluation to determine the suitability of IPT should always be completed before a Treatment Agreement is established. The Treatment Agreement to proceed with IPT is that last step of the Assessment/Initial Phase, and should be constructed only after the full evaluation, including the Interpersonal Inventory and Formulation, has been completed. Referrals for IPT, whether self-referrals by the patient or referrals from other professionals, should be managed by indicating that an evaluation for IPT will be conducted, rather than implying or directly stating that IPT will be definitively provided. The determination to proceed with IPT should not be made until the assessment is complete.

An evaluation for IPT need not be conducted hastily. There is no reason why the therapist cannot take several sessions to complete an evaluation if her clinical judgment suggests this should be done. It is naïve to think that an appropriate Treatment Agreement for IPT (or any other therapy) can be established for anyone after only one session – it takes time to listen and understand, not to mention to develop an inclusive therapeutic relationship.

Therefore, though assessment is an intrinsic part of IPT, it should not be framed in a way that obligates the therapist to proceed with IPT unless it is warranted. The assessment should set the stage, so to speak, for the conduct of IPT when indicated, but should not obligate the therapist to provide IPT, nor lead the patient to expect IPT, unless it is the most appropriate treatment.

The assessment should answer two simple questions:

1. Will this particular patient benefit from IPT?
2. Is IPT the best treatment for this particular patient?

The Assessment Process

Rather than reiterate the process of conducting a complete psychiatric assessment, this chapter will describe the elements of the assessment that are unique to IPT. This should not diminish the fact that conducting a thorough psychological assessment of each and every patient, including psychiatric history, family history, medical history, and a complete social assessment, is extremely important. The additional elements that should be included in IPT are an assessment of the patient's attachment and communication style, ability to provide narrative, motivation for treatment, and psychological mindedness. The empirical evidence supporting the efficacy of IPT for particular disorders should also be considered.

Assessing Attachment and Communication Style

A good psychological or psychiatric assessment allows the therapist to see both the forest and the trees. In IPT, this consists of a large-scale map of the route the patient has traversed to arrive at her current interpersonal circumstances, and a detailed blueprint of the specific interpersonal and psychological difficulties she is struggling with at the moment. The therapist can consider the patient's attachment style as the 'topography' of the map – a feature which inevitably dictates the general route to be taken, though there are many alternative paths along the way. The more detailed features – the trees – are the patient's current interpersonal relationships. These trees are either felled or nurtured by the patient's interpersonal communications.

There are several reasons why attachment must be examined during the assessment phase of IPT. First and foremost, the assessment should lead to a determination about whether the patient's attachment style renders her a suitable IPT candidate. Second, the patient's attachment style is closely correlated with her prognosis; a good assessment should allow the therapist to make a reasonable prediction about how therapy will proceed and conclude. Third, specific techniques and modification of structure follow directly from the patient's attachment style.

Attachment style can be assessed in four ways:

- The patient's description of her relationships
- A significant other's description of the patient
- The quality of the patient's narrative
- The quality of the patient–therapist relationship.

The patient's description of her relationships

The assessment of the patient's attachment style should begin with an evaluation of the patient's past and current relationships. Simply asking open-ended questions about her relationships is a good way to start. More specific inquiries can be directed towards what the patient does and communicates when distressed, ill, or otherwise seeking care. She should also be queried about her typical responses when asked to assist others. This information is easy to obtain, requires little in the way of inference, and is an obvious way to evaluate the patient's attachment style. Both directives and open-ended questions can be used to more fully understand the ways a patient functions in relationships.

The primary source of information is the patient's current relationships. This can be evaluated by asking both specific questions as well as those which require a bit more insight. For instance, the patient can be directly asked about any patterns that she has noticed in her relationships. Typical ways of beginning and ending relationships can be explored. The patient should also be asked about the ways she asks for help if it is needed, and the ways she communicates with others when feeling upset or angry. Both intimate and family relationships should be explored in detail, and work or school relationships covered as well.

Though IPT does not focus on reworking past relationships, information about past relationships should still be obtained. A full history of dating or sexual relationships is important, as the therapist can glean information about how the patient typically forms these types of relationships. Questions about the patient's interactions with important caregivers are also an excellent way to begin to solidify hypotheses about the patient's attachment style. Examples of specific questions that might be asked are provided in Box 4.1.

Box 4.1 Questions to assess attachment

Current relationships
- What are you like in relationships?
- What is it like for you when relationships end?
- What is it like for you to start new relationships?
- How do you perceive yourself to be around other people?
- What kinds of challenges are there for you in relationships with others?
- What things do you like about being in relationships?
- Describe one of your best relationships.
- Describe one of your worst relationships.
- What things would you like to change about yourself in your ability to connect with others?

Past relationships
- How did other people react when you accomplished something, such as good marks in school?
- How did other people react when you were hurt?
- How did other people react when you were angry?
- How did you go about asking for help if you needed it?
- Were there other people besides your parents who were primary care providers for you?
- How do you and your siblings get along?
- What were your relationships with your siblings like growing up?

The list of potential questions is endless – the point is to gather information directly from the patient to begin to develop hypotheses about her attachment style. Since attachment is the basis for the way relationships are formed and maintained, this information is crucial to develop an accurate Interpersonal Formulation, and to determine if the patient will do well with IPT. Of equal importance is the patient's *perception* of her style of relating to others. The interactions the patient reports and her perception of her interpersonal behavior may be congruent, or they may be entirely different. Both situations obviously provide a lot of information. Patients whose perceptions match their reported interactions generally have much more insight, particularly of the type useful in IPT. They are able to recognize the ways they are communicating, and can appreciate that their communications have an impact on others. Patients whose reports do not match their self-perceptions generally lack this kind of insight, and the therapist will have a longer row to hoe with such patients because they require that IPT be started at a more basic level. Consider the following two examples.

Case example 4.1: Congruent description and self-perception
Therapist: *Tell me how you and your wife get along.*

Patient: *Up until this fight about my mother-in-law, we got along pretty well. When I get mad, she just withdraws and gives me the silent treatment. Last week things came to a head, and we had* *a huge fight about whether to put her mother in a nursing home or have her come live with us. I have to say though, from her perspective, I would have been angry too – when I get mad, I tend not to listen, and I tend to be pretty tenacious. She doesn't really have much choice but to keep quiet, I suppose.*

Case example 4.2: Non-congruent description and self-perception

Therapist: *Tell me how you and your wife get along.*

Patient: *We have been having this huge fight about my mother-in-law. I have been furious because she hasn't considered my needs at all, and wants to have her mother live with us instead of going to a nursing home.*

Therapist: *When you get mad, how do you react?*

Patient: *I just get mad … you know … you'd be mad too if your wife did that to you.*

There are a lot of technical terms that can be used to describe factors which lead clinicians to consider patients to be good, or not so good, candidates for therapy. But they all boil down to one simple question, which is based more on intuition, experience, and clinical judgment than anything else, and that question is:

Would you want to work with this patient?

With respect to the specific examples above, it doesn't take a rocket scientist to figure out that the patient in Case example 4.1 is the best psychotherapy candidate. Technically speaking, he is already able, without prompting by the therapist, to recognize that his communications impact others. He is already acknowledging some responsibility for the problem, and appears to have at least an inkling that his communication style may be a problem. Narrative and self-perceptions are congruent.

It is important to keep in mind that the patient's description, though very helpful, is usually not a complete representative of the patient's style of interacting and her patterns of attachment. In any therapeutic situation, there is always information that is withheld, misrepresented, or conflated by the patient. This occurs for any number of reasons, but some of the salient ones are that the patient may want to present herself to the therapist in the best possible light; the patient may be motivated to blame others for her problem rather than taking responsibility herself; the therapeutic alliance and degree of trust in the therapist is not yet sufficient for the patient to be more revealing or open; the patient is looking to please the therapist and is reporting the 'right answer' that she thinks the therapist wants to hear; or the therapist hasn't asked the right questions or shown enough interest for the patient to take a risk with self-disclosure. It is simply human nature that people withhold or distort personal information at times, and the therapeutic situation is no exception.

As a consequence, the therapist should always be mindful of the fact that it is both *what* is said, and *how* it is said, that forms the basis for the assessment. This is a reflection of patients' tendencies to withhold or distort information that they give to their therapists. This withholding is most often a manifestation of the very difficulties which led to the patient's problems or led her to seek treatment. Bowlby[1] summarizes this concept well:

The fact is that much of the most relevant information refers to extremely painful or frightening events that the patient would much prefer to forget. Memories of being held always to be in the wrong, of having to care for a depressed mother instead of being cared for yourself, or the terror and anger you felt when father was violent or mother was uttering threats, of the guilt when you were told your behavior would make your parent ill, of the grief, despair and anger you felt after a loss, of the intensity of your unrequited yearning during a period of enforced separation. No one can look back on such events without feeling renewed anxiety,

anger, guilt, or despair. No one, either, cares to believe that it was his very own
parents, who at other times may have been kind and helpful, who on occasion
behaved in some most distressing way... (p. 425)

A significant other's description of the patient

If information from a significant other can be obtained, the therapist can ask that person the same
questions about the patient for additional information. This is frequently the case with adolescents,
whose parents are likely to be involved in treatment; it is less common but still possible with adults.
Couples IPT also presents an opportunity to get this information bidirectionally.

When asking significant others about the patient, the therapist must always be aware that
others also have biases, gaps, attachment quirks, and other agendas which may color their
report. Nonetheless, this is often helpful adjunct information.

The quality of the patient's narrative

In addition to collecting information directly about the patient's relationships, inferences
about the patient's attachment style can be drawn from the quality of the patient's narratives. In
simple terms, the quality of a narrative is nothing more than the patient's ability to tell a good
story. In thinking about how to assess this, consider what it is that makes a story compelling.
Better yet, think about those times when you have been really moved by a story that a patient
has told. Those that have affected you a great deal are usually prototypes for good narratives.

A good story should have a coherent plot.
>   It should make sense. It should come in context, rather than being told 'out of the blue'. The
>   story should make a point, and there should be a beginning and an end. In therapy, patients
>   who tell really good stories often add an anticipatory ending – a look ahead to the way they
>   want things to be when they finish treatment.

A good story or compelling narrative should have some action.
>   Something should be happening between the characters. Dialog should be occurring,
>   interpersonal interactions should be described. The more descriptive the action the better;
>   lots of affect, both in the content of the story and in the telling, make for a good tale.

There should be details which place the story in some kind of historical framework.
>   In therapy, stories should not be of the 'once upon a time' variety – they should specify the
>   time of the event and place it in a meaningful interpersonal context. For instance, a story
>   about a conflict with a spouse should be located in real time and space.

Consider the two following examples.

Case example 4.3: A less than compelling narrative
Therapist: *Tell me about your father's funeral.*
Patient: *I don't remember much about it really. It was a rainy day ... Most of my family had come,
and we had a wake at the church afterwards. I don't really remember talking to anyone. My father
and I weren't very close.*
Therapist: *How did your father die?*
Patient: *He had cancer ... prostate I believe. He was sick a long time.*

Case example 4.4: A compelling narrative
Therapist: *Tell me about your father's funeral.*
Patient: *There's not much to tell – it was a typical Irish affair ... actually, it was the kind of wake
that my father always wanted. He was a fun-loving man, and he had always talked about having*

a wake where everyone could come and remember the good times they had with him. He was an amazing man, really – even with the prostate cancer, which he suffered with for almost two years, he never lost his sense of humor. I remember visiting him in the hospital several days before he died. It seemed like we talked forever, and I think that we both knew that the end was coming. It's hard to describe what it was like – on the one hand, I don't think that I've ever felt as close to him as at that moment, when we both just held each other and said, 'I love you'. I still feel sad just thinking about it, because we'll never have any more time like that. As I was leaving, he said to me, 'Make sure your son knows how much you love him too'. I cried when I told that story during the eulogy …

The ability to relate narrative in a meaningful way is important for several reasons.

First, the ability to relate interpersonal narrative is essential in IPT. Every form of psychotherapy requires that the patient produce some material for discussion. It may be dreams, it may be cognitions, it may be free associations or reports about desensitization exercises, but every single therapy in existence requires that the patient has something to say. The more information the patient is able to produce, and the more accurate it is, the better the patient will do in treatment., as there is more material to be examined, and more information which can be used to understand the patient. An integral part of IPT is having the patient produce narrative information – the patient will be asked time and again to reproduce specific interpersonal interactions, complete with dialog, emotional content, and non-verbal information.

Second, the ability to relate narrative in a compelling or meaningful way is intimately connected to the patient's ability to communicate her experiences to others. This in turn has a profound impact on the quality of her social support network. Those patients who can describe their experiences in ways that draw others in to their stories generally have much larger and more intimate social support networks than those patients who do not have that capability.

Third, the patient's innate ability to describe her experience is connected to her ability to deal with specific individual conflicts. Those patients who can convey their experiences, emotions, and need for support effectively will be able to resolve specific conflicts more effectively than patients who cannot.

Fourth, the patient's ability to tell a compelling story makes a difference because it more effectively engages the therapist. Being more human than not, therapists are influenced by exactly the same factors which affect others in the patient's interpersonal world. Therapists are drawn to listen to compelling stories – those patients who tell good stories are fun to work with, and therapists are more invested in them. This does, of course, subtly but profoundly affect outcome.

In short, the more compelling the story, the better the outcome is likely to be. The more securely attached the patient, the more likely the story is to be compelling, and the more likely the patient is to be able to meaningfully engage others and share her experiences. Therefore, during the assessment, *the therapist should directly ask the patient to tell some meaningful or interesting interpersonal stories.*

In addition to the quality of the narrative in general, the way the patient describes other people in her interpersonal world illuminates her attachment style. As with stories, the therapist should directly ask for descriptions of others with whom the patient interacts. Those patients who are more securely attached are generally able to describe other people in 'three-dimensional' terms. In other words, they are able to portray other people as real, with good points and bad, altruistic and selfish motives, idiosyncrasies and strengths. This reflects a more accurate working model of relationships. More securely attached people are able to 'call it like it is' more precisely.

59

Those patients with more preoccupied attachment styles often portray others in more 'two-dimensional' terms. Because such patients are constantly concerned or preoccupied with getting their attachment needs met, they are hesitant to be critical of others who might provide them with care. Instead, an idealized, or on occasion, a devalued description of others will be provided. Hypochondriacal patients are classic examples of this kind of attachment and they provide corresponding descriptions: they idealize current and potential care providers while decrying those that have failed them. None of the figures in a preoccupied patient's world are complete – they have only good or only bad parts which are relevant only as they pertain to caring for the patient.

Patients with more fearful or dismissing styles of attachment, in contrast, will usually describe others in 'one-dimensional' terms. With these patients, there is literally no detail at all. There is literally nothing to hang one's hat on – no information, no details ... nothing. This is a reflection of the patient's interpersonal world, in which relationships carry much less meaning.

Consider the following three examples.

Case example 4.5: Secure attachment

Therapist: *Tell me about your mother.*

Patient: *My mother ... well, she and I get along pretty well now, though she certainly has her moments. When I was growing up, she was great. I remember when I was five and had the chicken pox, she took time off from work and stayed home with me. We played games, read books ... it was great. During my teen years ... well, that was another story. She was a bit old fashioned, and she and I got into some pretty loud arguments about what I was going to wear and how late I could stay out.*

I guess in general she has been pretty supportive. Like with my kids – she is always willing to lend a hand to help watch them, and is great with them, but she still has a tendency to be critical of some of the ways that we have decided to raise them.

Case example 4.6: Preoccupied attachment

Therapist: *Tell me about your mother.*

Patient: *My mother ... well she is just the greatest. She is always there to help, she's great with the kids ... frankly, I don't think I could have asked for a better mother. I can't think of a single thing I'd change about her.*

Therapist: *I thought just a minute ago you had mentioned that you and she were having a big conflict about how you were raising your children.*

Patient: *Oh that ... well, that hardly ever happens ... it wasn't really that important.*

Case example 4.7: Fearful attachment

Therapist: *Tell me about your mother.*

Patient: *My mother ... well, she's 56 years old.*

Therapist: *What is she like?*

Patient: *She's pretty nice, a good mom I guess.*

Therapist: *Any specific things about her come to mind?*

Patient: *No, not really. She was just a good mom.*

These examples demonstrate the types of responses that patients with varying attachment styles may give to direct inquiries about other people. In the first case, the securely attached patient is able to provide a well-rounded view of her mother. She has good and bad points, the patient is able to describe them, and the patient has integrated them into a coherent and meaningful whole person. Even better, she spontaneously produces narrative material that provides context and details for her description.

In the second case, the patient's description is idealized. When confronted by the therapist, she seems unable to integrate the two different aspects of her mother into a coherent whole. The threat of losing her mother and the limited support she provides leads the patient to idealize her. In addition to hypochondriacal patients, this unfortunately happens on occasion with victims of abuse, who despite severe trauma will continue to idealize the perpetrator of the abuse and blame themselves.

In the third case, the fearful patient is simply unable to provide much meaningful information at all. One can easily imagine that such a patient would be difficult to work with in any kind of therapy. This is not only because of the poor quality of information that she is providing, but also because she seems to have an inability to convey her inner experiences, feelings, and perceptions to others. To make matters worse, a patient like this will quickly be experienced as tedious by most therapists.

There is a great deal of overlap in attachment styles. All individuals have some combination of secure and insecure attachment traits. However, patients who are more secure have a better prognosis in therapy.

The quality of patient–therapist relationship

The last way to assess attachment is to examine the quality of the therapeutic relationship. As with the patient's report about relationships and the quality of the patient's narrative, the patient–therapist relationship has far-reaching implications about the patient's attachment style and prognosis in therapy. As the assessment proceeds, and for that matter, as all of therapy proceeds, the clinician should be finely attuned to the therapeutic relationship. In particular, the therapist should be keenly aware of her reactions to the patient. This is crucial because both attachment and communication can be assessed in this way.

Attachment can be assessed because the relationship that the patient develops with the therapist is a reflection of the attachment that the patient manifests in relationships outside of therapy. Given enough time in therapy, the patient's interpersonal working model will be imposed upon the therapist. With an insecurely attached patient, the working model will often be apparent in the first session, as it is so inaccurate that discrepancies are immediately evident. Borderline, narcissistic, and antisocial individuals are examples of such patients. On the other hand, those with more secure styles of attachment do not impose such distorted attributes upon the therapist, or at least don't do so quickly. They are cooperative, readily accept help, and are pleasant to work with.

Communication can be assessed because the patient's specific communications and metacommunications in therapy, just like all of their communications outside of therapy, elicit a characteristic response. In therapy, they obviously elicit a response from the therapist. Thus the therapist should be keenly aware of her reflexive responses to the patient. Does the patient make the therapist feel helpless? Angry? Bored? Effective and helpful? Each reflexive response is indicative of the patient's specific communication style.

In order to complete the assessment of attachment, the therapist should also conduct an assessment of the match between herself and the patient. The old adage to 'know thyself' cannot be overemphasized, for therapists, like patients, also have idiosyncratic styles of attachment and communication. Therapists who tend to be overly directive may have difficulty with fearful or dismissive patients, for example. Therapists who find it difficult to conclude treatment may encounter problems with patients with preoccupied attachment styles. Securely attached therapists, just like their patients, will more effectively utilize therapy.

Assessment of Attachment and Communication: Summary

The patient's attachment and communication style should be assessed in IPT using at least four different sources of information. First, the patient's direct descriptions of relationships should be examined. Second, reports from others about the patient's style of relating can be collected. Third, the quality of narrative, particularly in response to direct inquiries to 'tell a story', should be assessed. Fourth, the quality of the relationship between the patient and therapist should provide information. All of these coalesce to provide information about the patient's suitability for IPT and her prognosis.

The patient's attachment style therefore has direct implications regarding her ability to develop a therapeutic alliance with the therapist and the likelihood that treatment will be beneficial. Unfortunately, in IPT as in all other psychotherapies, the old saw about the 'rich getting richer' holds true. Those patients with relatively secure attachment styles are usually able to form a working relationship with the therapist, and because of their relatively healthy relationships outside of therapy, are also more likely to be able to draw upon their social support system effectively. Individuals with more preoccupied attachment styles can usually quickly form relationships with their clinicians, but often have a great deal of difficulty with the conclusion of treatment – a particular problem in time-limited therapy.

Those with fearful or dismissing styles of attachment may have difficulty trusting or relating to the therapist. Consequently, when working with fearful or dismissive patients the therapist may need to spend several of the assessment/initial sessions working on nothing more than developing a productive therapeutic alliance, waiting until it is established before moving into more formal IPT work.

In addition to evaluating therapeutic suitability, the therapist should use the assessment to forecast and plan for problems which may arise during the course of therapy. For example, since patients with preoccupied attachment styles may have difficulty in ending relationships, an astute therapist would modify the structure of IPT so that sessions are tapered in frequency as the conclusion of acute treatment draws near, and would discuss the conclusion of treatment early in the middle phase. Significant others may also be included in sessions more frequently to ensure that dependency on the therapist does not become problematic.

When working with fearful or dismissive patients, the therapist should plan to spend several sessions completing an assessment, taking great care to convey a sense of understanding and empathy to the patient. Soliciting feedback from the patient about the intensity of treatment is another tactic which may improve the therapeutic alliance.

Assessing Traditional Patient Characteristics for Time-limited Psychotherapy

In general, patients who have characteristics that render them good candidates for any of the time-limited therapies will be good candidates for IPT. A number of authors have described patient selection factors, and most stress that in short-term therapy, careful selection of patients is crucial to the success of the treatment.[2-5] The emphasis on these factors rests both on clinical experience and empirical data. The empirical evidence regarding patient selection for short-term therapy has identified several specific factors that have been associated with good outcome.[6-12] Though most of the research that has been conducted has investigated more psychodynamically oriented short-term treatments, the data are also useful in considering the suitability of patients for IPT.

The factors that are most commonly reported in the clinical and empirical literature and are integral to the selection of patients for IPT include:

- Severity of illness
- Motivation

- The ability to form a therapeutic alliance
- Ego strength
- Psychological mindedness.

Severity of Illness

The data on severity of illness as a predictor of outcome in short-term psychotherapy follow exactly the intuitively obvious conclusion that the more severe the psychopathology, the less suitable patients are for treatment of any kind.[13,14] This includes not only psychiatric symptoms such as psychoses, but also includes more severe personality disorders.[15-17] High levels of symptomatic severity in disorders such as depression also portend poorer outcomes in general.[6]

Motivation

The concept of motivation as it applies to time-limited therapy has been understood more as a desire to change as opposed to a simple desire to be rid of symptoms.[18] Elements of this kind of motivation include the patient's ability to recognize the psychological nature of the symptoms with which she is struggling, a willingness to participate actively in therapy, a willingness to explore new solutions to problems, and a willingness to extend herself in pragmatic ways, such as sacrificing time to come to appointments and paying fees[4] – the latter being paramount, of course, for therapists as well as patients. These factors are also intuitively obvious.

The empirical literature supports the importance of motivation as well.[19] Several authors, however, have suggested that motivation be assessed later in therapy as opposed to the initial session, as both the empirical evidence[20] and clinical experience indicate that later assessments of motivation may be more accurate.[21,22] This lends further credence to the fact that a thorough assessment is essential prior to developing a Treatment Agreement for IPT.

The Ability to Form a Therapeutic Alliance

The ability to form a therapeutic alliance is simply the patient's ability to work productively with the therapist. To do so, the patient must be able to both seek and receive help, to report feelings honestly to the therapist, and to trust the therapist. In IPT, this is conceptualized as the patient's ability to attach securely to the therapist. The empirical evidence supports the importance of this factor; as with motivation, the quality of the therapeutic relationship appears to be more clearly correlated with outcome when measured several sessions into therapy.[23,24]

The therapeutic alliance has also been correlated with outcome in IPT specifically. In the NIMH Treatment of Depression Collaborative Research Program (NIMH-TDCRP),[25] the quality of the therapeutic alliance was found to have a significant impact on outcome.[26] In particular, the patient's contributions to the alliance were found to carry great weight.[27] The patient's ability to engage in a productive therapeutic relationship was also found to have more impact upon the therapist's ability to competently conduct IPT than the severity of the patient's symptoms,[28] again emphasizing the importance of the therapeutic alliance.

Ego Strength

Ego strength has a long tradition as an important factor in psychotherapy. Ego strength has been defined as the capacity to withstand internal or external stress, the ability to experience distressing material during the therapy process, and the ability to constructively integrate affect and experience.[21,29] Specific objective measures which may serve as markers of ego strength include the patient's intelligence, work history, and level of education.[3] Given the abstract nature of the construct, specific empirical literature is sparse, although several authors have found support for the concept as a positive predictive factor.

Psychological Mindedness

Psychological mindedness includes a willingness to focus on internal processes, a capacity for introspection, and a curiosity about oneself with a willingness to explore thoughts and feelings. Closely connected to this concept is the ability to not only be aware of one's own thoughts and feelings, but to be able to communicate them effectively to others. This factor is crucial in any therapy, because if the patient is not able to describe her internal and external experiences, therapy cannot proceed. Communicating one's experience is essential to IPT, both in terms of the therapeutic process and the patient's ability to effectively engage her social support network.

While the empirical data regarding the importance of psychological mindedness are mixed,[10] clinical experience with IPT clearly indicates that it is an important factor in outcome. The relative lack of empirical support may be due to the fact that different qualities of psychological mindedness may be important for different types of therapies. For instance, in IPT patients need to make connections between interpersonal events and symptoms, while in cognitive behavioral therapy (CBT), the connections are between internal cognitions and symptoms. Dynamic therapies require yet again a different type of insight. These propositions remain to be empirically tested.

Most of the predictive factors common to all short-term psychotherapies are of the intuitively obvious type. In addition, most are abstract, which largely accounts for the relative lack of empirical research and absolute conclusions that can be drawn from the literature. The best way to assess patients for IPT is to use these criteria generally, operating under the principle that 'you know it when you see it' – in other words, patient characteristics such as psychological mindedness and motivation can be recognized without much difficulty, even though they often elude more concrete description.

It is important to note that diagnosis is not often cited as a primary basis for treatment selection. While the empirical data for all evidence-based psychotherapies are relevant to particular diagnoses, this is an artifact of the design of the studies. For example, most of the IPT studies have involved patients with major depression, as have many studies of CBT. This is because the diagnosis of depression is a specific inclusion criterion for these studies, and because empirically supported therapies must by definition demonstrate remission of symptoms and diagnosis. This is not to say, however, that a diagnosis is required for treatment, nor that patients who do not meet specific diagnostic criteria will not do well with IPT. Clinical experience suggests quite the opposite is true: patients with less severe distress or impairment (such as those who do not meet full criteria for a psychiatric diagnosis) are likely to do better in IPT than those who do have a diagnosable illness.

Patient Characteristics Specific to IPT

Characteristics specific to IPT which increase the likelihood that patients will benefit from IPT include:

- A relatively secure attachment style
- The ability to relate a coherent narrative
- The ability to relate specific dialogue from interpersonal interactions

- A specific interpersonal focus for distress
- A good social support system.

Secure Attachment Style

A secure attachment style is highly correlated with many of the factors that are associated with good outcome in psychotherapy. Patients with a more secure attachment style generally have more ego strength, are able to enter into therapy with a genuine desire to seek help, are able to trust their therapists, and can form productive therapeutic alliances more quickly. They also generally have both the internal and external resources to do well in therapy. They are more able to take risks and are more motivated to change, and their social support systems are usually much better than those of patients with insecure attachments. Attachment style is likely the most important factor in determining which patients are most suitable for IPT. There are accumulating empirical data that this is the case.[30,31]

Coherent Narrative

In addition to being able to recognize interpersonal issues and connect them with symptoms and distress, patients in IPT must be able to communicate their experiences in a coherent fashion. IPT rests largely on communication analysis, which requires that the patient be able to relate, in detail, the communication which occurs in incidents outside of therapy. Being able to re-create dialog, describe affect, and to literally be able to tell a good story is essential in IPT. Specifically asking the patient to tell several stories about important interactions during the assessment will allow the therapist to make a reasonable judgment about this factor.

Specific Interpersonal Focus

Given the time-limited nature of IPT, patients who present with more focal problems will generally do better in treatment. Those patients who begin therapy having already made a connection between their symptoms and interpersonal issues are even better candidates for IPT, as they will need no convincing that IPT is a plausible and applicable treatment for their specific problems. Patients who present for treatment with complaints such as 'I just don't feel well, but I don't know why', are not good candidates; those who present with complaints such as 'I am in the midst of a divorce which is leading me to have trouble functioning and making me feel depressed', are.

Patient aptitude for IPT is also important to consider. Patients who frame their problems in interpersonal terms are more likely to do better in IPT than those that do not. The patient's initial description of or attributions for her problems is quite telling in this regard. For example, a woman who describes her postpartum depression as due to 'difficulties with conflicts with my husband and problems dealing with going back to work after the birth of my baby' – classic Interpersonal Disputes and Role Transitions – is likely to do well with IPT. In contrast, a woman who describes her problems as feelings that, 'I don't measure up to other women as a mother, and I constantly worry that something bad may happen to my child' might do better with CBT, as her presentation is more consistent with distorted cognitive patterns. Research in this area is ongoing, but these distinctions have been found to be quite useful clinically.

Good Social Support

The better the social support, the more likely the patient is to improve. IPT in particular is focused on helping patients to utilize their social support systems to meet their attachment needs, hence the more resources that are available, the more likely that patients will be able to get their attachment needs met. Good social support is highly correlated with attachment security, because securely attached patients generally have better social support systems. The therapist should assess the intimacy of the patient's relationships – those who are able to engage in deeper and more emotionally close relationships will do well in therapy, as they will have others with whom they can share their experiences and call on for support. Those with more distant relationships will have more difficulty both in establishing a therapeutic alliance (their working model being that others are not trustworthy, including the therapist) and in developing and utilizing social support outside of therapy.

Empirical Support for IPT

There is a great deal of research relevant to the assessment of patients for IPT.[9] First, there are a number of efficacy trials investigating the use of IPT with specific diagnoses. Second, there are studies which have investigated the factors associated with good response to IPT. The data from these should inform the clinician about what is likely to be helpful for a given patient, but should by no means be the only factor in making this decision. The empirical studies are all based on populations of patients, not specific individuals; it is a unique individual with whom you will be working. In addition, all of the efficacy studies have limitations which restrict the conclusions which can be drawn about non-research use of IPT. Thus while the empirical data should be a major factor in making treatment decisions, final determination of appropriateness should also always include clinical experience and a good measure of clinical judgment.

Efficacy studies have been conducted using IPT to treat a number of specific diagnoses. IPT has been demonstrated to be of benefit with depression in general,[32,33] as well as depressed geriatric patients,[34,35] depressed adolescents,[36,37] and patients with dysthymic disorder.[38,39] IPT has also been used for perinatal depression, including postpartum[40] and antenatal depression.[41,42] In addition, it has been tested with patients with eating disorders.[43,44] Despite the extensive empirical testing of IPT with a variety of diagnoses, there are much less data regarding the use of IPT in general clinical (i.e. non-research) settings. This requires that clinicians utilize their judgment when working with patients who would not qualify for research, such as those with comorbid diagnoses or personality pathology, or more concisely put, the vast majority of patients who seek clinical care.

However, several studies have investigated patient factors which have been linked with better outcomes in IPT. The presence of a personality disorder has been associated with poorer outcome with treatment for depression. In the NIMH-TDCRP, depressed patients with personality disorders had poorer outcomes with respect to depressive symptoms and social functioning.[17] The suggestion that personality disorders are likely to be associated with a more difficult course in therapy certainly has intuitive appeal.[45]

As a consequence, special attention should be paid to patients diagnosed with personality disorders, both because of the empirical data and because of the clinical experience that has accumulated. Those with cluster A disorders including paranoid, schizoid, and schizotypal personality disorders may have difficulty forming effective therapeutic alliances unless the therapist works hard to convey a sense of understanding. Those with cluster B disorders such as narcissistic, histrionic, borderline, and antisocial personality disorders often require that therapists work to be empathic even in situations in which they are provoked to react with rejection or hostility. Patients with cluster C disorders probably require structural changes in IPT, such as the gradual tapering of session frequency with dependent patients. In sum, many patients with depression or anxiety superimposed upon a personality disorder are likely to benefit from short-term therapy with IPT if the therapist is adept at being flexible and adapting to the patient.

Additional data from the NIMH-TDCRP indicate that there are several other factors that are associated with a positive response to IPT.[46] These include a low level of social dysfunction at intake, as well as a high degree of interpersonal insight. Patients who report greater satisfaction with their relationships when they begin treatment are also more likely to benefit from IPT as compared with the other treatments. The NIMH-TDCRP results can be summarized by stating that those patients without severe personality pathology, who have a relatively good social support system, and who have an awareness of the way in which they communicate in interpersonal relationships, typically fare well with IPT.

Several personality characteristics have also been found to be associated with less optimal outcomes in IPT. Perfectionism has been shown to have a negative impact on outcome. Blatt *et al.*,[47,48] analyzing NIMH-TDCRP data, noted that perfectionism began to impede therapeutic progress in the latter half of treatment, and suggested that this may be due to the reaction of perfectionistic patients to an arbitrary, externally imposed termination date. This characteristic, however, is much less relevant to IPT in clinical settings, because the therapist and patient work together to set a flexible acute treatment schedule, and because IPT is concluded rather than terminated as was required in the NIMH-TDCRP research trial.

In the NIMH-TDCRP, patients with more avoidant traits were found to fare better in CBT than in IPT, while patients with more obsessive traits had better outcomes when treated with IPT as compared with CBT.[49] This finding seems rather counter-intuitive until one considers that a patient's coping mechanisms (avoidance or obsession respectively) are, when the stressor is great enough, causing more distress rather than being a functional way to cope effectively. Frank *et al.* also found that among women with recurrent depression who were treated with IPT, those with higher levels of self-reported panic and agoraphobic symptoms were less likely to respond to IPT.[50] Non-remitters were also found to have higher levels of somatic anxiety.[51]

Empirical data regarding biological predictors is limited, but studies investigating sleep parameters and their association with response to IPT have found that depressed patients with abnormal sleep electroencephalographic (EEG) profiles had significantly lower response rates than depressed patients with more normal sleep profiles.[52,53] More research regarding the predictive value of biological measures is clearly needed.

The empirical data regarding patient selection can be summarized as follows:

- There are good empirical data supporting the efficacy of IPT for a number of well-specified diagnoses, though the effectiveness data are limited.
- Social factors such as a good social support system have been associated with good outcome.
- The presence of personality disorders, although not a contraindication to IPT, may complicate its course and be associated with poorer outcomes.
- Treating patients with personality disorder comorbidity usually requires changes in structure, such as lengthening treatment, tapering treatment as it concludes acutely, and taking more time to develop an alliance early in therapy.

Conclusion

The selection of patients for IPT can best be understood to be on a spectrum, with highly suitable patients on one end and those who are less suitable on the other. While there are no absolute contraindications to IPT, there are patients who might benefit more from treatments other than IPT. Clinical judgment should be informed by an assessment of the patient's suitability for short-term treatment, the empirical evidence supporting efficacy of the various treatments available, and the clinical value of the treatment options.

In sum, the assessment process should assist the therapist to evaluate the patient's suitability for IPT, and it should be based on empirical data, clinical experience, and clinical judgment. An assessment of the patient's attachment style and communication patterns should be undertaken in addition to a thorough psychiatric assessment. The assessment should assist the therapist to anticipate and plan for potential problems in therapy, such as difficulty in forming a therapeutic alliance or dependency, and should direct the therapist to modify the therapeutic approach and structure so that these problems are minimized.

References

1. Bowlby J. The making and breaking of affectional bonds, II: some principles of psychotherapy. *British Journal of Psychiatry*, 1977, **130**: 421–431.

2. Malan DH. *The Frontier of Brief Psychotherapy*. 1976, New York: Plenum.

3. Marmor J. Short-term dynamic psychotherapy. *American Journal of Psychiatry*, 1979, **136**: 149–155.

4. Sifneos PE. *Short-term Dynamic Psychotherapy*. 1987, New York: Plenum.

5. Strupp HH and Binder JL. *Psychotherapy in a New Key*. 1984, New York: Basic Books.

6. Elkin I, *et al*. Initial severity and differential treatment outcome in the National Institute of Mental Health Treatment of Depression Collaborative Research Program. *Journal of Consulting and Clinical Psychology*, 1995, **63**: 841–847.

7. Calvert SJ, Beutler LE and Crago M. Psychotherapy outcome as a function of therapist-patient matching on selected variables. *Journal of Social and Clinical Psychology*, 1988, **6**: 104–117.

8. Carroll K, Nich C and Rounsaville B. Contribution of the therapeutic alliance to outcome in active versus control psychotherapies. *Journal of Consulting and Clinical Psychology*, 1997, **65**: 510–514.

9. Eaton TT, Abeles N and Gutfreund MJ. Therapeutic alliance and outcome: impact of treatment length and pretreatment symptomatology. *Psychotherapy: Research and Practice*, 1988, **25**: 536–542.

10. Lambert MJ and Anderson EM. Assessment for the time-limited psychotherapies, in Dickstein LJ, Riba MB and Oldham JM (eds) *American Psychiatric Press Review of Psychiatry*. 1996, Washington, DC: American Psychiatric Press, pp. 23–42.

11. Barber JP and Crits-Cristoph P. Comparison of the brief dynamic psychotherapies, in Crits-Cristoph P and Barber JP (eds) *Handbook of Short-term Dynamic Psychotherapy*. 1991, New York: Basic Books, pp. 323–356.

12. Demos VC and Prout MF. A comparison of seven approaches to brief psychotherapy. *International Journal of Short-Term Psychotherapy*, 1993, **8**: 3–22.

13. Luborsky L, Crits-Cristoph P and Mintz J. *Who Will Benefit from Psychotherapy?* 1988, New York: Basic Books.

14. Hoglend P. Suitability for brief dynamic psychotherapy: psychodynamic variables as predictors of outcome. *Acta Psychiatrica Scandinavica*, 1993, **88**: 104–110.

15. Shea MT. Some characteristics of the Axis II criteria sets and their implications for assessment of personality disorders. *Journal of Personality Disorders*, 1992, **6**: 377–381.

16. Shea MT, *et al*. Course of depressive symptoms over follow-up. Findings from the National Institute of Mental Health Treatment of Depression Collaborative Research Program. *Archives of General Psychiatry*, 1992, **49**: 782–787.

17. Shea MT, *et al*. Personality disorders and treatment outcome in the NIMH Treatment of Depression Collaborative Treatment Program. *American Journal of Psychiatry*, 1990, **147**: 711–718.

18. Lambert MJ. Psychotherapy outcome research: implications for integrative and eclectic theories, in Norcross JC and Goldfried MR (eds) *Handbook of Psychotherapy Integration*. 1992, New York: Basic Books.

19. Orlinsky DE, Grawe K and Parks BK. Process and outcome in psychotherapy noch einmal, in Bergin AE and Garfield SL (eds) *Handbook of Psychotherapy and Behavioral Change*. 1994, Wiley: New York.

20. O'Malley S, Suh CD and Strupp HH. The Vanderbilt psychotherapy process scale: a report on the scale development and a process-outcome study. *Journal of Consulting and Clinical Psychology*, 1983, **51**: 581–586.

21. Malan DH. *A Study of Brief Psychotherapy*. 1975, New York: Plenum.

22. Garfield SL. *The Practice of Brief Psychotherapy*. 1989, New York: Pergamon.

23. Strupp HH. Toward the refinement of time-limited dynamic psychotherapy, in Budman SH (ed.) *Forms of Brief Therapy*. 1981, New York: Guilford Publications, pp. 219–225.

24. Binder JL, Henry WP and Strupp HH. An appraisal of selection criteria for dynamic psychotherapies and implications for setting time limits. *Journal of Psychiatry*, 1987, **50**: 154–166.

25. Elkin I, *et al*. NIMH Treatment of Depression Collaborative Treatment Program: background and research plan. *Archives of General Psychiatry*, 1985, **42**: 305–316.

26. Krupnick JL, *et al*. The role of the therapeutic alliance in psychotherapy and pharmacotherapy outcome: findings in the National Institute of Mental Health Treatment of Depression. *Journal of Consulting and Clinical Psychology*, 1996, **64**: 532–539.

27. Zuroff DC, *et al*. Relation of therapeutic alliance and perfectionism to outcome in brief outpatient treatment of depression. *Journal of Consulting and Clinical Psychology*, 2000, **68**: 114–124.

28. Foley SH, *et al*. The relationship of patient difficulty to therapist performance in interpersonal psychotherapy of depression. *Journal of Affective Disorders*, 1987, **12**: 207–217.

29. Davanloo H. *Short-Term Dynamic Psychotherapy*. 1980, Northvale: Aronson.

30. McBride C, *et al*. Attachment as a moderator of treatment outcome in major depression: a randomized control trial of interpersonal psychotherapy versus cognitive behavior therapy. *Journal of Consulting and Clinical Psychology*, 2006, **74**: 1041–1054.

31. Ravitz P, Maunder R and McBride C. Attachment, contemporary interpersonal theory and IPT: an integration of theoretical, clinical, and empirical perspectives. *Journal of Contemporary Psychotherapy*, 2008, **38**(1): 11–22.

32. Elkin I, *et al.* NIMH Treatment of Depression Collaborative Research Program: I. General effectiveness of treatments. *Archives of General Psychiatry*, 1989, **46**: 971–982.

33. Weissman MM, *et al.* The efficacy of drugs and psychotherapy in the treatment of acute depressive episodes. *American Journal of Psychiatry*, 1979, **136**(4B): 555–558.

34. Reynolds CF, *et al.* Treating depression to remission in older adults: a controlled evaluation of combined escitalopram with interpersonal psychotherapy versus escitalopram with depression care management. *International Journal of Geriatric Psychiatry*, 2010, **25**(11): 1134–1141.

35. Reynolds CF, *et al.* Treatment of 70(+)-year-olds with recurrent major depression. Excellent short-term but brittle long-term response. *American Journal of Geriatric Psychiatry*, 1999, **7**: 64–69.

36. Mufson L, *et al.* A randomized effectiveness trial of interpersonal psychotherapy for depressed adolescents. *Archives of General Psychiatry*, 2004, **61**(6): 577–584.

37. Mufson L and Fairbanks J. Interpersonal psychotherapy for depressed adolescents: a one-year naturalistic follow-up study. *Journal of the American Academy of Child and Adolescent Psychiatry*, 1996, **35**: 1145–1155.

38. Markowitz J. *Interpersonal Psychotherapy for Dysthymic Disorder*. 1998, Washington, DC: American Psychiatric Press.

39. Browne G, *et al.* Sertraline and interpersonal psychotherapy, alone and combined, in the treatment of patients with dysthymic disorder in primary care: a 2 year comparison of effectiveness and cost. *Journal of Affective Disorders*, 2002, **68**: 317–330.

40. O'Hara MW, *et al.* Efficacy of interpersonal psychotherapy for postpartum depression. *Archives of General Psychiatry*, 2000, **57**: 1039–1045.

41. Spinelli MG and Endicott J. Controlled clinical trial of interpersonal psychotherapy versus parenting education program for depressed pregnant women. *American Journal of Psychiatry*, 2003, **160**(3): 555–562.

42. Grote NK, *et al.* A randomized controlled trial of culturally relevant, brief interpersonal psychotherapy for perinatal depression. *Psychiatric Services*, 2009, **60**(3): 313–321.

43. Fairburn CG, *et al.* A prospective study of outcome in bulimia nervosa and the long-term effects of three psychological treatments. *Archives of General Psychiatry*, 1995, **52**(4): 304–312.

44. Fairburn CG, Jones R and Peveler RC. Three psychological treatments for bulimia nervosa: a comparative trial. *Archives of General Psychiatry*, 1991, **48**: 463–469.

45. Shea MT, Widiger TA and Klein MH. Comorbidity of personality disorders and depression: implications for treatment. *Journal of Consulting and Clinical Psychology*, 1992, **60**: 857–868.

46. Sotsky SM, *et al.* Patient predictors of response to psychotherapy and pharmacotherapy: findings in the NIMH Treatment of Depression Collaborative Research Program. *American Journal of Psychiatry*, 1991, **148**: 997–1008.

47. Blatt SJ, *et al.* Impact of perfectionism and need for approval on the brief treatment of depression: the National Institute of Mental Health Treatment of Depression Collaborative Treatment Program revisited. *Journal of Consulting and Clinical Psychology*, 1995, **63**: 125–132.

48. Blatt SJ, *et al*. When and how perfectionism impedes the brief treatment of depression: further analyses of the National Institute of Mental Health Treatment of Depression Collaborative Research Program. *Journal of Consulting and Clinical Psychology*, 1998, **66**: 423–428.

49. Barber JP and Muenz LR. The role of avoidance and obsessiveness in matching patients to cognitive and interpersonal psychotherapy: empirical findings from the Treatment for Depression Collaborative Research Program. *Journal of Consulting and Clinical Psychology*, 1996, **64**: 951–958.

50. Frank E, *et al*. Influence of panic-agoraphobic spectrum symptoms on treatment response in patients with recurrent major depression. *American Journal of Psychiatry*, 2000, **157**: 1101–1107.

51. Feske U, *et al*. Anxiety as a predictor of response to interpersonal psychotherapy for recurrent major depression: an exploratory investigation. *Depression and Anxiety*, 1998, **8**: 135–141.

52. Thase ME, *et al*. Which depressed patients will respond to interpersonal psychotherapy? The role of abnormal EEG sleep profiles. *American Journal of Psychiatry*, 1997, **154**: 502–509.

53. Buysse DJ, *et al*. Pretreatment REM sleep and subjective sleep quality distinguish depressed psychotherapy remitters and nonremitters. *Biological Psychiatry*, 1999, **45**: 205–213.

5

The Interpersonal Inventory

Introduction

The Interpersonal Inventory is a register of the key contemporary relationships in the patient's life. It is a unique feature of Interpersonal Psychotherapy (IPT), and is extremely well-designed to structure the process of gathering information about social support and the Interpersonal Problem Areas while listening well. It embodies the essence of IPT: listening to the patient well while utilizing a structure that facilitates change. The Interpersonal Inventory is created during the Assessment/Initial Phase of IPT, typically during the first two to three sessions. It is best considered a 'work in progress' as most therapists and patients find that their perspectives of the patient's relationships and the interpersonal problems change during the course of IPT.

IPT is a focused intervention which requires that the patient and therapist maximize the use of the limited time available to achieve meaningful change in problematic relationships. The Interpersonal Inventory functions as the main structural component of this process by focusing the patient and therapist specifically on:

- Understanding contemporary relationships
- Exploring the background of the patient's current interpersonal problems
- Identifying communication styles and patterns of interaction relevant to the interpersonal problem
- Identifying specific IPT Problem Areas which will be foci of treatment.

The Interpersonal Inventory can be compiled in many different ways, but it is always in principle a thorough and extended social history with two significant differences. First, as befits the here-and-now focus of IPT, the emphasis of the Interpersonal Inventory is on current relationships that are relevant to the patient's current psychological distress (Box 5.1). Second, utilizing the inventory as a method of collecting interpersonal data at the beginning of IPT establishes the manner in which the patient and therapist will approach the therapy: collaboratively and with structure that facilitates listening well and provides opportunity for insight to develop.

Box 5.1 Features of the Interpersonal Inventory

- Includes significant current relationships, including recent losses
- Contains details about the development of problematic relationships
- Outlines general social support
- Includes current communication problems
- Includes current expectations about relationships
- Identifies specific Interpersonal Problem Areas
- Facilitates the planning of treatment interventions
- Evolves and changes during the course of IPT and serves as a monitor for progress
- Provides a reference point for reorienting during therapy

The Features of the Interpersonal Inventory

Includes Significant Current Relationships, Including Recent Losses

The Interpersonal Inventory should primarily focus on the patient's significant relationships in the here-and-now. Practically speaking, this usually limits the number of people to be discussed to seven or eight, though that too can be modified for cultural reasons or to better accommodate the attachment style of the patient. The idea is to get a bird's eye view of the patient's social support, not to extensively explore every relationship he has. Specific interpersonal problems which are identified during the inventory will be the focus of the middle sessions of IPT – the inventory is an assessment tool. By implication, the here-and-now emphasis literally pushes the patient to focus on current relationships and to work on changing them.

Contains Details About the Development of Problematic Relationships

The details that are obtained from the patient should be a reflection of his experience of current problems rather than an exhaustive history. More details about the identified relationship problems will be obtained in the Middle Phase. The therapist must ensure, however, that the information gathered in the inventory is accurate, as some patients are prone to leave out details which might implicate them as being responsible for their problems. Past history is relevant as far as it illuminates the patient's actions in the present, and the extent to which past history is collected must be determined using clinical judgment, while being mindful of the short-term nature of IPT.

Outlines General Social Support

In addition to particular problematic relationships, the therapist should collect information about the patient's social support in general. One of the primary goals of IPT is to help the patient more effectively utilize his social support, so an accurate appraisal of the available resources is crucial. This information will also help the therapist to understand more about the patient's attachment style and ability to enlist the support of others.

Includes Current Communication Problems

The Interpersonal Inventory should note the patient's attempts to deal with his particular problems as well as his associated affective response to those problems. The therapist's inquiries regarding disputes or transitions should also elicit examples of problematic communication and specific interactions with others, as these frequently lead directly to IPT interventions.

Includes Current Expectations About Relationships

In addition to examples of specific communication, the therapist should also collect information about the patient's expectations of others in his social network. How does he expect others to provide support? Are the expectations realistic? Are they reasonable? What is the patient's perception of the expectations others have of him? This information will also direct IPT interventions – frequently techniques to help change communication should be coupled with those which foster changes in the patient's expectations of others.

Identifies Specific Interpersonal Problem Areas

One of the primary goals of the Interpersonal Inventory is to identify the specific Interpersonal Disputes, Transitions, or Grief and Loss issues that are relevant and connected to the patient's distress. The collection of information about relationships will facilitate this. The goal at this point is simply to identify the salient problems; more information and details will be gathered in the Middle Phase when the identified interpersonal problems are discussed at much greater length.

Facilitates the Planning of Treatment Interventions

The issues highlighted in the Interpersonal Inventory will not only help the therapist and patient understand his relationship problems and the extent of his social support, but will also provide a guide to which particular interventions are likely to be helpful. For example, if the patient is in the midst of an Interpersonal Dispute and, during the development of the inventory, describes what appears to be poor communication within the relationship, the therapist should anticipate that the best techniques to use are those focused on improving communication. Techniques such as communication analysis (Chapter 9) and role playing (Chapter 12) are well-suited for this. From these initial points of intervention the progress of the interpersonal work will follow logically.

Evolves and Changes During the Course of IPT and Serves as a Monitor for Progress

The Interpersonal Inventory is best considered an evolving story or 'work in progress' by the patient and therapist. The Interpersonal Inventory as it initially unfolds may be incomplete or distorted by the patient, sometimes by intent, as the patient wishes to avoid portraying himself in a negative light, and sometimes because the patient is either unable to organize the information fully or because he may be avoiding difficult issues. However, as treatment progresses, the patient's perceptions often change, more information typically emerges, and the patient's situation changes as a result.

Near the Conclusion of Acute Treatment, the patient and therapist should refer back to the initial Interpersonal Inventory and compare it to its current state in order to review the progress that has been made, as well as to discuss the work that remains to be done. The review of this material at the Conclusion of Acute Treatment reinforces the patient's gains, and can help him better understand the changes within his entire social network. The Inventory can also be used as a tool to subjectively examine outcome in IPT.

Provides a Reference Point for Reorienting During Therapy

As IPT proceeds, particularly with a patient with multiple or complex interpersonal problems, the patient and therapist may find themselves confused about which direction the treatment should progress. In these circumstances it is useful to refer to the Interpersonal Inventory for reorienting IPT. Rather than digressing or moving tangentially, the therapist can literally remind the patient (and himself) about the specific Problem Areas that were illuminated in the Inventory and Interpersonal Formulation. The Interpersonal Inventory is like a beacon or lighthouse that can illuminate the path of the therapeutic process when displacement of the interpersonal focus of IPT is threatened (Figure 5.1). As such, it can help the therapist to navigate a clear path between listening well and maintaining therapeutic structure, rather than straying into the Scylla of rigidity or the Charybdis of loss of focus.

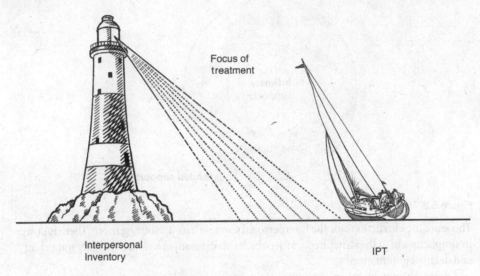

Focus of treatment

Interpersonal Inventory

IPT

Figure 5.1 The Interpersonal Inventory as a guide for IPT

Constructing an Interpersonal Inventory

In principle, the Interpersonal Inventory is a structured method of collecting interpersonal data. In practice, the Interpersonal Circle, a paper and pencil tool developed to collect the information needed for the inventory, can be used. The Interpersonal Circle is a tool which is both simple and immensely powerful – a way for the therapist to listen well while encouraging the patient to think. As with all of the tools used in IPT, the structure of the Inventory and the Interpersonal Circle should be used to:

- Facilitate listening well
- Direct the patient towards greater insight about his relationships and his communication style
- Facilitate change.

All of the paper and pencil tools in IPT are structured to open the therapeutic conversation further, to help the patient organize his thoughts and feelings, and to help the therapist listen well. The Interpersonal Circle, like the other tools, should be used flexibly and creatively.

The Interpersonal Circle is nothing more than a series of concentric circles drawn on a piece of paper (Figure 5.2). Using a blank piece of paper, the therapist draws three circles and then asks the patient to imagine that they are in the center of the innermost circle. The therapist then asks the patient to write down the names of seven to eight people in his social support network – people relevant to the presenting problem specifically. The innermost circle should include people with whom the patient feels intimate; the middle circle people with whom the patient feels close; and the outermost area those who are extended supports. The therapist should then hand the paper to the patient and ask him for a brief description of each person as he writes their names on the diagram (such as husband, wife, father, co-worker, etc.). Once seven to eight people are placed on the Interpersonal Circle, the therapist and patient will go back to each one and collect much more detailed information about them.

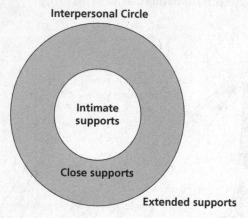

Figure 5.2 The Interpersonal Circle

Those are the instructions for the Interpersonal Circle. That's it. Nothing more. There is power in simplicity and in the structured way in which this diagram can elicit extremely important and detailed information.

There are no right or wrong answers; no right or wrong places to put other people on the diagram. The exercise is designed to facilitate more openness and description by the patient, and to facilitate a structured way of organizing information so that the therapist can listen well. Many times patients will ask where a particular person should be placed on the diagram: for instance, should a spouse with whom he is in conflict be placed on the intimate circle, or in the outermost circle since she isn't being supportive right now? The best therapeutic response is simply to ask the patient to decide.

Should the patient put people where they would like them to be ideally, or where they are right now? Let the patient decide. Should the patient put people in family groups, or should they be grouped in some other way? Let the patient decide. Should someone who has died be placed on the circle? Absolutely, but let the patient decide where: open up the discussion rather than closing it down by imposing unnecessary, rigid rules from a manual. There are few things that will damage the therapeutic alliance more than conveying that you aren't interested in your patient's perspective – telling your patient that people must be or cannot be included in the Interpersonal Circle because 'the protocol says so' is conveying exactly that. Be flexible, listen well, and during the inventory, encourage more information, not less.

Some Interpersonal Circles are simple, others are not. There are no right or wrong ways to construct it. For example, in Figure 5.3 the patient has written down his important interpersonal supports rather simply. Ron, Hermione, and Ginny are intimate supports (Albus and Sirius, noted in italics, have unfortunately died but remain highly significant); Neville, Fred, and George are close supports, while Arthur and Molly, also important people, are perceived to be at greater distance.

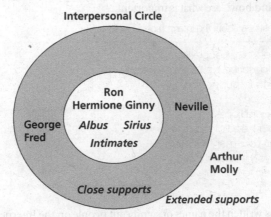

Figure 5.3 Example of a completed Interpersonal Circle (1)

In contrast, in Figure 5.4, the patient has a more complex circle, with italics indicating a significant person who has died but still has an important influence, along with arrows indicating the movement that the patient would like to occur in the relationships. The idea is that Charles, though at somewhat of a distance now, would ideally move closer, while Camilla, who apparently is intolerable, would exit the scene entirely. These are the kinds of conflicts that are often revealed only in confidence to a therapist; a stiff upper lip must be maintained in public.

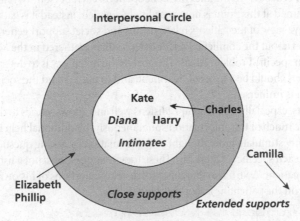

Figure 5.4 Example of a completed Interpersonal Circle (2)

As noted, there are no right or wrong answers or ways to draw the Interpersonal Circle. In fact, the more the patient wrestles with it, draws on it, modifies it, and marks it up, the better – it is an indication that he is thinking and invested. The process of struggling a bit to decide where to place people (Where should my partner go? Where should my father go? Where should my estranged child go? Where should my boss go?) is crucial in starting the patient to think about his relationships, and to develop some insight into how he forms and maintains them, and the contributions that he is making to good and bad ones.

To start the process, the therapist can, if additional instructions are needed, ask the patient to consider some of the questions listed in Box 5.2 to get the conversation going. These are sample questions only – you should develop your own. The spirit of the questions, and the depth of the questions which influence the patient to be introspective, such as 'Who has loved you well and how?' are what is important.

Box 5.2 General questions about the Interpersonal Circle

- Who are the important people in your life?
- How would you describe your social support system?
- Who do you go to for support?
- Who do you support?
- Who do you depend on?
- Who is inside your head at the moment?
- Who is taking up your mental energy?
- Who has loved you well and how?
- Who do you need to tell that you love?

Once the patient has written the names of significant people on the Interpersonal Circle, then the therapist and patient should go back and review each of those relationships in detail. It is vastly better to invite the patient to decide where to start. This both facilitates collaboration (as opposed to the therapist dictating which person the discussion will start with) and also allows the patient to work his way gradually into the process. For example, if his relationship with Camilla or Charles is emotionally fraught and difficult to talk about, then he can choose to start with an easier relationship to describe, such as his new wife Kate.

The patient should describe each of the relationships in detail, particularly the support received, the support wished for or desired, the support expected, and a brief history of the relationship. Perhaps 8–10 minutes might be spent on each person. To reiterate, the information obtained at this point is not exceedingly detailed; instead it is gathered to develop a bird's eye view of the patient's relationships and social support generally. Much more information about the conflictual relationships will be gathered in the Middle Phase when working on specific Problem Areas. The goal in the inventory is to determine which of the relationships should be a focus of treatment, and to understand the social context in which the patient is immersed.

Many patients, especially if the therapist listens well and allows stories to develop, will be able to provide much of this information spontaneously. If additional help is needed, the therapist can gently stimulate more thought and information by asking questions like those in Box 5.3 about each specific relationship. These too are suggestions, not a list that must be asked of each patient. A virtuoso therapist will develop questions of his own and modify them depending on the patient he is working with.

Box 5.3 Specific questions about the individuals on the Interpersonal Circle

- How often do you see this person?
- What do you like about the relationship?
- What don't you like about the relationship?
- What has changed in the relationship?
- How would you like the relationship to be different?
- What kind of support do you get from this person?
- How do you support them?
- How would you describe an argument?

The Interpersonal Circle is a tried and true method of collecting information from patients in a way which is non-judgmental, encourages detailed information, gives a visual representation of relationships, and best of all, literally *requires the patient to be introspective* when determining where to place others on the circle. Patients have given amazingly positive feedback about it; many find it was one of the most helpful things they did in therapy.

Be creative as well as flexible – the Interpersonal Circle is not set in stone. If you prefer, you can use triangles, or squares, or four circles instead of three. When working with adolescents we have had patients who used different colors for different relationships; we have had patients who included pets, and a few who have put God, on the circle. All the better: this simply speaks to the power of the simple tool to engage people in the process of thinking about their relationships.

There are two caveats to creative modification. The first is that the Interpersonal Circle should always be done in session, never as homework. The reason for this is that if the patient takes it home and fills it out, you'll miss all of the non-verbal nuances and struggles the patient has when doing the exercise. The therapist needs to see and talk with the patient about why a particular person is in a particular place, and to see the scribbles and erasures, and to see the emotions that accompany the process.

Second, the therapist should always give the paper with the blank circles to the patient to fill in. This is collaboration in action. Moreover, if the therapist fills in the names, all of the spacing and placement of the people on the Interpersonal Circle will be lost. This is very important information, and it works in a fashion similar to family modeling. Finding out who is next to who, the people that are at a distance, and the groupings of people will all be lost if the therapist writes down the names. And experience is clear that giving the patient control and listening well will ultimately result in much more extensive and helpful information. Let the circle be the structure – the therapist's job once the circle is introduced is simply to facilitate the discussion and listen well.

Using the Interpersonal Inventory During the Course of IPT

In the Assessment/Initial Sessions of IPT the Interpersonal Inventory is used to gather information. The Interpersonal Inventory also has conceptual utility, as the patient's descriptions of relationships will provide a wealth of information about his attachment and communication styles. Inconsistencies in the patient's accounts of events, or the lack of detail about an interpersonal problem, are often very informative about his perceptions or expectations about a relationship. The patient's reports of his communication style or attempts at problem solving are also informative. Moreover, the Interpersonal Inventory may highlight problematic communication that is consistent across a number of relationships but which is only apparent when they are scrutinized as a whole. In other words, the Interpersonal Inventory should provide a good view of both the forest and the trees.

When compiling the Interpersonal Inventory, the therapist should be thinking about questions such as:

How does the patient engage social support?

How does the patient resolve interpersonal problems?

How does the patient deal with loss?

How does the patient deal with attachment disruptions?

How does the patient care for others?

The answers to these questions will help to identify the patient's strengths and vulnerabilities, and should guide the entire course of IPT so that specific interpersonal problems can be addressed. It is the principal way in which specific interpersonal problems are identified, and these should be noted in the Interpersonal Formulation as topics to address in detail in the Middle Phase. The Interpersonal Inventory serves as a reference point throughout treatment to keep IPT on track and focused on specific interpersonal issues.

The Interpersonal Inventory also often serves as a measure of the patient's progress through treatment. At the Conclusion of Acute Treatment, it is helpful to review the original circle with the patient to discuss the changes that have occurred. This includes not only the resolution of identified problems, but also changes in the patient's conceptualization of relationships and problems. For instance, at the Conclusion of therapy the patient may see an Interpersonal Dispute less as an irreconcilable conflict and more as a problem with communication. Emphasizing areas in which the patient has gained insight into his contribution to the problems that were discussed is very helpful, as is a review of the steps that the patient took to solve them.

The Interpersonal Inventory also serves as a guide to identify potential future problems. If the initial version of the inventory indicates that a particular interpersonal problem arose consistently or was present for a long time – for instance, a pattern of preoccupied attachment and communication – this should suggest a focus for the future when problems in other relationships may lead to exacerbations of the patient's distress. The Interpersonal Inventory also has great utility with maintenance IPT. The focus of maintenance treatment is usually upon ongoing work in one or two Problem Areas. The Interpersonal Inventory serves to preserve the interpersonal focus of maintenance treatment and to optimize the use of the time available.

Case example 5.1: Lana

Lana was a 34-year-old married woman who was receiving IPT in combination with anti-depressant medication for an episode of depression. She presented for help with a conflict with her husband which she described as one of the main contributors to her distress. She completed an Interpersonal Circle (Figure 5.5) in session 2; her husband was notably placed in the outer circle. Lana described wishing that he were closer but not know-ing how to facilitate that. In the initial sessions of IPT, she appeared well engaged in the therapy, participated in the process of the inventory and formulation (Figure 5.6; described in detail in Chapter 6) and identified an Interpersonal Dispute with her hus-band. She seemed to be motivated to address her interpersonal problems.

During a session in the Middle Phase of IPT, Lana asked the therapist to advise her about whether she should disclose a previous indiscretion to her husband. The therapist sug-gested that rather than telling Lana what to do, it would ultimately be more helpful for her to decide, though he was very willing to spend time discussing the options and the benefits and costs of the choices. He also stated that his role in IPT was to assist her to determine what the best decision was rather than to make the decision for her. The therapist also felt that this position was more ethical, and was certainly more consistent with the approach to treatment used in IPT.

Lana became very angry as a result of the therapist's refusal to tell her what to do, but did not communicate this directly to the therapist. Instead, she began to withdraw from the therapeutic relationship by becoming increasingly silent and withholding. Recogniz-ing that this was likely to be what happened in her relationships outside of therapy, the therapist planned to move the discussion to situations when this occurred with Lana's husband, and to explore the ways she dealt with her anger with others. However, the therapist also recognized that Lana's reaction to him was causing the therapy to move from the established focus on Lana's conflict with her husband, as the problematic patient–therapist interaction was standing in the way of progress.

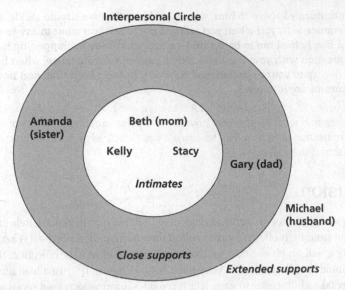

Figure 5.5 Interpersonal Circle – Lana

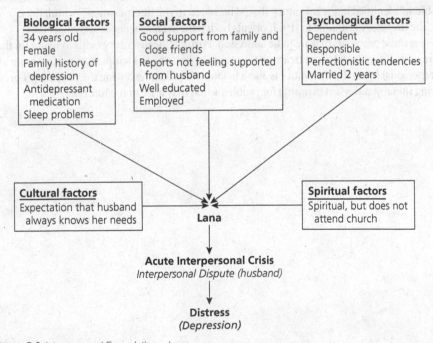

Figure 5.6 Interpersonal Formulation – Lana

At the beginning of the following session the therapist chose to use his experience with Lana to get more information about the style of communication that she likely used with her husband. Rather than explore the implications of the conflict within the therapeutic relationship, however, he shifted the discussion to similar conflicts Lana had experienced with her husband.

> Lana, if we go back to the Interpersonal Inventory, we determined that the main problem was a dispute with your husband. When we did the inventory we identified that some of your expectations of your husband, and the way

you communicated these to him, were a problem that we should tackle. I think my experience with you when you wanted me to tell you what to say to your husband has helped me to better understand what may be happening in your communication with your husband. What happens, for instance, when he doesn't live up to your expectations? How do you feel about that, and how do you communicate it to him?

Lana began describing an incident in which she felt her husband had been unresponsive to her requests, and went on to relate how she had 'shut him out' as a way of communicating her frustration with him. The treatment was effectively refocused on the dispute with her husband thereafter.

Conclusion

The Interpersonal Inventory is a critical element of IPT. The Interpersonal Circle in particular is a simple but stunningly effective way to collect the information needed – it is a structured way of listening well, and is also designed to influence the patient to be reflective. The inventory should be collected in the Assessment/Initial Phase of IPT, usually in session 2 or 3, and may take a full session to complete. It provides information about social support generally, and also helps to identify foci for treatment in the Middle Phase. The interpersonal problems identified in the inventory should be added to the Interpersonal Formulation.

The inventory is unique to IPT. It orients both patient and therapist to the specific interpersonal problems that are to be addressed. Further, the inventory helps to maintain the therapeutic focus throughout treatment, and aids in resisting the temptation to stray from an interpersonal focus. The inventory is also a helpful tool when reviewing the patient's progress during therapy and when planning for problems that may arise in the future.

The Interpersonal Formulation

Introduction

The ability to develop an accurate and concise psychological formulation of a patient's problems is an invaluable skill for all clinicians. The Interpersonal Formulation synthesizes information about an individual's biological and psychological makeup, attachment style, personality, social context, culture, and spirituality, creating a plausible hypothesis explaining her psychological symptoms. The formulation should lead to:

- An understanding of the patient's experience
- A plausible and personally meaningful hypothesis explaining the origin of the patient's distress
- A validation of the patient's experience
- A plausible rationale for treatment with Interpersonal Psychotherapy (IPT)
- A mutually determined focus for intervention based on the three Problem Areas
- A guide to the therapeutic stance to be taken in treatment
- A guide to the use of specific therapeutic techniques
- An accurate assessment of prognosis.

The Interpersonal Formulation is a theoretically grounded working understanding of the unique individual with whom the clinician forms a relationship in therapy. Because IPT is based on Attachment and Communication Theory, the formulation is an approximate understanding of the patient's experience from that perspective. It bridges the gap between a general theory of human behavior and the patient's specific and unique problems.

It cannot be emphasized enough that *working to understand the unique individual who is seeking help* is the most important therapeutic task in IPT. The formulation is not a definitive interpretation of the patient's problem by an omniscient therapist; it is a collaborative process that addresses the following questions:

- How did the patient come to be the way she is?
- What factors are maintaining the problem?
- What can be done about it?

If effectively and collaboratively developed, the Interpersonal Formulation should enhance the therapeutic alliance and convey the therapist's genuine attempts to understand the patient.

The Interpersonal Formulation is *not* a diagnosis to be presented to the patient. Instead, it is a collaboratively developed explanation of the patient's distress which describes how her symptoms have developed and are being maintained. The formulation emphasizes both the interpersonal factors involved in the origin and context of the problem, as well as how IPT will help the patient overcome her symptoms. It is a pivotal part of IPT, as the successful collaboration between patient and therapist to provide a valid formulation sets the scene for the conduct of treatment.[a]

The Biopsychosocial/Cultural/Spiritual Model

The Biopsychosocial/Cultural/Spiritual model of mental illness asserts that biological, psychological, social, cultural, and spiritual factors coalesce within an individual to produce a unique diathesis or response to stress. When faced with a sufficient interpersonal crisis, vulnerable individuals are likely to have psychological difficulties. The Biopsychosocial/Cultural/Spiritual model therefore frames psychological difficulties as the response of a unique and multifaceted individual to a unique stressor rather than as categorical illnesses.

The utility of this model in clinical practice has become increasingly evident as movement towards a dimensional view of mental health has continued. This dimensional view of Biopsychosocial/Cultural/Spiritual functioning incorporates states of 'good' mental health as well as illness, acknowledging both strengths and symptoms rather than simply identifying pathological syndromes. As a consequence, the model offers both the patient and therapist a simple and clear way of organizing and understanding the complex and multiple determinants of psychological symptoms and interpersonal distress.

In contrast to the medical model of mental health which requires that an individual's problems be categorized as medically based syndromal diagnoses, the Biopsychosocial/Cultural/Spiritual model emphasizes the whole person and her suffering rather than focusing exclusively on a diagnosable disease. This by no means diminishes the importance of diagnoses, but rather emphasizes the uniqueness of the individual who is suffering. This is vastly more congruent with the aim in IPT that the therapist should work to understand the patient in the context of her unique personal and social circumstances, and that the patient is helped to appreciate the influence of these factors as well. The value of the Biopsychosocial/Cultural/Spiritual model is that it conceptualizes distress as being determined by many factors, none of which alone can explain the patient, the specific manifestations of her distress, or its course.

The Biopsychosocial/Cultural/Spiritual model as it is applied to the Interpersonal Formulation in IPT acknowledges:

- *Biological factors* – such as genetic vulnerabilities, physical illness, substance abuse, medication side-effects, and injuries to the central nervous system
- *Psychological factors* – such as attachment style, temperament, psychological defense mechanisms, cognitive style, intelligence, personality, psychological development, and ego strength
- *Social factors* – such as available social supports, financial resources, education, and work environment
- *Cultural factors* – such as family structure, cultural meaning, and culturally recognized ways of coping with distress
- *Spiritual factors* – such as religious communities, spiritual practices, and spiritually based meaning.

---

[a] The Interpersonal Formulation is one of the concepts and tools in IPT which can be used with any psychotherapeutic approach. The collaborative development of an understanding for the patient's distress will be helpful with all patients.

The Elements of the Interpersonal Formulation

The Interpersonal Formulation is built upon the foundation of the Biopsychosocial/Cultural/ Spiritual model. In addition, there is a strong emphasis on both attachment and interpersonal theory. The formulation includes hypotheses regarding the patient's current functioning, and it is not static or fixed – it should be continually modified by the collaborative efforts of the patient and clinician as therapy proceeds. The formulation will evolve and change emphasis over time as the patient and therapist come to better understand the patient's unique circumstances and experience of distress.

Step 1: Development of the Interpersonal Formulation with the Patient

At the end of the Initial/Assessment Phase, once the full clinical and IPT assessments are complete, including the Interpersonal Inventory, the therapist should ask for the patient's assistance in collaboratively developing an Interpersonal Formulation. The best way to do so is to rely once again on the ever-ready blank piece of paper and pencil. The therapist can either draw five boxes or five columns, labeling them Biological, Psychological, Social, Cultural, and Spiritual factors, respectively (Figure 6.1). As with all of the other IPT tools, the paper should then be handed over to the patient to fill in.

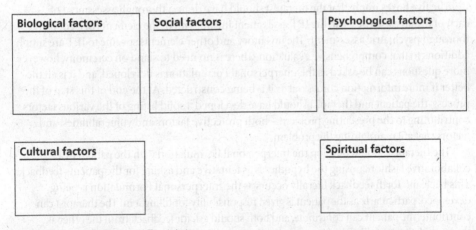

Figure 6.1 The Interpersonal Formulation

The therapist should then ask the patient to help develop a summary of the various factors that are contributing to her problems. Examples can be given if necessary to get the work underway. As the various factors are listed, the patient (*not the therapist*) should write them on the paper in the columns that make the most sense to the patient. If prompting is needed, the therapist can offer a few thoughts about what is likely to be contributing to the problem – often the patient may not be aware of some of the Biological factors (for instance, a past or current problem with autoimmune or thyroid functioning), so the therapist can offer these for inclusion if needed. Both the patient and the therapist should contribute to the Interpersonal Formulation, ideally with the patient taking the lead, but with plenty of input from the therapist.

Both strengths and vulnerabilities can be listed. Some obvious examples of strengths are an absence of a family history of psychiatric problems, a strong social support network or intimate relationships, a deep spiritual faith, or being well-educated or insightful. The best way to proceed is to use the patient's own terms as much as possible. This not only helps to understand the way the patient explains her distress, but will also make the Interpersonal Formulation more meaningful for her.

The use of the patient's own words is particularly important in the Psychological area. While the therapist may be thinking in technical terms, such as the description of the patient's attachment style or personality traits, the patient's own words can and should be used to develop the Interpersonal Formulation in this area. The therapist can keep the technical terms in mind, but the formulation should be in terms the patient can identify and understand.

For example, the patient may describe her personality as being 'perfectionistic and detail oriented'. While the therapist may understand this as obsessive-compulsive personality traits, the better terms to put on the Interpersonal Formulation are the patient's. They will be more meaningful and almost certainly more accurate – after all, the patient has spent a lifetime with herself, the therapist only a few hours. Another example might be a patient who describes herself as a 'people person' or as someone who 'doesn't like crowds'. Better to put that on the Interpersonal Formulation rather than some technical jargon or interpretation. The patient might describe herself as 'outgoing' – that should be put on the formulation as well. The therapist can hold the more technical terms; the point of the Interpersonal Formulation is to develop a meaningful explanation that both the patient and therapist have contributed to and that has meaning for the patient.

The five boxes imply that the therapist should have done a thorough assessment of each of the areas. To be clear, the IPT assessment includes *all* of the elements of a good and thorough psychiatric assessment. The inventory and other elements specific to IPT are simply additions to that comprehensive evaluation. There is no need to stand on ceremony, however: more questions can be asked as the Interpersonal Formulation is developed, and it is all the better if more information comes out as it is being constructed. At the end of this step of the process, the patient and therapist should have developed a solid listing of the various factors contributing to the presenting problem – both protective factors and vulnerabilities, and factors that are maintaining the problem.

The therapist should develop the Interpersonal Formulation with the patient in a collaborative fashion, posing the hypotheses as tentative and asking for the patient's feedback. This back and forth feedback literally occurs as the Interpersonal Formulation is being developed, particularly as the patient is given responsibility for filling it in. The therapist can contribute, the patient can contribute, and both should ask for feedback from the other as the formulation unfolds. The Interpersonal Formulation, like all of the tools used in IPT, is a structured way of listening well. Figure 6.2 gives a brief overview of some of the various factors that might be included in each area. This list is neither comprehensive nor required – the primary point is to develop a formulation which is relevant for the unique patient. It is, however, a good starting point for questions and for developing a solid formulation. The following sections describe these in more detail.

Biological Contributions to Distress

Genetic factors

Documented or suspected illnesses or symptoms in family members are of clear significance. A common oversight is to take at face value a negative family history. The therapist should

Biological factors	Social factors	Psychological factors
Age	Intimate relationships	Attachment
Genetics	Social support	Personality
Gender	Employment	Temperament
Substance use	Education	Defense mechanisms
Medical illnesses	Health care system	Trauma history
Medical treatments	Means of communication	Stigma

Cultural factors	Spiritual factors
Tradition	Tradition
Family	Social support
Cultural meaning	Spiritual meaning

Figure 6.2 Some factors that may be included in the Interpersonal Formulation

not merely inquire about diagnoses or treatments, but should also ask about the presence of symptoms or behaviors suggestive of illness in family members.

Drug and alcohol use

These may not be reported by the patient, as recreational drug and alcohol use is common in many societies. Heavy use may not be reported for fear of reprisals or because of denial. The therapist should help the patient understand the subtle effects of even moderate psychoactive substance use, which may disturb psychological health and interpersonal functioning in ways that may not be apparent to the patient. Both the contribution of these factors and the interpersonal determinants of drug and alcohol use should be included in the Interpersonal Formulation.

Medical illness

A comprehensive medical history must be obtained during the evaluation. Some illnesses will be readily acknowledged by the patient, though they may not be recognized as connected to psychological difficulties. The formulation should also include the patient's means of coping with the illness and its interpersonal significance. Physiological changes such as menarche or menstrual changes may be significant biological factors that are not recognized by the patient as relevant to her distress.

Effects of medical treatments

Many medications have psychological sequelae and are relevant to the Interpersonal Formulation. Corticosteroids, for instance, are often in this category, as are medications which produce sexual side-effects, such as those used for hypertension or to treat depression. These may also lead to significant interpersonal difficulties in marital or other intimate relationships. The issue of compliance with psychotropic medications that create these kinds of problems should also be addressed – an antidepressant medication which causes fatigue and sexual dysfunction is apt to have both physical and interpersonal consequences that may affect usage.

Diet and exercise

These may be protective or may be vulnerabilities. Often they are used as coping strategies during times of stress.

Psychological Contributions to Distress

Recall that though these are the elements that should be assessed, the patient's words and descriptions are much better to use in this section of the Interpersonal Formulation. The therapist can obsess about the technical terms on her own.

Attachment style

The patient's attachment style is usually evident in the ways the patient has functioned in previous and current relationships. In addition to the patient's own description of herself in relationships, the therapist can extrapolate a lot about attachment style from the information collected in the Interpersonal Inventory. The therapist's experience of the patient should also help her to understand how the patient's attachment style has contributed to the current problems. The therapist may find it difficult to 'connect' with the patient, or may find that the patient frequently challenges her; these behaviors or evoked responses are important data regarding attachment style.

Temperament

Temperament can be considered to be the genetically and biologically determined manner in which an individual responds to her environment. The therapist can evaluate the patient's temperament in a manner similar to that used to examine the patient's attachment style.

Cognitive style

The patient may display problematic cognitive processes such as generalizations or selective abstraction, particularly when discussing her relationships. Statements such as 'This always happens to me', or 'He only stays because of the children', may be very informative, as the patient's cognitions about her relationships are often the most strongly held. The therapist should attempt to establish whether this type of thinking pattern pervades other interpersonal aspects of the patient's life. Although cognitions are not a primary focus in IPT, they certainly may be addressed. What makes IPT unique is the primary focus on interpersonal issues outside of therapy. Methods of dealing therapeutically with these unrealistic expectations (the IPT jargon for cognitive sets) is described in subsequent chapters, but the primary tactic in IPT is to deal with the interpersonal aspects and ramifications of such expectations.

Psychological coping mechanisms

The way in which a person deals with intrapsychic stress is a key determinant of mental health. The therapist can develop an impression of the patient's coping mechanisms by considering how the patient describes her attempts to deal with current interpersonal problems. Consider, for example, a patient who is dealing with an impending divorce. She may describe frequent physical symptoms or a preoccupation with her health. She may describe behavior such as physical aggression or substance use. While discussing the breakdown of her marriage, she may exhibit a lack of affect, or perhaps may endow her estranged husband with all manner of personal faults that seem more her own. In a situation like this the therapist can infer that the patient probably relies on more immature or neurotic coping mechanisms such as projection, acting out, or isolation of affect. This not only helps the therapist to understand how the patient has come to be in her current situation, but also how she is likely to deal with the challenges of IPT, and the type of obstacles that she is likely to present to the therapist during the treatment.

Jargon such as 'isolation of affect' are the therapist's terms, however. While they are important and carry meaning for the therapist, they do not carry meaning for the patient.

They should not be used in the collaboratively developed formulation. Instead, factors like this can be included in the Interpersonal Formulation by literally asking the patient questions such as 'What are you like when you get angry? and 'What are you like when you get distressed?' Her descriptions, such as 'quick tempered' or 'I tend to hold in anger', can be written verbatim in the psychological box.

Social Contributions to Distress

The patient's current social milieu should be summarized and included in the Interpersonal Formulation; a thorough assessment of it should have already occurred during the Interpersonal Inventory. The absence of support, or of people who can provide secure attachment relationships, usually has a profound effect on the patient's current distress. Conversely, those patients who have extensive social support systems will be less vulnerable to psychological difficulties when faced with crises.

Employment status and education should be included. Access to healthcare is a huge factor for many patients, and may have led them to defer seeking care, or limit the care that they can obtain. Means of communication has become a much greater issue, particularly for younger patients, since the first iteration of this text. Many people now communicate primarily through cell phones, text, or Facebook with many of their social supports. Assessing whether that support is meaningful and helpful, and whether more of it would be a help or hindrance to recovery, is an important part of the Interpersonal Formulation.

Cultural Contributions to Distress

Cultural factors may greatly influence the patient's willingness to seek care, to engage in particular treatments, and the value she places on professional mental healthcare. Family structure is heavily influenced by culture, as are role stereotypes based on age or gender.

Spiritual Contributions to Distress

Religious organizations can provide great support, or can be barriers to care. Spiritual meaning and traditions should be assessed, particularly with grief and loss issues. Social support from spiritual and religious groups should be evaluated, as should early experiences of religion which may have caused alienation.

Step 2: Completing the Interpersonal Formulation with the Patient

The length of the Interpersonal Formulation will vary depending on the particular patient. With complex patients with extensive medical and psychiatric histories and chaotic social situations, it may include a dozen or more factors in several of the boxes. With others who are less complex, there may only be a handful of factors, with many of them in the social and psychological boxes. The formulation should be comprehensive, but need not be exhaustive. As a rule of thumb, it may take 8–10 minutes to complete as a summary of the information collected during the assessment/initial sessions of IPT.

Once the Biopsychosocial/Cultural/Spiritual boxes are completed, the therapist can summarize them by stating that these factors are strengths and vulnerabilities that have led the patient to react to interpersonal crises in a particular way. Lines are often drawn from the boxes to another box drawn in the middle of the page representing the patient as a unique individual (Figure 6.3). The therapist should go on to explain that the particular interpersonal crises described by the patient have interacted with these vulnerabilities to cause her distress, and can at this point add a psychiatric diagnosis as one of the results of the crises if a diagnosis is warranted. If not, the therapist can simply work with the patient to fully describe the symptoms and dysfunction which are part of her distress. In either case, the distress is literally linked by the therapist to the patient's interpersonal problems; this is further emphasized by the Interpersonal Formulation diagram, which reinforces their direct connection.

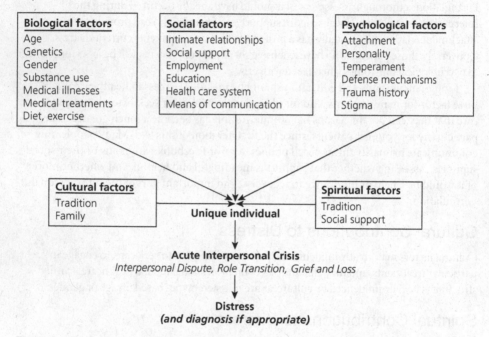

Figure 6.3 A complete Interpersonal Formulation

The completion of the formulation should set the stage for the Middle Phase of IPT, in which the focus will be directly on the acute interpersonal crises, that is, the three Problem Areas as they apply to the particular patient. Only after the completion of the Interpersonal Formulation should the therapist move to developing a Treatment Agreement with the patient regarding the treatment focus, the approximate duration of treatment, and other logistical issues. Done well, the treatment plan – what is to be done to help the patient – flows naturally and obviously from the formulation. It will be no surprise to the patient, given her presenting complaints and organized understanding of her distress and diagnosis, that the IPT approach will be of benefit. The logical and easy-to-understand focus of IPT, flowing from a solid assessment and formulation, is one of the great strengths of IPT.

Case example 6.1: Penny

Penny, a 32-year-old legal secretary, was referred to a psychiatrist for assessment of an episode of depression that followed the birth of her daughter 3 months earlier. She complained of irritability, poor concentration, self-reproach, loss of interest in her usual activities, and excessive tearfulness. She recognized that these symptoms were a marked departure from her usual self, and had resulted in an ongoing conflict with her husband. Penny told her therapist that she and her husband had discussed the arrangements for the arrival of the baby, and had agreed that she would take maternity leave for a year while her husband, Brad, continued to work full-time. According to Penny, Brad was also supposed to contribute to the running of the household and had agreed to take care of the baby on weekends in order to give Penny some 'time to herself'. Penny had also discussed babysitting arrangements with her mother, who had agreed to offer a day a week to look after the baby in order for Penny to keep up with things at work, even though she was officially on maternity leave.

Penny described being physically well throughout her pregnancy. She stated that during the pregnancy she felt 'terrific', but since the birth had experienced a major 'let down', which she felt was hormonal. She reported having intermittent mood swings during the latter half of her menstrual cycles, though she had not sought any treatment for this previously. The decision to have a child was, according to Penny, based largely on her age. She stated that she had determined that if she were going to have children, it had to be now, as it would be much more risky if she were any older.

After the arrival of the baby, Penny described that 'she had found that she had less time to spend with her husband' as the demands of childcare left her tired. When asked for more details, she disclosed that their sexual intimacy was virtually non-existent, and that she had not felt close to him at all. Moreover, in order to keep up with the finances, Brad had started working longer hours to offset the drop in income created by Penny's maternity leave. Penny found also that her mother was increasingly unreliable in fulfilling her childcare agreement.

Penny was an only child. Her mother had suffered from depression throughout Penny's childhood, apparently with postpartum onset. Penny's relationship with her mother during adolescence was described as conflicted, and she reported feeling closer to her father during that time. She described her mother currently as helpful at times but unreliable in general. In contrast, she stated that since she had gotten married, she had little contact with her father.

Penny said that throughout her schooling she excelled academically, although she did not pursue tertiary studies. She stated that as a student she was always noted for her impeccable bookwork as well as her dedication to her chosen sport of swimming. She described her working life as highly satisfying as she felt she was a valued member of the team at her legal firm. She pointedly mentioned that the partners always asked her to assist with their cases. She enjoyed work, and stated that she missed the social support she received there.

Penny had been married for eight years. She described being happy in her married life, although she felt that the lack of time she and her husband had together, as well as her inability to regularly see her friends and colleagues, was 'taking its toll'. Her description of her relationship with her husband was interesting: Penny said they had gotten married because, 'they worked well together'. She reported that her husband had complained on occasion that their relationship lacked intimacy, and was frequently dissatisfied with their sexual relationship, but Penny stated that she was quite satisfied with both of these aspects of her marriage.

Penny described herself as a perfectionist and told the psychiatrist that her self-esteem was related to her ability to achieve things. She reported being 'in control' of her life prior to the arrival of her baby, but the lack of structure and continual demands of motherhood coupled with the lack of definite goals was difficult. She reported some difficulties in breastfeeding her child in the first few weeks, which she said made her feel 'even less in control of things'.

Penny's Interpersonal Circle, developed in the second session, is depicted in Figure 6.4.

The mutually determined factors contributing to the Interpersonal Formulation of Penny's interpersonal distress and the development of her postpartum depression included the following.

Biological factors:
- Gender
- Postpartum

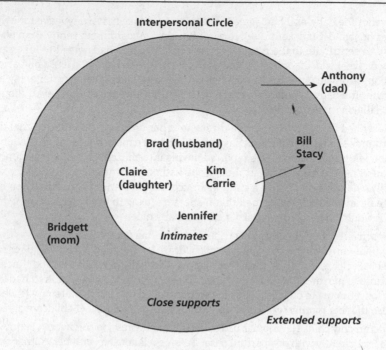

Figure 6.4 Interpersonal Circle – Penny

- History of depression in her mother
- Predisposition to hormonally influenced mood swings

Psychological factors:
- Self-reliant
- Hard worker
- Perfectionist
- [*Dismissive attachment traits* – therapist's thoughts]
- [*Obsessive-compulsive personality traits* – therapist's thoughts]

Social factors:
- Poor support from family
- Fair support from husband
- Good support from work colleagues

Cultural factors:
- Pressure to be perfect mother, wife, and employee
- Little expectation for childcare help from extended family

Spiritual factors:
- Regular church attendance

Interpersonal Problem Areas:
- *Role transition* into motherhood – adjusting to the physical and psychological demands of having a baby, as well as the loss of the benefits of full-time work
- *Interpersonal dispute* with her mother – unmet expectations of childcare and support as well as difficulty communicating her needs

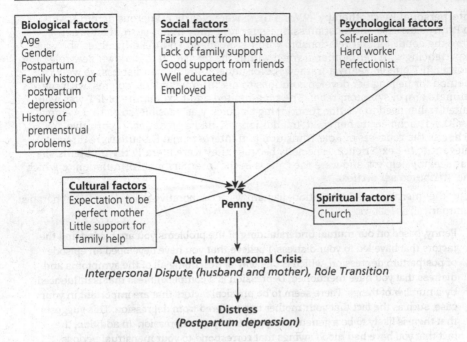

Figure 6.5 Interpersonal Formulation – Penny

- *Interpersonal dispute* with her husband – unmet expectations between Penny and her husband

Penny's Interpersonal Formulation is depicted in Figure 6.5.

This conceptualization of Penny's distress and depression was compatible with several treatment options:[b]

Cognitive behavioral therapy – Penny described a degree of perfectionism and in her history highlighted a number of thoughts that seemed to reflect dysfunctional cognitive schema. Her need for perfectionism and her tendency to 'all-or-nothing thinking' would provide material for focal cognitive interventions.

Self-psychology – Penny described a distant relationship with her mother, and there was evidence that this was re-emerging as a significant issue in the context of her own motherhood. Self-psychology would offer Penny a therapeutic relationship that offered opportunities for 'mirroring' or 'idealizing' transference. This would potentially improve Penny's symptoms and functioning, but would be primarily focused on facilitating the evolution of her 'disorganized selfhood.' Despite the fact that Penny did not show evidence of severe personality disturbance, there would likely be benefits to this approach, although its long-term nature would be problematic, particularly considering the logistical limitations imposed by her new parenting responsibilities.

Family therapy – Penny and her extended family system appeared to be in crisis largely because of the introduction of a baby as a new member in the family system, with clear changes in the relationship between Penny and her husband and mother. There would potentially be benefit in bringing the family into therapy in order to deal with the difficulties that the family system encountered since Penny's transition into parenthood.

[b] We ask the reader for some latitude in our descriptions of treatment options – we have an obvious bias towards IPT, but certainly acknowledge that other approaches are also of help, and encourage the reader to make his or her own determination about the best treatment for a given patient. Most important is to have several options and therapeutic tools in one's toolbox.

Interpersonal Psychotherapy – While there were clearly numerous determinants to Penny's distress, the most pressing issues for Penny in her current situation were the conflict in her relationship with her husband and the difficulties she was experiencing with her mother, framed within the transition to her own new role of mother. IPT offered Penny a framework for understanding her distress, as well a method for helping her develop solutions to her interpersonal problems, with the ultimate aim of symptom relief. The time-limited and focal nature of IPT was well suited to her need to resume functioning as quickly as possible, so as to develop a healthy attachment to her child. In addition, IPT had a great deal of intuitive appeal to her as the concepts of Role Transition and Interpersonal Dispute were directly relevant to her experience, especially because they were literally the problems she was seeking help for, and were the causes in the Interpersonal Formulation to which she attributed her distress.

After the Interpersonal Formulation diagram was collaboratively developed, the therapist summarized as follows:

> Penny, based on our mutual understanding of the problems you are having and the factors that have led to your distress, I believe that you have developed an episode of postpartum depression, which is one way of describing all of the symptoms and distress that you have mentioned. Depression is a complex illness that is influenced by a number of things. There seem to be physical factors that are important in your case, such as the fact that your mother has suffered from depression. This suggests that there is likely to be a genetic component to your depression. In addition, the fact that you have had mood swings that correspond to your menstrual periods suggests that there may be hormonal factors involved as well.
>
> There also appear to be factors within your psychological makeup which are contributing to your problems. You've usually been able to deal with life very successfully by working hard and being a high achiever, and that feeling of being in control of your life has been very important to you. No doubt that sense of control has been changed with the arrival of your daughter – babies are experts at keeping their parents on an irregular and unpredictable schedule. It's been difficult to use your normal style of getting organized and working harder to cope with all of the changes since she's been born.
>
> In going through your transition to parenthood, it seems that other relationships have been affected as well. You were quite clear that your relationship with your husband, which was good before Claire was born, has been affected by the new responsibilities that you both face. It sounds like your relationship with your mother has become more of a problem since Claire was born as well.
>
> All of these factors are important, and it seems to me that you became depressed after the birth of your daughter because of a combination of all of these things. The transition to becoming a mother has clearly brought about major changes in your life – both the good and the stressful – and has challenged your ability to cope with things as you normally have in the past.
>
> I believe that it will help a great deal to work on the transition you are going through, and on the relationship conflicts you described with your husband and mother. I think that IPT is a natural fit – the primary focus of treatment is to help people resolve interpersonal conflicts and adjust to major life changes like having a child. Using IPT will also allow us to get a handle on your symptoms without needing to use antidepressant medication, since you're concerned about the effect that medication might have on your baby.
>
> What are your reactions to this summary?

The summary of the Interpersonal Formulation need not be technical – it should be framed in terms that are readily understandable to the patient, just like the terms in the formulation diagram. Further, it is extremely helpful to emphasize the patient's strengths. In this case, Penny had a number of strengths; the magnitude of the transition to parenthood was simply too great for her to deal with given her typical coping style and interpersonal resources. One can imagine, for instance, that if she had a better relationship with her mother, she may have weathered the postpartum period with fewer problems, or if she had been less obsessional and less driven to be in control of everything, she may have been able to adjust more easily to the chaos of a new baby. Framing her difficulties as a temporary reaction to a difficult situation both reinforces her usual ability to cope with stress and implies that the difficulty is time-limited and will be overcome.

The discussion about the formulation and treatment planning should always be collaborative. The therapist should always ask the patient for feedback, be receptive to it, and be willing to incorporate the feedback. New information that emerges during the Middle Phase of therapy can also be incorporated into the continually evolving formulation.

Conclusion

The Interpersonal Formulation in IPT is the result of a collaborative process in which the patient and therapist arrive at an understanding about the causes of the current problems the patient is experiencing. The formulation is the product of an integration of the Biological, Psychological, Social, Cultural and Spiritual factors that create a vulnerability to psychological distress, and the interpersonal crises that precipitate it at a given point in the patient's life. This process ultimately validates the patient's experiences and links these factors to her interpersonal distress. The formulation also provides the rationale for the use of IPT as a therapeutic intervention, as well as providing information to the therapist about which specific IPT techniques are likely to be most beneficial.

7

The Treatment Agreement

Introduction

Interpersonal Psychotherapy (IPT), like all other psychotherapies, requires a Treatment Agreement: a collaborative establishment of a set of guidelines for its conduct. Also like all other psychotherapies, IPT simply does not work as well if a treatment contract is unilaterally imposed by the therapist. The agreement should be the result of a collaborative process.

The Treatment Agreement in IPT is for the benefit of both the patient and the therapist. For the patient, it establishes expectations for the treatment along with the obligations of both the patient and therapist. For the therapist, it provides a practical guide to treatment, particularly with patients whose maladaptive attachment communication styles are likely to require structural accommodations in the therapy. Since both the patient and therapist have important contributions to make to the agreement, it should be collaboratively negotiated rather than being rigidly dictated by the therapist.

While it may seem a matter of semantics, the use of the term Treatment Agreement instead of 'treatment contract' is critical in IPT. The term 'contract' implies that the terms cannot be changed, and that if a specific number of sessions are contracted for at the beginning of treatment, exactly that number – no more and no less – must be delivered. Instead, IPT is far better delivered flexibly using a dosing range of sessions that can be agreed on not in the first session, but after the formulation at the end of the Assessment/Initial Phase of treatment. The term 'contract' also implies that the therapist dictates the terms, and the patient has to agree to them if he wants treatment; if he does not agree, he is wished good luck and shown to the door. In contrast, listening well to the patient, developing a strong therapeutic alliance, and working collaboratively with him, all point clearly to negotiating a flexible agreement for treatment.

The term 'contract' also implies, incorrectly, that any attempts on the part of the patient to modify the arrangement can be conceptualized as resistance. For example, if the patient asks to meet for an additional session or two, a therapist can dogmatically interpret the patient's resistance to termination as pathological, rather than carefully and honestly working with him to understand the patient's request and collaboratively deciding whether additional sessions might actually be more helpful. Resistance is a helpful concept in understanding electrical circuits; in psychotherapy it is simply a way to label a patient rather than working hard to understand his point of view.

Developing the Treatment Agreement

Unlike human relationships outside of a clinical setting, the therapeutic relationship is constrained by ethical and practical concerns (although one might well argue that it would be desirable if all relationships were bound by similar ethical concerns). The concept of clinical 'boundaries' is one of the best examples of this. In addition to the practical necessity of agreeing to a specific time and place to meet for therapy, therapeutic relationships nearly always have limits to things such as contact with the therapist outside of therapy, arrangements for emergencies, payment for services, and so on. Ideally these are established clearly and *a priori* rather than emerging as problems later in the therapy. Setting these boundaries both preserves the integrity of the therapeutic relationship and protects the patient and therapist from exploitation. The patient and therapist should establish the boundaries of the therapeutic relationship as part of the Treatment Agreement. Like all of the components of IPT, developing the Treatment Agreement is a collaborative process between the patient and therapist. The option to revisit and renegotiate it should remain throughout the treatment. Clinical judgment should guide this process.

The negotiation of the Treatment Agreement is an interpersonal process between patient and therapist. As a consequence, the agreement should be negotiated after the therapist has had the opportunity to thoroughly assess the patient's clinical presentation, attachment style, and social situation. The therapist should have a fairly well-developed sense of the therapeutic relationship after this assessment. This means that the agreement comes after the development of the Interpersonal Formulation at the end of the Assessment/Initial Phase of IPT – it is the last task to be completed in this phase.

The agreement should include mutually negotiated therapeutic goals. If the patient and therapist develop an agreement with a shared vision, the likelihood of the treatment being successful is greatly increased. As a result, the therapist should help the patient to articulate his specific goals – the outcomes in the relevant Interpersonal Problem Area(s) – as clearly as possible. This mutual determination of goals is an intrinsic part of the development of the Interpersonal Formulation.

The patient's attachment style should also influence the process of developing a Treatment Agreement. Patients with more secure attachment styles are more likely to tolerate the therapist 'taking the lead' in setting goals, while those with more insecure styles of attachment will likely feel alienated or rejected if the therapist is too directive in setting the agenda. This a catch-22 experience in all types of therapy, as securely attached patients, though able to tolerate more directiveness from the therapist, are also more capable of taking the initiative or working collaboratively; with the securely attached, the development of an agreement is quite easy. In contrast, those less securely attached are more sensitive to the therapist being too directive, while at the same time they are less likely to be able to take the lead themselves. This is yet another reason why patients with more secure attachment styles fare well, and those with less secure attachment styles require flexibility in IPT structure and techniques, along with more attention to the therapeutic alliance.

The Components of the Treatment Agreement in IPT

The core components of the Treatment Agreement in IPT are shown in Box 7.1. Depending upon the therapist's clinical judgment, it can be either written or verbal. Providing a written description of the conduct of IPT and a description of the patient's role in treatment is extremely helpful with some patients, but is unnecessary and cumbersome for others. Flexibility is the key – the way in which tools such as the agreement are used should be determined to a large degree by the characteristics of the individual patient rather than being dogmatically applied to everyone. Patients who are more securely attached are likely to do quite well in therapy without the need for a written agreement, while those patients with evidence of insecure attachment and more problematic interpersonal styles may benefit from a clearly written description of the conduct of IPT and their specific goals. Whether written or verbal, the agreement in IPT should specifically address the points in the following sections.

Box 7.1 The core components of the IPT Treatment Agreement

> ○ The number, frequency, and duration of sessions
> ○ The Problem Areas to be addressed
> ○ The expectations of the patient and therapist
> ○ Contingency planning (e.g. emergencies and rescheduling)
> ○ Treatment boundaries

The Number, Frequency, and Duration of Sessions

These should be determined primarily on the basis of the severity of the patient's problems and his attachment style. Sessions may also vary with the style and availability of the therapist, but in general will be within a dosing range of 6–20 sessions, usually of 50 minutes duration. Issues of cost and payment should also be clarified.

The Problem Areas to Be Addressed

This should include the Problem Areas and relationship issues which have been identified by the patient and therapist in the Interpersonal Inventory and Interpersonal Formulation.

The Expectations of the Patient and Therapist

The patient is expected to take responsibility for utilizing the sessions well – being open, honest, and on time – and for working between sessions on problems that are identified in his social environment and interpersonal relationships. Patients frequently have the incorrect assumption that the bulk of change in IPT will take place in the sessions rather than in their interpersonal environment outside of therapy. The bottom line in IPT is changing the patient's functioning in his social environment; hence he must do some work between sessions. The amount of work and effort the patient puts in is highly correlated with the outcome of the therapy.

Contingency Planning

This includes matters such as missed sessions, lateness, or illness. In general, if the therapist is late or misses a session, the time should be made good at a later time. If the patient misses a session or is late on several occasions, the reasons should be discussed. Often there are legitimate reasons, such as transportation problems, child illness, or even problems with parking. Common sense suggests that sometimes a cigar is just a cigar, and needs no further smoking.

In the case of repetitive problems with missing appointments or lateness, the IPT therapist should frame the lateness or absence as an overt interpersonal communication, rather than examining the psychodynamic underpinnings of such behavior directly with the patient. The therapist can also use this information about the patient's behavior to further develop his hypotheses about the patient's interpersonal relationships and attachment style. The therapist can then draw attention to other circumstances in which the patient has been late or not met obligations with others in his social network, as opposed to discussing such issues within the therapeutic relationship.

Treatment Boundaries

'Boundaries' in IPT are best defined as the ethical and practical constraints that distinguish the therapeutic relationship from other non-professional relationships. Relevant boundary issues include clinical and non-clinical contact outside of working hours, appropriate arrangements for emergencies, and expectations regarding substance use and aggressive or inappropriate behavior. While many (including us) would argue that these are implicit in any therapeutic relationship, it is worthwhile with more complex patients to discuss these formally and negotiate them explicitly. An ounce of prevention is worth a pound of cure: it is better, particularly with more complex patients, to discuss potential problems before they arise rather than having to deal with them after the fact.

Practically speaking, these boundaries can be established by asking more complex patients questions such as, 'What are we going to do if you cut yourself?' or 'What are we going to do if we happen to meet in public?' or 'Are we going to use email to communicate, and if so, what are the expectations we have about it?'

Maintaining the Treatment Agreement

Violations or breaches of the agreement may occur even with explicit *a priori* discussion. These may range from simple matters such as lateness or delayed fee payments to more significant problems such as inappropriate behavior in sessions or inappropriate contact outside of therapy. While all of these problems can be viewed as having psychodynamic and transferential significance, the focus of the IPT therapist's responses to such occurrences is to address them as interpersonal behaviors in the here and now.

Agreement violations, conceptualized as conscious interpersonal behaviors, often provide valuable information about the patient's experience of the therapeutic relationship as well as his behavior in relationships outside of therapy. In some cases the behavior may have a simple explanation such as logistical difficulties (time off work, childcare, etc.) or financial limitations that are best dealt with by the therapist pragmatically. In others, they reflect the patient's attachment style and corresponding difficulties with communication, and may also reflect personality difficulties and psychological defenses. It is the therapist's task to analyze this information, integrate it into a coherent understanding of the patient, and use it to help the patient improve his communications with others and relationships outside of therapy.

Agreement violations in IPT should generally be dealt with using a three-step process. First, the therapist should state directly to the patient that a violation has occurred. A brief discussion should follow to ensure that the patient recognizes this, and that there is continuing agreement on the limits in future sessions. Second, the therapist should clearly communicate his expectations to the patient. In other words, the therapist should direct the patient to the specific kind of behavior that the therapist would like instead of the patient's disruptive behavior. Third, the therapist should direct the discussion towards problems that similar behaviors may have caused the patient in relationships outside of therapy. For example, if a patient has been calling the therapist too frequently between sessions, the therapist should directly point out to the patient that they had agreed that calls would be limited. Next, the therapist should direct the patient to new behavior – calling the emergency room after hours, or having the patient call at a specific time during the week as opposed to the out-of-hours calls. The therapist should ensure that the patient understands both the problematic behavior and the way it should be modified.

After this, the therapist can then use the information gleaned from the violation to begin asking questions about the patient's relationships outside of therapy. For instance, the therapist might ask the patient how he typically asks others for help when distressed. What happens when he calls other people frequently? Has he ever gotten negative feedback from others about being too persistent? How has the patient dealt with this?

In IPT, most agreement violations can be dealt with very directly in this way. All provide important information to the therapist about potential problems that the patient may be having in his social relationships. Rather than using agreement violations to focus more on the patient–therapist relationship, in IPT the discussion should be quickly turned to similar problems outside of therapy.

Practical Reasons for Agreement Violations

Many patients have legitimate reasons for missing appointments, payments, or for not fulfilling other parts of the Treatment Agreement. As an advocate for the patient, it is certainly within the purview of the IPT therapist to actively assist the patient to seek out and utilize resources in the community that might be available. Referrals for assistance with payments for treatment, housing resources, childcare resources and the like can be provided by the therapist. Though this is clearly not the primary goal of IPT, if the patient is unable to come to sessions because of practical reasons such as these, treatment will obviously not be successful. The patient is fully responsible for utilizing the resources, but the therapist can direct the patient to them, rather than interpreting and labeling the patient's inability to find and use such resources as resistance to therapy.

In some cases, the agreement violations arise as a result of a misunderstanding by the patient, which may merely reflect his problems in communication. Reframing the problem as a consequence of poor communication between patient and therapist may therefore reinforce the need for clear communication in other relationships as well, and examples from these can be discussed in therapy. When the problem arises as a consequence of unrealistic or unreasonable expectations on the part of the patient, this too can be addressed as a process that may be typical of the patient's other relationships.

The Implications of the Agreement Violation for the Patient's Social Relationships

It is axiomatic in IPT that whatever occurs in the therapeutic relationship parallels processes in other relationships. The therapeutic relationship is a real relationship influenced by the same factors that affect all of the patient's relationships. The patient's attachment style and experience of other relationships will affect the way he experiences the constraints of the therapeutic agreement. If problems emerge in the therapeutic relationship, they therefore shed light on these factors, and on the relationships that the patient is involved in outside of therapy. The patient's experience of, and reaction to, the Treatment Agreement is therefore extremely valuable information about his interpersonal relationships.

Managing Agreement Violations within the Therapeutic Relationship

In some cases, the patient's reactions to the therapist and the Treatment Agreement may be so extreme or difficult to manage that the therapeutic relationship must be directly addressed. The preservation of the therapeutic relationship must be the primary consideration in IPT – without it, therapy cannot proceed. If the therapeutic relationship is threatened, the therapist may choose to renegotiate the agreement with the patient. Doing so may have additional therapeutic benefits for the patient as he may experience this process as a new way of behaving and communicating that generalizes to other relationships. If this fails, the therapist should strongly consider moving to another form of therapy in which the patient–therapist relationship is more directly addressed as the focus of treatment.

In many circumstances, the patient may be unaware of the impact of his interpersonal behaviors. Such 'blind spots' or communication problems may become apparent to the therapist when they are examined against the background of the Treatment Agreement. Using this information, the therapist can then begin to examine other situations in which the patient's lack of insight about the consequences of his communication may be a problem. The therapist can address this by hypothesizing that others are likely to respond to the patient in the same way that the therapist has, and that situations that provoke or elicit similar responses from others occur in the patient's relationships. Discussing these kinds of interactions and reflecting on the likely responses from others, informed by the therapist's experience with the patient in a similar interaction, is a potent way to help the patient develop insight into his communications and what follows in their wake.

In summary, the therapist's actions should always reinforce the agreement by implication, and by explicit reminder if needed. Interventions regarding the agreement should first and foremost be pragmatic: a gentle reminder, and then discussion of the patient's social relationships in which similar communication problems are likely to be occurring.

Case example 7.1: Barry

Barry was a 21-year-old man who had been referred by his local physician for management of depression. Barry described experiencing difficulties in his relationship with his girlfriend and had suffered periods of dysphoria, leading to vague suicidal ideation. Barry's local doctor had started antidepressant medication, which had provided some benefit in relieving his symptoms. His Interpersonal Circle is shown in Figure 7.1.

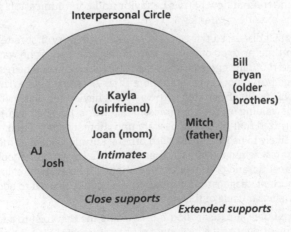

Figure 7.1 Interpersonal Circle – Barry

At the end of the Assessment/Initial Phase of therapy, after developing an Interpersonal Formulation (Figure 7.2), Barry and his therapist negotiated a Treatment Agreement and agreed to meet for 10–12 more sessions of IPT. They agreed that the frequency of the latter sessions would likely be tapered. They also agreed to focus on an Interpersonal Dispute with his girlfriend and an Interpersonal Dispute with his mother.

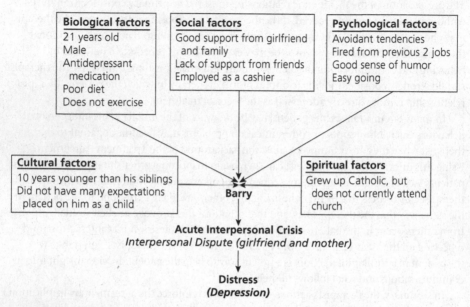

Biological factors
21 years old
Male
Antidepressant
 medication
Poor diet
Does not exercise

Social factors
Good support from girlfriend
 and family
Lack of support from friends
Employed as a cashier

Psychological factors
Avoidant tendencies
Fired from previous 2 jobs
Good sense of humor
Easy going

Cultural factors
10 years younger than his siblings
Did not have many expectations
 placed on him as a child

Barry

Spiritual factors
Grew up Catholic, but
 does not currently attend
 church

Acute Interpersonal Crisis
Interpersonal Dispute (girlfriend and mother)

Distress
(Depression)

Figure 7.2 Interpersonal Formulation – Barry

Barry arrived 10 minutes late for session 4, citing problems getting off from work. The therapist conducted a shortened 40-minute session and highlighted the benefit of taking full advantage of all of the time set aside for treatment. Barry arrived on time for session 5, but canceled session 6, 2 hours prior to its scheduled time. The therapist first arbitrarily and unilaterally decided that the session would not be made up as Barry had not provided 24-hour notice prior to cancellation. After consideration, however, the therapist thought better of it, recognizing that this was not a particularly collaborative way to proceed, and also recognizing that doing so would miss an opportunity to understand how Barry's behavior and communication played out in similar situations outside of therapy.

Instead, the therapist discussed this series of events with Barry, first reiterating the need for Barry to be on time, as to do otherwise was limiting the benefit he was getting from therapy. They then mutually agreed that in the future, Barry would be responsible for paying for sessions he did not cancel with more than 24 hours' notice. The therapist recognized that he was feeling frustrated with Barry's behavior and was irritated that Barry did not seem to be valuing his time or professional efforts. Being an astute therapist, however, he recognized that his reactions were undoubtedly a reflection of the ways in which Barry was likely to be interacting with others. Putting aside his frustration and annoyance, the therapist reminded himself that any course of action he took in IPT should be gracious, therapeutic, and of benefit to the patient. The therapist realized that his reactions were important 'diagnostic' information, and could be used to address problems in Barry's relationships outside of therapy.

Barry arrived 10 minutes late for session 7, prompting the therapist to address the Treatment Agreement right at the beginning of the session. He planned to move from there to a discussion about other relationships in which Barry had difficulty in maintaining his commitments.

Therapist: Barry, over the last several sessions you have had problems keeping your appointments or being here on time. I want to remind you that we had agreed that we would meet for 50-minute sessions, and when you are late we aren't able to meet for that long. While you might still get some benefit from the time that is left in the session, I don't think that you are getting the full benefit of treatment by being late. It's almost like taking half of a dose of medicine – you might feel somewhat better, but the effect isn't as great as the full dose.

Barry: I can see your point ... I have just had trouble getting everything organized to get here on time.

Therapist: We had also agreed that you would call at least 24 hours ahead of time if you had to miss an appointment, and I want to remind you of that as well.

Barry: I'll try my best, but the time I missed I had a real emergency at work.

Therapist: I appreciate that things come up, but I do want to make sure that we are clear on our expectations of each other. Barry, since this has happened several times during our work together, I wonder if this is a problem in other relationships you have. What are your thoughts about that?

Barry: Well, my girlfriend is always getting on me about being late. She says that is one of her main complaints with me – that if I'm late, it means that I don't take things seriously enough.

Therapist: What's your reaction to that?

Barry: I've tried to convince her that my being late has nothing to do with her – it's just a bad habit that I've gotten into. I wish she wouldn't take it so personally.

Therapist: It sounds like she is interpreting your being late in a way that you aren't intending.

Barry: That's right. But I haven't been able to convince her otherwise.

Therapist: May I give you some direct feedback?

Barry: Sure.

Therapist: I think it's important for you to know that nearly everyone you interact with is going to react to you being late by being irritated or upset. I have had that reaction myself when you missed the appointment and the times you have been late. Other people do take that personally, whether you intend it or not. That's going to have a big impact on your relationships, and I wonder if it's a big factor in the disputes you're having with your girlfriend and your mother. Were you aware that people react to you that way?

Barry: I'm not late that much ... I still don't see why people take it that seriously, but I guess maybe you have a point. That has probably had something to do with my jobs too – one of my bosses got pretty mad at me for not showing up a couple of times ...

Barry reluctantly agreed that some of his behavior was frustrating, and then began to explore ways he might be able to more effectively manage his behavior, recognizing that it was a problem for others, and was not communicating what he intended. This became a major focus of treatment.

Additional Thoughts About the Treatment Agreement

We have written a great deal about potential violations of the Treatment Agreement. When violations do occur, they present real difficulties in treatment and challenges for the therapist. However, these kinds of problems just aren't that common. They aren't that common in general, and they are even less common when IPT is done well. If the therapist listens to the patient, and honestly tries to understand him, then there are not that many times when disagreements occur. And if the patient truly feels understood, he will make every effort to be on time.

These kinds of problems also aren't that common because of the flexibility inherent in IPT. If the therapist unilaterally insists that the therapy must terminate after a fixed number of sessions, the patient is likely to object. A poor therapist will remain intransigent and label the patient as difficult or resistant; a virtuoso therapist will discuss problems with the patient and come to an agreement to extend therapy if both agree it would be of benefit. Violations just aren't that common if IPT is conducted well and collaboratively.

As a corollary, if the therapist finds that agreement violations occur with several of his patients, it is worth carefully examining where the problem is originating. Therapist rigidity will provoke patient 'resistance' as a reaction; therapist flexibility and listening well will facilitate a strong therapeutic alliance.

Conclusion

The Treatment Agreement is an essential part of IPT. It should be negotiated after the Interpersonal Formulation is completed at the end of the Initial/Assessment Phase of IPT. Establishing a clear and consistent agreement is crucial because it is a reference point both therapist and patient can return to if therapeutic boundaries are threatened. Since addressing the therapeutic relationship directly is not a focus of IPT, the agreement carries even greater weight because it allows boundary problems to be addressed *a priori*, ideally without recourse to discussions of transference.

Section 3

IPT Techniques

8

Clarification

Introduction

Clarification is one of the most frequently used techniques in Interpersonal Psychotherapy (IPT). It is the 'heart and soul' of the Assessment/Initial sessions, but should be used frequently at all times during the course of IPT. Clarification is nothing more than:

- Asking good questions so that the therapist can better understand the patient's experiences
- Asking very good questions so that the patient can understand his own experiences better
- Asking extraordinarily good questions so that the patient is motivated to change his behavior.

Clarification is a 'non-specific' psychotherapeutic technique, and its use is not unique to IPT. As with all IPT interventions, clarification should facilitate the IPT therapist's understanding of the patient, the patient's understanding of himself, and increase the therapeutic alliance.

The process of collaboratively exploring – clarifying – a particular aspect of a patient's interpersonal experience is therapeutic in a number of ways:

- It provides the therapist an opportunity to validate the patient's experiences and distress
- It provides an opportunity for the patient to explore and reflect upon his interpersonal experiences within a supportive therapeutic relationship
- It helps the patient to more clearly communicate his experiences to others, as practice in doing so occurs first under the therapist's guidance
- It helps to consolidate the therapeutic alliance by emphasizing that the patient and therapist are involved in the collaborative process of exploring the patient's experiences.

Despite the apparent simplicity of clarification, asking questions is a real art. It requires that the therapist take a genuine interest in the patient, and that the therapist be able to convey this interest to the patient. This is not a platitude. It is a very real and very critical part of the therapy. To do IPT well requires – literally – that the therapist listen well, listen with genuine empathy, and listen with genuine caring for the patient. Nothing less will do.

Patients who are less securely attached are apt to be particularly vigilant for therapists who are less than genuine, so clinicians will need to work diligently and creatively to use clarification to foster a productive therapeutic relationship with them. With such patients, clarification as a means of conveying a desire to understand the patient and to help him feel less isolated is critical in developing the alliance. With such patients the structure of IPT can be changed as well, so that an additional assessment session or two can be used to listen well and work on the alliance before introducing more structure.

When in doubt, listen well. When in doubt, clarify more.

Clarification in IPT

Clarification as a technique is best considered an integration of the following:

- **Directive questioning**: The therapist should gently guide the patient towards pertinent interpersonal issues during the clarification process. The primary focus on interpersonal issues is an aspect of clarification that is unique to and characteristic of IPT.
- **Empathic listening**: The therapist should validate the patient's experiences and concerns regarding his interpersonal problems.
- **Reflective listening**: The therapist should work to ensure that he is correctly understanding the patient, often using statements such as, 'So what you've said is . . '. to check his comprehension of the patient's description.
- **Encouragement of spontaneous discourse**: The therapist should use verbal and non-verbal cues to encourage elaboration by the patient.

Clarification and the Patient's Attachment Style

During the process of clarification, the therapist can gain valuable insight into the patient's attachment style by evaluating the way he responds to open-ended questions about relationships. This is particularly helpful during the Interpersonal Inventory. Such inferences may help the therapist understand the patient's experience of interpersonal problems, as well as helping to anticipate potential problems in the therapeutic relationship. It should also guide the therapist in determining to what degree close or open-ended questions should be used, and the degree to which the questions should be directive. More securely attached patients can generally tolerate more directiveness on the part of the therapist, while those that are less securely attached may need more empathy and reflection from the therapist in order to develop and sustain a good alliance, particularly early in therapy.

The Art of Clarification

The use of clarification requires a balance between encouraging spontaneous narrative by the patient and using more directive questions to keep the discussion focused. The therapist should be prepared to allow some degree of drift, as it may lead to the disclosure of new material, but the general focus should be interpersonal and based on the Problem Area under discussion.

The artful use of clarification can be compared with a damper on a fireplace. More directive questions can be used to 'open the damper' and generate a more intense fire, while less directive and more empathically driven questions can be used to 'close the damper' so the fire doesn't get out of control. Enough heat is needed to keep the patient motivated to change; too much and the patient will (psychologically) spontaneously combust. More securely attached patients can generally tolerate more affective heat than those less securely attached. The therapist's job is to keep the fire burning at the most efficient level by directing the interview in this way.

As an example, consider a patient in distress after being diagnosed with cancer. Opening the damper would be asking questions such as: 'What was it like for you when you received the diagnosis?' or 'What do you imagine the surgery and chemotherapy will be like?' Closing the damper would be asking questions or making statements such as, 'What's been helpful to you in coping with this?' or 'How have others been supportive to you?' Empathic comments such as 'I'm sorry that you're struggling so much' will close the damper even more.

The directive clarifications get right to the point, and ask in open-ended fashion questions about the patient's experience. They are the 'What is that like for you?' questions. The less directive clarifications ask more about support, coping, and how the patient can manage more effectively. Both are important. Balancing them well is to conduct virtuoso IPT.

In contrast to IPT, therapists using more 'expressive' and psychodynamically based treatments often encourage the patient to produce narrative that is free-flowing and at times may be circumstantial or discursive. While this may be useful for uncovering latent or unconscious psychological content, it is not so useful in IPT. There are several reasons for this. First, expressive orientations distract from the focus on the rapid resolution of the patient's symptoms and distress. Allowing an open-ended focus over a longer time period is likely to move the treatment to a transference-based therapy. That's fine if you are doing long-term psychodynamic work, but not so good if you are doing a short-term acute treatment such as IPT. The acute time limit in IPT requires a more specific focus for discussion than longer and less structured treatments. Efficiency is key in IPT.

Second and most importantly, using more directive clarifications in IPT allows the therapist to encourage the patient to make changes in his communication and to resolve the problems he faces outside of therapy. This is because when the patient reflects upon and responds to the 'What is the experience like for you?' questions, he is learning to communicate his experiences differently. And he's getting practice in talking about them, and in helping others understand them. This happens first with the therapist, then with others outside of therapy. The goal is to get the patient to articulate his experiences, struggles, distress, and need for help to others in a way that they can better understand and better respond to.

Using Clarification to Begin Sessions

Mindful[a] of the need in IPT to maintain an interpersonal focus and to direct the patient's attention to the specific problem at hand, the therapist should typically begin sessions by avoiding general non-directive statements such as 'How are things since we last met?'

More appropriate and directive questions to start sessions include those that draw the patient's attention to the interpersonal problem last discussed, and those that clearly convey to the patient the expectation that work is to be done on these issues between sessions. Examples of directive questions like this are:

Over the last few weeks we have been discussing the problem you are having with your partner. Can you update me how this has been progressing?

Last week we decided that you would take on the homework assignment of talking with your partner about finances. How did it go?

Initial questions like the above establish a focus for the discussion of interpersonal problems, direct the patient's attention to the specific problem at hand, lead naturally into a continuing

---

[a] You can and should be mindful in IPT just like you can focus on interpersonal issues in mindfulness oriented therapies – both will be the better for it.

discussion of the problem in the current session, and reinforce the therapist's expectation that the patient will work on the problem between sessions.[b]

Potential Difficulties with Clarification

The Patient Who Continually 'Wanders off Subject'

The therapist must be constantly attentive to the direction of the discussion. If the patient begins to wander off, redirection or a gentle but direct request to return to the interpersonal topic are helpful. The therapist should highlight the need to remain on task, and if needed can review the Interpersonal Formulation with the patient to emphasize the specific Problem Areas that were determined to be therapeutic foci. The use of more closed-ended questions may be helpful to redirect the discussion to interpersonal areas, with a return to more open-ended questions once the focus of discussion is firmly refocused upon the interpersonal problem.

Patients who are vague at times or who have trouble organizing their thoughts well tend to engender digression in the therapy. When a therapist finds himself following a divergent lead, it is best to regroup by consulting the Interpersonal Inventory or Formulation. Returning to the original Problem Areas allows the therapist and patient to refocus the discussion.

It is also useful to examine the disorganization or digression as an interpersonal communication, and to discuss the ways it might cause problems in the patient's extra-therapy relationships. For instance, the therapist might comment:

> There have been a few times now when our discussion has led us to areas that seem to be a little off the track. This seems to have made us both a bit confused about where we are heading in working with your problems. Do you find that this happens when you are discussing this problem with others? How does it seem to affect your relationships with other people?

The Therapist Who Continually 'Wanders off Subject'

There are occasions when even the most experienced IPT therapist finds himself moving into more intrapsychic work with the patient. Many times this is because the patient's psychodynamic processes are just too intriguing, and the therapist falls prey to the temptation to ask about dreams or even the patient's fantasies about the therapist simply because it is so fascinating (and narcissistically gratifying). This is particularly difficult for therapists who come from a more psychodynamic background, because there are times the therapist may feel that he has to 'hold back' and not follow transferential leads that might be used in less structured approaches. Recognizing this temptation when it occurs is the best way to prevent drift, and if the patient begins to share a fascinating dream, the therapist can simply ask him whether he has told anyone else about it, and how the meaning in the dream and its ramification for relationships might be communicated to significant others.

---

[b] Can you set a formal agenda at the beginning of each IPT session? Yes. IPT is flexible and can accommodate that. But use your therapeutic judgment carefully in doing so. The reason is that setting an agenda does not reflect real interpersonal relationships. If you are conducting a psychotherapy workshop or an administrative meeting, you set an agenda. If you are sitting down to coffee with a friend, it would seem artificial and awkward to set an agenda – you don't say to a friend, 'I'm going to spend 5 minutes talking about my divorce, 10 minutes on the death of my beloved uncle, and 7 minutes talking about my State Fair photo exhibition. Then you can talk.' Therapy is not a friendship, but it is designed in IPT to facilitate the goal of helping the patient communicate better with his social supports. This should be practiced in therapy, then extended to the patient's social relationships, where there is no agenda.

Case example 8.1: Henry

Henry was a 36-year-old legal assistant who presented with worsening anxiety in the context of a marital problem. Henry had received some benefit from cognitive therapy, although his ongoing relationship difficulties had continued to result in symptoms. Henry complained to the therapist that his wife, 'did not understand him', and that he 'didn't want to be in the marriage anymore'. Henry gave an account of his relationship with his wife that implied a great degree of indifference about its survival. They had been together only 6 months before getting married; his wife had suggested marriage; Henry described that he simply 'went along'. The therapist asked if Henry recalled any of his thoughts at the time of his wife's suggestion that they get married, to which Henry rather pointedly replied, ' I don't really know, and I haven't really given it much thought.' His other relationships seemed to be equally 'unimportant' to Henry, which was also clear in his Interpersonal Circle (Figure 8.1).

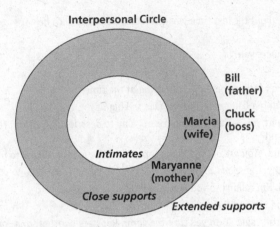

Interpersonal Circle

Bill (father)

Chuck (boss)

Marcia (wife)

Intimates

Maryanne (mother)

Close supports

Extended supports

Figure 8.1 Interpersonal Circle – Henry

While constructing the Interpersonal Inventory, the therapist attempted to clarify the dispute between Henry and his wife further:

Therapist: *Henry, tell me more about your wife.*

Henry: *Well, um … there isn't really much to say.*

Therapist: *Well, perhaps you could tell me how the relationship started.*

Henry: *Not a lot to say really – we met, she proposed, I didn't think too much about it, we got married.*

Therapist: *Tell me more about how you met.*

Henry: *Like what?*

Therapist: *Well … how you felt about her then for instance.*

Henry: *Much the same as now really.*

Based on Henry's responses and the pattern of relationships he described, the therapist hypothesized that Henry's style of attachment was rather fearful and a bit dismissive, and that this was leading to his difficulty in describing any details about his relationships and feelings. Henry's tendency to be dismissive of relationships was clearly a potential threat to the therapeutic relationship, just as it was to his relationship with his wife.

It soon became apparent that the therapist needed to do two things, and to do them skillfully. First, the therapist needed to direct the therapy so that more specific information about Henry's interactions with his wife could be obtained. At the same time, the therapist needed to make sure that the therapeutic alliance was strengthened so that Henry wouldn't literally dismiss the therapist and bail out of therapy. An artful mix of directive questions, empathy, warmth, and a genuine effort to understand Henry was required.

Therapist: *Let me slow down the pace a bit – I really want to understand as best I can what your experience with your wife has been like for you.*

Henry: It's hard to describe really, but it's been quite frustrating.

Therapist: *It sounds like it has been – it's hard for me to imagine what it must be like for you. Could you tell me more about your experience?*

Henry: Nothing I do seems to make any difference to her. She doesn't seem to appreciate that I have feelings too, even though I may not be quite so direct about it as she is. I really hate it when she says that I never talk about my feelings. I think that she just doesn't listen.

Therapist: *That does sound frustrating. If we could, I'd like to focus a bit more on one or two specific interactions you have had with her, so that I can understand the details a bit better.*

Henry: Uh huh.

Therapist: *Tell me about the last time you had a disagreement with her.*

Henry: OK.

Therapist: *Where were you?*

Henry: At home.

Therapist: *What was it that you were both doing at the time?*

Henry: I was watching a ball game and she was talking at me.

Therapist: *'Talking at you' – that's an interesting way to describe it. Can you remember some specific things she said?*

Henry: Yeah, she said, 'You are always doing something else except talking to me!'

Therapist: *How did you respond to that?*

Henry: I said, 'Well, I'm talking to you now, aren't I?'

Therapist: *What did she say then?*

Henry: Well, I think she said, 'Can you turn the damn Roosters game off and commit to the conversation?'

Therapist: *OK, and how did you respond.*

Henry: I didn't really respond, I just kept watching the game – it was the Grand Finals after all.

The therapist continued to clarify the specific aspects of Henry's interpersonal dispute with his wife. He remained mindful of Henry's attachment style, and continued to artfully use both open and directive questions to elucidate Henry's interpersonal experiences. The therapist's genuine interest in understanding Henry, his real curiosity, and his empathy was able to carry the therapeutic alliance, and ultimately to help to create a relationship in which Henry could learn to connect better with his wife.

This was also reflected in the adaptations the therapist made to the structure of IPT. Rather than rushing to develop a formulation, the therapist elected to spend several sessions on the inventory. He also asked Henry to bring in some photos to help gather more information about his relationships. They looked at these together, and then Henry simply explained what was going on in the photos.

In addition, the therapist made sure to be as collaborative as possible. Henry was very sensitive to not being heard, so the therapist not only listened well but acted on what he heard by specifically asking for Henry's input about how often they should meet, what they should focus on, and about how long they should tentatively plan for therapy to continue. To do otherwise would have quickly destroyed the therapeutic alliance and would have caused Henry to dismiss the therapist as yet another person who didn't listen to him or understand him.

Conclusion

Clarification is much more than merely asking questions. Clarification involves a delicate balance between directive queries and encouragement of narrative. That balance will vary depending on the patient's attachment style. Clarification is a fundamental method for establishing and maintaining an interpersonal focus in IPT. The aims of clarification are to foster the therapeutic alliance and to develop an understanding of the patient's interpersonal experiences, helping both the therapist and patient to develop insight into his problems and ultimately motivating him to change.

Communication Analysis

Introduction

The basic premise of Interpersonal Psychotherapy (IPT) is that individuals have difficulties because they are faced with an overwhelming stressor in the context of insufficient social support, both in their intimate relationships and in their general social network. Though the lack of sufficient social support is frequently due in part to deficits within patients' support systems, it is also frequently due in part to poor communication. Patients – people – often do not communicate their needs clearly, nor in a way to which their social support system can productively respond. As a direct consequence of these maladaptive styles of communication, patients do not get their attachment needs or their needs for emotional and physical support met adequately, and they become distressed.

The Goals of Communication Analysis

Communication analysis is simply a formal technique for investigating the hypothesis that the patient's difficulties are being caused, perpetuated, or exacerbated by poor communication. The goals for communication analysis are:

- To help the therapist identify the patient's communication patterns
- To help the patient identify her communication patterns
- To help the patient to communicate more effectively.

To do this, the therapist should work sequentially with the patient through the following steps:

1. Collect information about the patient's interpersonal relationships and samples of the communication that occurs within them
2. Develop hypotheses about why the communication is going poorly
3. Present the hypotheses to the patient as feedback about her communication
4. Solicit responses from the patient about the therapist's feedback
5. Revise the hypotheses if needed
6. Problem solve to develop and practice new ways of communicating.

A strong therapeutic alliance must undergird this process, as the patient must be able to tolerate feedback from the therapist for it to have any impact, and for it to lead eventually to change. The specific ways of giving feedback must also be selected wisely, carefully considering the patient's attachment style and insight.

Sources of Examples of Communication

The obvious requirement for communication analysis is that there must be communication to analyze. In IPT, the therapist relies on five potential sources of information:

1. The patient's description of her communications, both generally and specifically
2 The quality of the patient's narrative
3. The patient's in-session communication with the therapist
4. Reports from or interactions with the patient's significant others
5. Interpersonal Incidents.

Each of these provides extremely important information, and can literally be thought of as providing different perspectives on the patient's communication. Communication analysis must be preceded by an extensive social history, a detailed description of the patient's relationships, and her expectations of others, all of which should be collected during the IPT assessment. This means that communication analysis should be used primarily in the Middle Phase of IPT to gather more detail about specific interpersonal problems.

The therapist should also explore the patient's perceptions of the expectations that others have of her – this will have been done to some degree in the Interpersonal Inventory, but should be done in more detail in the Middle Phase. The rule rather than the exception is that interpersonal difficulties are caused not only by poor communication but by expectations that are unrealistic or non-reciprocal.

Most patients are able to give a fairly accurate accounting of their expectations of others, although this will be colored to some degree by their ability to relate narrative and their insight. Unfortunately, a patient who has difficulty in communicating directly to others in her social network will usually also have difficulty communicating directly to the therapist. Further, a patient who misperceives the communication or intent of others will often report a biased view of the communication she has with others. Such patients may attribute malevolent or uncaring motives to others when their attachment needs are not met, despite the fact that the significant other may be communicating clearly and may be invested in the relationship. The therapist should therefore explore the possibility that the problems in communication arise from any or all of the following:

- The patient is not communicating her needs clearly
- The patient is not communicating her needs in a way to which her social support system can respond
- Individuals in the patient's social support system are not communicating clearly to the patient
- Individuals in the patient's social support system are not communicating in a way to which the patient can productively respond.

The Patient's Description of Her Communications

During the initial history and the construction of the Interpersonal Inventory, most patients will spontaneously provide the therapist with a great deal of information about their communication patterns. This may involve direct descriptions of communication by more insightful patients, or may come in the form of general complaints such as, 'My husband never understands me,' or 'My wife never listens to me'. Being able to draw the inferential conclusion that communication is not going well is not difficult in the latter cases, and does not require years of psychotherapy training. The IPT therapist should make lots of direct inquiries about communication throughout the therapy. These direct questions might include those listed in Box 9.1.

Box 9.1 General questions about communication

- What kinds of patterns do you see in your relationships?
- What kinds of patterns do you see in your communications with others?
- What kinds of things do you have difficulty talking to others about?
- What is it like for you to express anger or displeasure to others?
- How do you respond when others get angry with you?
- What kinds of relationships do you have trouble with?
- What do you do when you are under stress?
- How do you communicate your needs to others when under stress?
- How do you typically respond to others when they ask you for help?
- What feedback have you gotten from others about your relationships?
- How well do you think others understand you?

The patient's responses to these questions should lead the therapist to develop hypotheses about the specific communication difficulties that the patient is having. This information is particularly useful in judging a patient's insight and her ability to be empathic and to understand others' points of view. For instance, if a patient recognizes when responding to these questions that she is contributing to the communication difficulties, and if she can understand the kinds of responses that are being elicited, therapy will be much less difficult than with a patient who blames others for all of her problems.

The direct report provided by a patient is colored by a number of factors that the therapist should take into consideration. These include the patient's insight, motivation, ability to disclose personal information, and ability to be empathic. The patient's attachment style also dramatically affects her presentation. Patients who are more securely attached are more trusting early in therapy, more able to readily disclose information, and are generally more understanding of others' points of view. Conversely, those with less secure attachments have more difficulty forming an alliance, understanding their contributions to communication problems, and in receiving feedback from the therapist. In the latter cases, the pacing of IPT should be slowed to accommodate this, i.e. more sessions with more of a focus on clarification rather than on using directive techniques early in the therapy.

Another piece of information the therapist should be attentive to is the degree to which the patient generalizes descriptions of her communications. Patterns which are described in absolutes, such as 'My boss *never* recognizes my accomplishments', or 'My spouse *always* criticizes me', signify much more entrenched and less insightful ways of understanding communications and relationships. When met with such generalizations, the therapist should move to the use of Interpersonal Incidents (described below).

In general, the concept that the 'rich get richer' applies in communication analysis as in other areas of therapy. Patients with better communication skills are better able to describe the relationship problems they are having, better able to listen and to understand other's reactions to them, more insightful, and more accepting of feedback from the therapist. In contrast, those whose communication skills are poor manifest that communication style in therapy, making it more difficult for the therapist to understand the problem, to give feedback about it, and to assist the patient to develop insight. Consider the following examples from the Assessment/Initial Phase of treatment with two patients with marital conflicts.

Case example 9.1

Therapist: *Tell me how you react when others are critical of you.*

Patient: *In general, I don't like it. I tend to take criticisms very personally ... even though I know that the other person may be trying to give me some feedback I can use, I often see it as critical. And then when I feel criticized, I withdraw from the other person. I remember one time when I was getting dressed for work several days ago, and my wife said, 'That tie doesn't look quite right with that shirt.' Intellectually I knew that she was just trying to help, but it felt like she was criticizing my competence and trying to put me down. And I was mad because she was probably right about the tie, so I felt even worse.*

Therapist: *What did you do after your wife's comment about the tie?*

Patient: *I reacted like I usually do – I just kind of looked at the floor and pouted. She's got to the point that she's pretty fed up with that, so she started to leave. But as she was going downstairs, I walked into the hall after her and said, 'I know you were just trying to help, but I can't stand it when you criticize me.' We talked about it for a few minutes, but then we both had to leave for work.*

Case example 9.2

Therapist: *Tell me how you react when others are critical of you.*

Patient: *Boy, that's a good question. My wife criticizes me all the time for no reason. She has a real bad habit of losing her temper – you just can't reason with her.*

Therapist: *Tell me about a specific time when you felt she was critical of you.*

Patient: *Happens all the time ... last week, yesterday, next week for sure. Maybe you should be seeing her instead of me.*

Therapist: *What do you do when you feel she's being critical?*

Patient: *I react like anyone would – I tell her to cut it out. In a reasonable way, of course ... I don't yell and scream like she does ...*

As a means of making concepts such as insight and empathy more concrete, simply consider which of these two patients you would prefer to work with. The first recognizes his communication pattern of withdrawal under fire, has insight into his own reactions as well as his wife's motives, and even better, has already attempted to address the conflict directly with his wife. In contrast, the second patient has externalized the problem, has not recognized how he might be contributing to the communication problem and presents his wife as completely at fault, and has no motivation to change his own behavior. There is a long line of therapists waiting to work with the patient in Case example 9.1 instead of Case example 9.2.

The first patient provided a very good description of the way in which communication occurs in his relationship. The therapist can use this information directly to give feedback to the patient, and to help him modify his communication patterns. While the therapist must draw some inferences about the way in which the second patient is communicating, hypothesizing that he has difficulty communicating directly, tends to be critical, and tends to generalize, is quite reasonable and is supported by the patient's presentation.

The art of IPT is in helping the patient to gain insight into his communication, and then to make changes. This is not so difficult with patients like the first securely attached, insightful, and motivated one. But it takes a therapist who is able to modify her approach to accommodate the patient's attachment style and lack of insight, and one who is able to modify the structure of IPT, knowing that the pace will need to be slower and more time will need to be spent understanding the second patient's experience and developing a therapeutic alliance before more structured and directive interventions can be used.

The Quality of the Patient's Narrative

In addition to the information provided by the patient in response to the therapist's direct questions about communication, the quality of the patient's descriptions also reflects her communication style. The patient's ability to produce a coherent narrative, for example, is a reflection of the way she communicates outside of therapy. If the patient is unable to present a clear picture of the problem to an empathic therapist who has been *trained* to help the patient tell her story, it is certain that she has trouble when trying to communicate to others in her social environment. The therapist should attempt to answer the following questions about the patient's narrative:

- To what degree does the patient spontaneously produce narrative?
- How compelling is the narrative? In other words, how well does the patient engage the therapist in the narrative?
- How well are emotions conveyed by the patient?
- How specific is the information presented? Is it simply a generalization, or can the patient describe specific interactions?

The quality of the narrative is also important because it directly affects the patient's ability to engage others for support. A clear and compelling description of the patient's plight will tend to effectively draw in others to help; a brief and boring description will not. A good story is interesting to listen to and to relate to; a poor story is not. Consider another comparison, this time new mothers with newborns in the hospital intensive care unit (ICU).

Case example 9.3

Therapist: *What has the experience of having your baby in the hospital been like for you?*

Patient: *It's almost impossible to describe really ... I think about her all the time, even when I'm not in the room with her. To see all of the tubes coming out, and on the machine ... sometimes it seems like it's just a dream, and I'll wake up and I'll still be pregnant and deliver a healthy baby. I never thought that I could care for someone else as much as I love her. Several days ago I finally got to hold her – she's big enough now that she can come out of the incubator for a little bit, and it was like my heart just melted, like nothing else mattered. And then I had to put her back in after a few minutes ... I've missed so much, so much of having a normal baby, but I'm so blessed that she's alive; that the doctors are taking care of her ... that was probably more than you wanted to hear ...*

Therapist: *Quite the contrary – that was a beautiful story. Tell me more about the words you'd use to describe how you have been feeling.*

Case example 9.4

Therapist: *What has the experience of having your baby in the hospital been like for you?*

Patient: *It's been really hard.*

Therapist: *Tell me more.*

Patient: *I'm not sure what else to say. I worry a lot about her.*

Therapist: *Tell me about a day or two that sticks out as difficult for you. What were they like?*

Patient: *Oh, mostly all days are the same. I just hang out in her room, hold her when I'm allowed to ...*

Therapist: *What is that like when you get to hold her?*

Patient: *Pretty good; she's getting healthier I guess since they let her out.*

The therapist in Case example 9.4 has to work very hard to get information, persisting despite a desire to ask about something else, or even to do something else. This patient will have an incredibly difficult time engaging other people for support, because it is difficult for her to pull them into her experience. Her poor narrative is a hindrance to getting the support she needs.

The Patient's In-session Communication with the Therapist

The patient's communication with the therapist is another extremely important piece of information. Since the patient–therapist relationship is typically not directly addressed in IPT, this information is usually gathered by the therapist experientially rather than by direct inquiry. A slightly different way of understanding this source of information is to think of it as derived from the process which occurs during the therapy. In other words, how does the patient 'work' with the therapist, and within that framework, how does the patient specifically communicate to the therapist?

For instance, when the therapist is negotiating the Treatment Agreement or constructing the Interpersonal Inventory with the patient, how capable is she of participating in the process? Does the patient simply passively accept the therapist's suggestions, does she immediately complain that there won't be enough sessions, or is she able to productively engage in the discussion, give input, and compromise? When discussing homework, does the patient have the capacity to work productively with the therapist and to offer her own suggestions, or does she resist suggestions passively or even aggressively? All of the interactions in therapy are potential sources for this kind of information.

One of the basic tenets of IPT is that the patient behaves and communicates consistently across relationships, including the therapeutic relationship. Simply put, *people just can't help but be themselves*. Thus the information gleaned from the therapeutic relationship has direct implications about the patient's relationships outside of therapy. Questions about those outside relationships should be directly informed by the therapist's experience with the patient in session.

Reports from the Patient's Significant Others

Some of the best sources of information about the patient's communications are her significant others. While it may not always be possible, in IPT it is strongly encouraged to meet with the patient's partner or spouse during the therapy. This serves as a means of providing psychoeducational information about the treatment to the partner, serves to demystify therapy, and also helps to enlist the partner in the recovery of the patient. Most important, however, is the opportunity it gives the therapist to observe the couple's communication '*in vivo*' and to get information from an outside observer. In fact, given all of the advantages of having the patient's partner participate in therapy if the issues involve them (a Dispute or Transition involving the partner for example) there is every reason to include the partner as much as possible. That way the communication can be directly addressed with both parties present.[a]

The advantage of including a significant other can best be illustrated by noting the experience that most therapists have had when meeting the spouse of a patient two or three sessions into a course of individual therapy. The patient may have described her spouse in great detail, but when the therapist has the opportunity to meet the spouse in person, rarely does the description do justice to the reality. A patient may describe a spouse who is distant and uncaring, only to have the therapist find after meeting the spouse that he is quite reasonable and not at all like the patient's description. Conversely, a patient may describe her partner in glowing terms, with the therapist only later discovering upon meeting the spouse that the description is completely inaccurate, and that the spouse is in reality a wolf dressed in the sheep's clothing of the patient's over-idealized description.

[a] There is accumulating evidence supporting the use of IPT with couples. Approaches currently being studied include couples work in the context of perinatal depression, and partner-assisted IPT in which the partner is included as a support for the patient when they are not directly involved in the conflict. We have found a couples approach to be extremely effective – the opportunity to see and hear communication as it occurs is immensely helpful in understanding communication problems and in helping both partners to communicate more clearly and effectively.

Communication analysis is based on the premise that communication problems are directly involved in the patient's symptoms and interpersonal difficulties. However, an important caveat is that the therapist must be mindful that the individuals who are the recipients of the patient's communications almost certainly also have limitations in their own ability to communicate. If so, improvement in the patient's communication skills may still be met with rejection or misunderstanding by others.

In addition, the motivations of others with whom the patient is communicating may be very different from the patient's. For instance, a patient may be attempting to get her attachment needs met in a romantic relationship in which the other person has little or no investment. More direct communications on the part of the patient may continue to be met with responses that are negative. This being the case, it is nearly always helpful for the therapist to meet with the significant others who are involved in the patient's social support system, particularly those which are involved in marital or intimate relationships. This is even more desirable in an Interpersonal Dispute. Doing so allows the therapist to:

- Observe the communication in the relationship '*in vivo*'
- Obtain information from the significant other about his perception of the problem
- More accurately gauge the investment of the significant other in the relationship
- Provide psychoeducational information to the significant other
- 'Demystify' the therapy experience for the significant other
- Assign communication homework to the couple.

Interpersonal Incidents

As noted above, one of the explicit and overriding goals of IPT is to help patients improve their interpersonal communication. The therapeutic aim, given an individual patient's underlying attachment style, is to help the distressed patient more closely meet her attachment needs by communicating them more effectively to others. One of the specific techniques unique to IPT to help do this is to collect information about particular Interpersonal Incidents. The technique allows the therapist to more thoroughly understand the communication that is occurring, and it is also helpful in assisting the patient to begin to appreciate the ways she is not communicating effectively with others. Interpersonal Incidents are frequently used in IPT, and are often the first step in the more formal process of communication analysis.

An Interpersonal Incident is an episode in which communication occurs between the patient and a significant other. An Interpersonal Incident is a description by the patient of a *specific* interaction with her attachment figures or social contacts – it is not a description of a general pattern of interaction. For instance, if the identified dispute is a conflict between partners, the therapist might ask the patient to 'Describe the last time you and your partner got into a fight,' or to 'Describe one of the more recent big fights you had with your partner'. The therapist should direct the patient to describe in detail the communication which occurred in each of the specific incidents, taking care to re-create the dialog as accurately as possible. The patient should also be directed to describe her affective responses as well as both verbal and non-verbal responses, and to describe observations of her spouse's non-verbal behavior. The purpose of collecting and discussing an Interpersonal Incident is fivefold:

1. To collect information regarding the miscommunication that is occurring
2. To help the therapist recognize the patient's style of communication and its consequences
3. To help the patient recognize her style of communication and its consequences
4. To motivate the patient to change her communication
5. To help the patient develop new ways to communicate more effectively.

The Interpersonal Incidents process involves three steps:

1. Collecting information about a specific Interpersonal Incident
2. Analyzing the Interpersonal Incident
3. Changing communication.

Step 1: Collecting Information About a Specific Interpersonal Incident

In psychotherapy, patients will often describe interactions with significant others in very general terms, leaving the therapist with little information about the specific communication which has occurred. For instance, a patient may say that her husband 'never listens to her'. This statement strongly implies that the patient believes two things: (1) the problem is pervasive – her husband literally never listens to her, and there are no exceptions; (2) the situation is permanent and unchangeable – her husband not only doesn't listen to her now, but will continue to ignore her in the future. Given these expectations, it is no surprise that the patient feels a sense of hopelessness. If her statement and the implications are true – if in fact her husband never listens to her and never will – the only options left to the patient are to put up with the relationship and continue to suffer, or to end the relationship. No middle ground, compromise, or improvement in communication is possible.

A general statement like this should not be allowed to stand unchallenged in therapy. Irrespective of the approach taken, the therapist must work on the patient's sense of frustration and helplessness, or the relationship problem will continue, along with the psychological distress the patient is suffering. Direct, focused, and externalized attributions of problems by the patient must be challenged by the therapist.

There are several different ways of approaching a patient who makes a general statement like this. First, the therapist might choose to challenge the veracity of the patient's statement. For instance, the therapist might ask if it is really true that her husband always ignores her all of the time and under all circumstances. Exceptions would be sought – perhaps there were times in the past that were different. A cognitive therapist might challenge the distorted and absolute thinking of a patient who made a statement like this, perhaps assigning homework with the specific intent of challenging her cognition and determining whether her husband did in fact always ignore her.

In contrast to an approach which questions the accuracy of the patient's cognitions, the IPT therapist is focused on the way the patient communicates her attachment needs. Rather than addressing internal processes, the IPT therapist is concerned with examining the interpersonal communication which is occurring in the relationship. In IPT, this begins with collecting detailed dialog from a specific interaction.

The hypothesis guiding the way an Interpersonal Incident is collected and analyzed is that the 'problem' presented by the patient is the result of poor communication. Something is not going well in the communication between the patient and her husband. This does not presuppose blame; rather, it is assumed in IPT that the communication within the *system* is maladaptive. In fact, in a situation in which there is a clear-cut dispute between two individuals, it is preferable to meet with both in therapy to observe the communication '*in vivo*'. Unfortunately, it is often not possible to do so – in marital disputes one partner may not be willing to attend the sessions; in conflicts at work only one party may attend. There are a variety of situations in which only one of the people involved in the conflict is willing or able to come to therapy. The principle in IPT in such a situation is to work with the person who does come, with the hope that as that individual changes her communication, the system as a whole will change as well.

Thus the basic hypothesis with which the IPT therapist begins is that the patient (and her husband) are not communicating well and that the patient's attachment needs are not being met. (It is, of course, quite likely that her husband's interpersonal and emotional needs are not being met either.) The IPT therapist works from the position that both parties are communicating ineffectively, and that both likely have unmet needs. Both may also be assuming that their communication is being understood and that they understand the other person, when in fact this is almost certainly not the case.

A general statement such as 'My husband never listens to me' also conveys a great deal about the patient's reluctance to address her own behavior and her possible contributions to the problem. Absolute statements are at one level an attempt by the patient to influence the therapist, so that the therapist will come to share the same absolutist view as the patient – i.e. that 'blame' for the problem is external to the patient. Such a statement literally 'pulls for' a response from the therapist in which she is drawn to sympathize with the patient and to say something such as: 'If I had a husband like that, I'd feel frustrated too.' Thus the patient's statement is in part an attempt to enlist the therapist as an accomplice in blaming her husband for the problem. Consider, for example, the differences in the presentations below. In Case example 9.5, the patient makes a general statement about her husband which indicates a complete externalization of the problem – it is all her husband's fault. The first patient is literally attempting to elicit a response from the therapist which confirms her worldview and which absolves her from responsibility for change. Conversely, in Case example 9.6, the patient exhibits some insight, an openness to change, and enlists the therapist to help to create that change.

Case example 9.5: General statement

Patient: *It's all my husband's fault – he never listens to me!*

(Note that blame is placed on the husband with no acknowledgment by the patient of any responsibility for the communication problem. Insight is very limited. The therapist can respond by accepting the patient's statement as fact, by challenging it, or by asking for more information about the situation.)

Therapist: *Tell me more.*

Patient: *Well, he has a bad habit of always ignoring people, and as soon as he thinks anyone is being critical, he simply walks away. He'll never change.*

(The patient attempts to elicit a sympathetic response from the therapist, hoping to gain an accomplice in blaming her husband. An IPT therapist would move here into an Interpersonal Incident to get more information about the communication that is occurring and to begin to examine the patient's specific communication with her husband.)

Case example 9.6: Specific statement

Patient: *My husband and I have been having some problems lately in talking about things. I feel really frustrated.*

(Note the absence of absolute conditions, the framing of the problem as mutual and systemic, and the inclusion of a description of feeling state by the patient. The patient moves to enlist the therapist as an expert in helping her solve the problem.)

Therapist: *Tell me more.*

Patient: *Well, over the last several months when we try to talk about money, both of us end up getting really frustrated. He has a tendency to withdraw when he thinks that I am getting critical, but he doesn't seem to understand how worried I am about our finances right now.*

(The patient recognizes her husband's response to her communication, has some insight into her contribution to the problem, and also understands that there is a mutual communication problem. This patient will be much easier to work with because she is open to change, in stark contrast to the first patient.)

General statements such as 'My husband never listens to me', although containing a grain of truth, almost always represent only one (very biased) side of the story. What is more likely is that while the patient's husband may indeed be insensitive, some of his non-responsiveness is due to the patient's communication style. She may, though intending otherwise, come across as critical or uncaring, or may simply be trying to communicate at a time when it will not be well received. She may also be unwittingly ignoring important communications from her husband.

The general statement in Case example 9.5 does not contain any of this information. More detail must be obtained. Therefore, when eliciting Interpersonal Incidents, the therapist's task is to have the patient re-create, in as much detail as possible, a specific interaction between herself and her husband. This should not be a *typical* interaction, which will allow the patient to continue making general statements – it must be a *specific* incident. As this is not usually what patients spontaneously talk about, the therapist must direct the patient to produce this material. The goal is to use this 'step-by-step' (or perhaps better put, 'blow-by-blow') report to understand the way the patient conveys her attachment needs, acting on the hypothesis that she is communicating in such a way that she is being misunderstood and is therefore not being responded to as she would like.

Case example 9.7: Maude

Maude was a 42-year-old woman who sought treatment for a marital conflict. She had been married to her husband Harold for 11 years, and had two children aged 5 and 7 (Figures 9.1 and 9.2). She reported that things with Harold had been deteriorating over the last two years, culminating with his decision to quit his job and become a day trader in stocks. She reported that she was very concerned about their finances, and that he had not been willing to talk to her about them. By her report he got very defensive when she questioned him about their financial situation. She reported that she felt that the family was essentially living off of her salary while Harold was 'gambling' with the family's future.

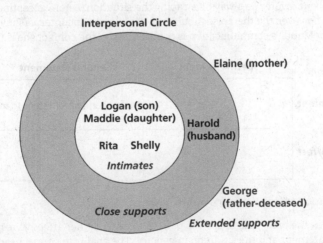

Figure 9.1 Interpersonal Circle – Maude

Early in the Middle Phase of IPT, Maude and her therapist were discussing her conflict with Harold. Her description of the conflict was a classic general statement about the relationship:

Therapist: *Tell me about your relationship with your husband.*

Maude: *He never listens to me. I am getting very worried about the finances, and he will never talk about it. He just gets defensive. To be honest, I came to therapy in part to try to decide if it would be better if the children and I left him.*

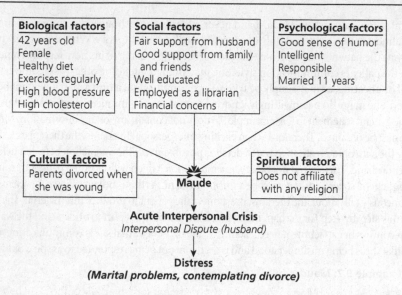

Figure 9.2 Interpersonal Formulation – Maude

A grid can be used to graphically display the process which drives the exploration of an Interpersonal Incident (Figure 9.3). The patient's communications can be divided into general statements and specific statements, and the emotional descriptions of events can also be either general or specific. The process with Maude began with her general statement about her husband: 'He never listens to me.' If this was true, and if the situation is as she describes, her concerns are quite warranted, and it is quite understandable that she would think about divorce as a way of escaping the situation. Before accepting heading in this direction, however, the therapist should move into a specific Interpersonal Incident to determine how Maude's communication is contributing to the conflict she is describing.

	Specific incident	General statement
Content		My husband never listens to me
Affect		

Figure 9.3 Interpersonal Incidents: general statement

The next step in the process is to ask the patient to describe her affective responses to the general statement and the situation in general. The goal is to connect symptoms and distress with the interpersonal problem, and to help the patient become more affectively engaged in the process – it is important because it is causing distress. In this case, Maude described feeling very hopeless, frustrated, and angry (Figure 9.4).

After obtaining information about the emotional content of the conflict and connecting it to the interpersonal problem, the therapist should specifically ask the patient to describe an Interpersonal Incident. This can be done by asking her to describe either a recent conflict, or to describe a specific incident that is a good example of the conflict problems. The patient should not, however, describe the 'typical' pattern of interaction, as this is simply reiterating the general statement of the problem. The therapist must

	Specific incident	**General statement**
Content		My husband never listens to me
Affect		I feel depressed, frustrated, angry

Figure 9.4 Interpersonal Incidents: general affect

direct the patient to present a specific interaction so that the specific communication can be examined in detail. Directives such as 'Tell me about the last time you and your husband got into conflict' or 'Tell me about one of the big conflicts you have had recently' are good ways for the therapist to do this.

Once the patient begins to describe the interaction in detail, the therapist must then direct the patient to produce, as accurately as possible, the exact dialog that occurred. In addition to the spoken communication, the patient should also be asked to describe the emotional content of the communication in detail. The task of the therapist is to get the patient to re-create, in as much detail as possible, a precise description of the interactions that occurred during the conflict. The therapist should ask not only about the verbal interactions that occurred, but also the non-verbal communications that took place, such as using silence in a hostile fashion, slamming doors, leaving the situation in the middle of an interaction, etc. This should include a detailed description of what the patient said to begin the interaction, how her husband responded, what she understood him to say, how she responded in turn, and so forth until the end of the interaction. The whole interaction. In detail. Everything that was communicated. Special note should be made of the end of the interaction, as many conflicts may carry over to the next day, or may be brought up again in subsequent disagreements. The end is also a time when one or both people may act out by leaving angrily, slamming doors, giving the silent treatment, or turning to look at an interesting app on their cell phone.

The following dialog ensued when the therapist asked about a specific interaction:

Therapist: *Tell me about the last time that you and Harold had a disagreement about the finances.*

Maude: *Oh, we fight about it all the time.*

Therapist: *It would be most helpful if you could tell me about a specific time – perhaps one that has happened recently or is clear in your mind. I'd like to know about the specific details as much as possible.*

Maude: *Well, the last time that comes to mind is a fight we had last Tuesday after dinner. We were eating late, and had put the kids to bed.*

Therapist: *What happened?*

Maude: *I asked him how his day was, and then we got into a fight.*

Therapist: *Tell me more about what exactly was said.*

Maude: *I think I said something like, 'I suppose you've been making loads of money again today.'*

Therapist: *That's the way it started?*

Maude: *Yes, and then he said, 'Don't start that up again.'*

Therapist: *What did you say next?*

Maude: *I said, 'We've got to talk about this sometime, so quit trying to avoid it.'*

Therapist: *What happened next?*

Maude: *He got up and left.*

In contrast to Maude's general statement, the additional information suggested that there was much more to the story. Asking about a specific incident allowed the therapist to more clearly examine the communication that was occurring, and to draw more accurate conclusions about what was causing the conflict and what might be done to resolve it. Maude's responses are shown graphically in Figure 9.5.

	Specific incident	General statement
Content	Tuesday evening we had a fight after dinner	My husband never listens to me
Affect		I feel depressed, frustrated, hopeless

Figure 9.5 Interpersonal Incidents: specific incident

The next step is to connect emotional responses to the specific incident. In addition to the spoken words, the emotional content of the communications should be examined. Asking questions about what kinds of emotions were conveyed, how the patient felt about specific statements, and even the way in which she perceived her husband to be responding emotionally are crucial. The following interaction occurred as the specific incident was discussed further:

Therapist: *Tell me about your emotional reactions during that specific interaction.*

Maude: *I was furious. You know, I guess I was really already mad going into the discussion – it had been building up for a long time, and I really wanted to let him know how angry I was with him.*

Therapist: *What was the tone of voice that you used when you made the statement about him making loads of money?*

Maude: *I was furious. I'm sure there was an edge to my voice, though I don't usually yell. In fact, I know that there was – I really want him to know how angry I am.*

Maude's specific affective responses are shown graphically in Figure 9.6.

	Specific incident	General statement
Content	Tuesday evening we had a fight after dinner	My husband never listens to me
Affect	I felt angry, hopeless	I feel depressed, frustrated, hopeless

Figure 9.6 Interpersonal Incidents: specific affect

The purpose in clarifying the specific communication and the affect involved is to examine the ways in which the communication is going poorly or is ineffective. This should help the therapist to draw some tentative conclusions about what is not going well, and what the patient might do differently to communicate more effectively. The next steps involve helping the patient to recognize this by reanalyzing the incident, and then brainstorming with the therapist to figure out how she can communicate more effectively.

Step 2: Analyzing the Interpersonal Incident

Step 2 in the process of communication analysis is to help the patient understand how she is communicating, and how her communication is keeping her from getting her needs met. When the therapeutic alliance is strong and the patient securely attached, the therapist may be able to give direct feedback to the patient about her ambiguous communication or suggest specific ways to improve it. In most cases, however, an intermediate step is needed.

After the dialog is clear, the patient and therapist can go through the incident once more in detail. This time, however, *the emphasis is on determining what the patient was trying to communicate*. The premise is that what was intended is not being communicated clearly. Asking the patient what she intended to communicate, and what her husband may have heard, in contrast to what was actually spoken or emoted, make the discrepancies more apparent to the patient, or at least easier for the therapist to identify to the patient.

It is at this point that the therapist should ask the patient *how well she felt understood.* Asking this simple question is literally the most important intervention in all of IPT. It is a concrete application of the basic principles of communication analysis specifically and of IPT generally, namely that the patient is not getting her attachment needs met because her communication is unclear. She is not being understood. And she is distressed and feeling alone and isolated and hopeless and depressed because she is not being understood.

Asking 'How well do you feel understood?' requires that the patient reflect upon this. Almost invariably patients in conflict will reply that they don't feel understood at all. That is the core communication and attachment issue in IPT: feeling misunderstood and alone. Asking this question serves another purpose. Since nearly all patients reply that they don't feel understood at all, the therapist can then respond by stating 'That is what we are going to work on! – helping you communicate more clearly so that you are better understood.' And that is what IPT is designed to do – help people communicate their attachment needs and needs for support more clearly, and to develop and utilize a social support system that can respond to those needs.

The patient's response to the question 'How well do you feel understood?' literally allows the therapist to get her foot in the door to influence the patient to change her communication, and to state directly that this is the goal of IPT. While it should be communicated much more artfully and gracefully, the bottom line is for the therapist to respond by telling the patient:

> Since you don't feel understood, let's do something about it. And that something is figuring out how you can communicate more effectively.

In this second step of working with an incident, the goals are to collect more information and to generate some insight and motivation on the part of the patient. The idea is to move the patient from a feeling of anger, sadness, or hopelessness to a feeling of being *misunderstood*. This allows the therapist and patient to reframe the situation as one that she can do something about – if her communication is being misunderstood, then a change in communication may help resolve the problem. In addition, the therapist can often (if the alliance and patient's attachment style can tolerate it) ask questions about how well the patient understands the other person's point of view or feelings about the interaction. Most patients who are honest and non-defensive will confess that they really don't know or understand what the other person is thinking and feeling. Again, this leads to an opportunity for the therapist to highlight that the communication within the dyad is unclear or ambiguous, and that the patient may want to find out from her partner what he is thinking and feeling.

To clarify Maude's intent and help her understand the lack of clarity in her communication, the therapist returned to the specific dialog and asked questions about what

Maude intended to communicate, and how well she felt understood. He also asked questions about how well Maude understood Harold's reactions and motivations, which were designed to help Maude reframe the situation as a problem within the relationship rather than externalizing it entirely to Harold. The therapist's hope was that as Maude realized she didn't understand his position well, or if she at least became motivated to find out more about how he was reacting, the communication would be improved.

The therapeutic interaction continued:

Therapist: *I'd like to go back through the interaction you described if we might. What I'm interested in is understanding more about what you were trying to communicate to Harold. When you started the conversation with him – made the comment about him making 'loads of money' – what were you trying to get him to understand?*

Maude: *That's easy. I was trying to convey that I wanted to talk to him about our money situation. I'm worried, and it feels like he is taking risks with our future.*

Therapist: How well do you feel that he understood what you wanted in that moment?

Maude: *[pausing for a moment] I guess not at all. I don't think that he really understands my point of view at all. If he did, he would take it seriously – he'd listen and stop gambling with our money.*

Therapist: *It sounds like he didn't understand your point of view well at all. That's what I think we can work on: helping you to communicate more effectively so that he can understand better what it is you want and need from him.*

Maude: *That would be nice, but I'm not sure he's capable.*

Therapist: *[consciously deciding to stay on task with the incident] You mentioned that he got up and left after you started the conversation. What do you think he was trying to communicate to you?*

Maude: *[pausing again] You know, I'm not sure. I hadn't really thought about it that way. I just assumed he was refusing to change, and that he wasn't interested in listening. But I don't really know what he was trying to communicate.*

Therapist: *How well do you think you understand his point of view, and what he is trying to communicate to you?*

Maude: *[longest pause yet] I don't know. I guess not very well. I'm not sure what he's thinking ... he's not the best communicator you know ...*

Therapist: *It sounds like both of you had pretty strong feelings, including feelings of being misunderstood. I suspect that neither of you really got across what you were intending. You told me that you were trying to let Harold know how angry you were – to talk about the finances – but I wonder if he really understood that. His reaction – walking away I mean – would sure suggest that he didn't understand what you wanted. That's what I'd like to focus on: figuring out ways you can communicate more effectively, so that the two of you can begin to bridge that misunderstanding gap and begin to come to an agreement about what to do.*

Maude's responses are shown graphically in Figure 9.7.

Step 3: Changing Communication

At this point, the therapist elected to move on to changing communication. This is simply working with the patient to find better ways of communicating by brainstorming and coming up with a reasonable and feasible way of communicating differently. More of the same communication will get the same results: the patient has to try something different. A great

	Specific incident	**General statement**
Content	Tuesday evening we had a fight after dinner	My husband never listens to me
Affect	I felt misunderstood	I feel depressed, frustrated, hopeless

Figure 9.7 Interpersonal Incidents: identifying misunderstandings

analogy to use is to suggest to the patient that the conflict has arisen and been perpetuated in part because the communication is not going well. It's as if she's speaking German and her husband French. Yelling louder in German is not going to solve the problem; the couple has to develop a common language – a common understanding – to make any progress.

Maude seemed to appreciate that her communication wasn't getting her what she wanted, and was also beginning to realize that her husband was communicating something too, although it wasn't entirely clear to her what that was. Changing communication was focused on two issues: first, to assist Maude to find some different ways to talk about her concerns so that she could get a response from Harold closer to what she wanted; and second, to motivate her to collect more information about what Harold was trying to communicate.

Therapist: *Let's do some brainstorming about how you might communicate more clearly so that Harold can better understand what you are intending to communicate to him.*

Maude: *Well, I suppose I could ask him directly to spend some time talking – the last several months I've been so angry I've just made snide remarks to get his attention. Still, it's such a hot topic for us that I don't know if that will work.*

Therapist: *It may not work, but the results probably won't be any worse than what is happening now.*

Maude: *That's certainly true – we don't seem to be getting anywhere now.*

Therapist: *How could you find out more about what he is really feeling?*

Maude: *I guess I'll just have to ask him.*

Therapist: *When would be a good time to ask him about it, and to have the conversation?*

Maude: *Tuesday evenings are the best – we have dinner late, and the kids are in bed – I hope we haven't set a precedent with our last fight!*

Therapist: *Tuesday it is then. You'll have to let me know next week how it went.*

Maude: *I'm a bit more optimistic now – he's not such a bad guy, you know.*

At the end of the discussion of the Interpersonal Incident, Maude had a different picture of the interaction between herself and her husband. Rather than viewing the problem as intractable, Maude now saw some hope that things could be different. By changing her communication, it was possible that she could get her needs met more effectively. Further, it was possible that her husband would do likewise in response if she were able to take an interest in what he was feeling and thinking instead of being critical. Finally, Maude and the therapist developed a plan of action designed to specifically address the problem, also giving her a sense of hope that things would improve.

The interaction can be depicted graphically – Maude's general statement began with an absolute assertion that her husband never listened to her. The associated affect was that she felt depressed, frustrated, and hopeless. When discussing the specific Interpersonal Incident, she initially described feeling angry and hopeless. As the interaction was discussed in detail, her views changed as she began to see that she was not being understood, and that she didn't really have a good idea about her husband's perspective either. She also began to realize (or at least a seed was planted) that she could change her communication and perhaps bring about different results. Her affect shifted to more of a feeling of hopefulness, and the hope that she felt about the specific interaction was then generalized, so that the absolute statement, 'He never listens to me' was transformed into a qualified 'He doesn't listen to me when I approach him critically'. Maude's more insightful concluding statements (Figure 9.8) contrast sharply with her initial general statement (Figure 9.3).

	Specific incident	General statement
Content	Tuesday evening we had a fight after dinner because I started the conversation being critical	My husband doesn't listen to me if I am critical of him
Affect	I felt misunderstood	I feel HOPEFUL that things can change

Figure 9.8 Interpersonal Incidents: affective shift

Maude attempted some of the communication changes that she and her therapist discussed over the next week. Though she and Harold continued to have some conflict, she felt that the continued refinement of her communication was quite helpful. Maude and her therapist continued to review additional Interpersonal Incidents to explore what was working, and what was not working, in the couple's communication. After 8 sessions, Harold, recognizing the changes that were occurring with Maude, relented and came in for several sessions. He also reported that he felt the marriage had improved.

Working with Interpersonal Incidents is an extremely useful specific form of communication analysis. It is a formal means of investigating the hypothesis that the patient's difficulties are being caused, perpetuated, or exacerbated by poor communication. The technique of examining Interpersonal Incidents expands upon this concept by focusing on specific key interactions. It is particularly useful when dealing with Interpersonal Disputes, and in helping patients with less secure attachments understand how their style of communication may be contributing to their relationship problems.

The Process of Communication Analysis

To reiterate, there are five potential sources of information for communication analysis:

1. The patient's description of her communications, both generally and specifically
2. The quality of the patient's narrative
3. The patient's in-session communication with the therapist
4. Reports from or interactions with the patient's significant others
5. Interpersonal Incidents.

Irrespective of the source of the communication samples, the general process of communication analysis is quite simple technically: *It is nothing more than developing a hypothesis about what is causing the patient's communication difficulties, and reflecting that hypothesis back to the patient in a way in which she can respond to the feedback and use it to make changes.* However, while the technical aspects are straightforward, the art of giving useful feedback is much more complicated, as the therapist must be able to modify her style to account for the idiosyncrasies of the individual patient.

The feedback to be given is simply a synthesis of all of the information gathered from the patient about her communications, applied to a specific situation. Data from the patient's direct report of communications, the therapist's impressions of the patient's narrative, the therapeutic alliance, information from others if available, and from Interpersonal Incidents should all be included. These should all be integrated and summarized for the patient, presented in the context of a specific interpersonal relationship. For instance, with Maude, the therapist might comment on the marital dispute as follows.

Therapist: *Based on what you have told me about your relationship with Harold, it appears to me that he doesn't understand why you are so upset. And it sounds like you really don't understand his position well either – the miscommunication is going in both directions. My impression is that when you try to talk to him, your anger leads you to start the conversation by making indirect criticisms of him, and then he just disengages or leaves. Both of you end up feeling even more angry and misunderstood. I don't think that way of communicating your anger to him is going to work well. I think it would be helpful to think about different ways of starting the conversation and being more direct about how you feel and what you want. What are your thoughts about that?*

Rather than viewing the hypotheses regarding the patient's communication difficulties as set in stone, the therapist should always see them as works in progress that take into account additional information as it is developed. IPT continually revolves around the gathering of more and more detailed information about relationships and communications; thus the hypotheses that are developed by the therapist should be under constant revision, and always open to input from the patient.

Further, the presentation of the formulation of the patient's communication difficulties is not a one-off occurrence. It is a continuing process in which a tentative hypothesis is offered, the patient responds to it, and more information is collected. This forms the basis for yet another, more precise hypothesis, which is then discussed again. Wrapped into this process are discussions about how the patient's communication could be modified and the problem resolved.[b]

Giving Feedback to the Patient

Once the therapist has gathered information from some or all of the sources noted above, and has developed a preliminary hypothesis about the patient's specific communication difficulties, the interactive process of giving feedback to the patient should begin. The most crucial aspect of this process is the therapeutic alliance. In Kiesler's terms,[1] the patient–therapist relationship must have a high degree of *inclusion* in order for the therapist's feedback to the patient to make a difference. In simple terms, the therapeutic relationship has to be important to both patient and therapist. The patient must attach importance to the therapist's

---

[b] This, among many other instances in IPT described in this text, is a superlative example of the way in which psychotherapy is a science. That the data are based on single case examples rather than randomized controlled trials makes it no less valid, and in contrast to the conclusions drawn from groups of patients in controlled trials, the hypotheses the therapist tests with her patient and the data she gathers has immediate relevance to the work with that patient. Thus our conviction that the clinical judgment and experience of IPT scientist-practitioners is at least as valuable and valid as any conclusions drawn from randomized trials.

feedback – it has to have an impact on the patient. If the relationship is tenuous, or if the feedback is given prematurely, the therapist's comments to the patient will be easily dismissed.

The ideal outcome of the feedback process is that the patient responds to the therapist's feedback by literally replying, 'You really think so?' The emphasis is on the 'you' – the therapist – who is valued and whose opinion has meaning for the patient. The degree of importance, respect, and expertise that the patient attributes to the therapist – i.e. the quality of the therapeutic relationship – will be the primary factor which determines how the feedback is received. The therapist should establish this kind of relationship with the patient by conveying warmth, empathy, genuineness, and unconditional positive regard[2] – all of the factors which, though not sufficient for change in IPT, are necessary for change in IPT.[c]

As in all aspects of IPT, the therapist must modify her style to accommodate the attachment style of the patient. More securely attached patients are able to tolerate more direct feedback, and their security allows them to tolerate it earlier in therapy. In contrast, those patients with preoccupied attachment styles should be encouraged to develop their own ideas about their communication problems rather than having the therapist give them a lot of direct feedback. They need to take ownership in order for the changes to occur. Less directive interventions are usually warranted with them so that passivity or dependency does not become a major issue. Those patients who are more dismissive or fearful in attachment style require more time to develop a strong therapeutic alliance, so feedback should be delayed until the alliance allows them to tolerate it. They too should be encouraged to develop their own ideas, with the therapist encouraging the fearful patients and complimenting the dismissive ones in order to facilitate the process even more.

An important part of giving feedback to the patient is soliciting her verbal responses to the therapist's hypotheses. This means that the conceptualization developed by the therapist is not a definitive 'interpretation' of the patient's problems, in which the therapist provides the patient with the 'correct' understanding which she must accept in order to gain insight. Instead, the therapist should literally offer her conceptualizations as hypotheses – concepts that offer a reasonable explanation but which are open to further investigation and exploration. The therapist should frame feedback to the patient in a way which reflects this. Statements such as 'The information you've given me about your relationships seems to suggest ...' or 'I wonder if you are having problems with ...' should be used, rather than more definitive statements. And each should be followed by an invitation to the patient to respond: 'What are your reactions to this?'

The more ownership the patient has of the conceptualization of the problem the better. Thus patients should be asked to develop their own ideas about their communication problems. Questions such as, 'What do you think are the major patterns in your communications?' or 'How do you see all of these things coming together?' may be very helpful. Input from the patient should be encouraged as much as possible.

In IPT, communication analysis does not necessarily require an understanding of the psychological or historical factors involved in the communication problem. While it is of great benefit if the patient appreciates the historical precedents to the problem, it is not necessary. *What is required in IPT is that the patient recognizes her current communication patterns, appreciates the kinds of responses that she elicits from others, and that she makes changes in her communication to resolve the problem.*

---

[c] 'You really think so?' really is the best response, because it indicates that the patient is engaged in the process and thinking about the feedback. If your patient responds to you by saying 'You know, you're absolutely right', you should forgo the narcissistic gratification and run for the hills.

The implications of this statement are profound. What this means is that even though patients who are less insightful, less motivated, and less securely attached are more difficult to work with in therapy, they are still amenable to treatment because the IPT approach does not require deep psychological insight. It simply requires that the patient recognize that there is a communication problem and that by changing her communication, it can be improved or resolved. In fact, it is even possible that the patient can still see the problem as being external to herself (i.e. the fault of another person) but can recognize that changing her communications will cause others to respond differently and will improve the situation. Even very insecurely attached or difficult patients can come to this realization.

This is not to say that insight and intrapsychic change should not be encouraged in IPT – it is always better that these happen than not. However, IPT can be used with patients who appear to lack the capacity for insight, who are not psychologically minded, or who for other reasons are poor candidates for more insight-oriented therapies. Perhaps the best example of this is the work in IPT that can be done with patients with somatization disorders.[3-5] In general, such patients are very poor candidates for therapy because they have maladaptive attachment styles, very poor insight, a distrust of the medical system, and are poorly motivated. Moreover, they are often hostile towards caregivers, and most importantly, are quite fixed in their beliefs that their problems are physical rather than psychological. They are, to state the obvious, not optimal candidates for psychotherapy.

Nonetheless, even if such patients continue to blame their problems on a medical care system that doesn't respond to their needs, they can often come to recognize that changing their communications leads to better provision of medical care. The goal in IPT is to help such patients to recognize that changing their communications will result in more effective responses to their attachment needs. For instance, a patient who frequently visits the emergency room for physical complaints may come to realize in IPT that this is not an effective way to get her physical problems addressed. Emergency rooms are very busy, so the patient will have to wait; she is likely to see a different physician at every visit, and is clearly not going to get the personal attention that she desires. Scheduling regular appointments with a family physician who knows her well and is able to give more personal attention is likely to get her attachment needs met more effectively.

Somatizing patients may not develop any understanding of the dynamic processes that drive their care-seeking behavior. They may continue to externalize the problem, blaming the medical system or even individual emergency physicians who 'don't give patients the time they deserve'. But most will grudgingly agree that they are more satisfied seeing a doctor who knows them well rather than sitting for hours in an emergency room. They are able to recognize that changing their communication results in better care.

Case example 9.8: Fred

Fred was a 32-year-old man who sought treatment for complaints of marital dissatisfaction. He described that frequent fights with his wife Sandra were causing him to have trouble sleeping, were making him more irritable, and were also affecting his work. He stated that he was 'fed up', and was particularly upset about the fact that Sandra had not been willing to go to therapy with him. He reported no previous history of psychological treatment, and denied any problems with substance abuse.

In the first session and then again during the construction of the Interpersonal Inventory (Figure 9.9), Fred described that his attempts to be more intimate with his wife had all been met with rejection. He reported that she, 'never wants to talk, and consistently rejects any attempts I make to be affectionate.' He felt that the relationship was coming to an end, but was willing to give it one last try.

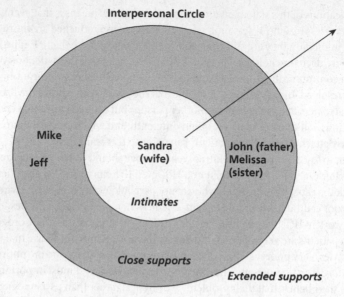

Figure 9.9 Interpersonal Circle – Fred

After identifying the conflict with his wife as a focal point in the Interpersonal Formulation (Figure 9.10), the therapist asked Fred in session 3 to describe his relationship with his wife in detail.

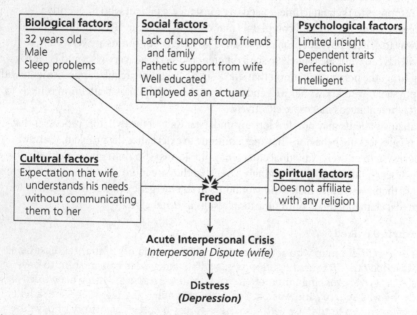

Figure 9.10 Interpersonal Formulation – Fred

Therapist: *Fred, tell me more about your wife in detail.*

Fred: *Well, when I first met her, I thought she was the greatest thing since sliced bread. We had a really close relationship. Over the last several years, things have gotten really bad. I don't think she really cares about me anymore.*

Therapist: *What kinds of patterns do you see in your relationship with her?*

Fred: *Patterns? I hadn't really thought about that … I guess the main one I would say is that I don't get enough affection from her. Yeah, that's pretty consistent.*

Therapist: *What about patterns in the way you communicate with her?*

Fred: *She thinks that I am too demanding – I don't agree though – but it's been a consistent complaint of hers. She grew up in a home where there was hardly any physical affection, and I think that has affected her a lot.*

Therapist: *How do you ask her for affection or let her know that you want to be closer?*

Fred: *Usually I feel much closer to her when we are, you know, when we get together – you know, sleep together.*

Therapist: *It sounds like your sexual relationship is very important to you.*

Fred: *That's right! And she hasn't been willing to do anything at all recently – she says that she doesn't feel close to me and won't even consider sex.*

Therapist: *How have you responded to that?*

Fred: *I figure that if she really cared about me, she'd know how important the sexual part of our relationship is. After all, as long as we've been married, she ought to know me by now.*

Therapist: *So how do you tell her that you are upset about it?*

Fred: *I tell her that if she really loved me she'd take better care of me and pay attention to what I need.*

Therapist: *How is that said exactly – I mean, tone of voice for instance.*

Fred: *I just say it to her in a very matter of fact way – I hardly ever get angry – so she should certainly be aware of how I feel. It would sure be helpful if you could see her so that you could talk some sense into her!*

The therapist was able to draw several tentative conclusions from this interaction and other information provided by Fred. The direct report that Fred gave indicated that communication was occurring, but it appeared that Fred was making several assumptions about what his wife understood. He was assuming that she should understand his needs without communicating them when he stated that 'She should know how important the sexual part of our relationship is.' He also assumed that she would behave in a particular way 'if she loved me'. Assumptions that one's partner should literally be able to 'mind-read' and respond appropriately are quite common in disputes between intimate partners.

The narrative that Fred produced was fairly coherent, but notable for what appeared to be a dichotomous presentation of his wife. His description of her when they met was glowing, but he described their current relationship in very negative terms. There did not appear to be any balance in Fred's description of her. A two-dimensional picture was emerging, with Fred's wife being either idealized or devalued. Further, his entire narrative was framed by his complaints that his wife was not caring for him. Rather than a dispute over a particular issue, Fred's problems seemed to be related to a general or diffuse sense that his needs were not getting met.

Fred's insight appeared to be quite limited as well. He made clear that his wife was to blame for his problems, and he presented his own communications in the best possible light: 'I just say it to her in a very matter of fact way – I hardly ever get angry – so she should certainly be aware of how I feel.' Based on the other parts of Fred's history, the therapist strongly suspected that this was not the case, and that Fred's communications to his wife were neither clear nor presented in a 'matter of fact' way. More likely there was a lot of emotion being communicated by both Fred and his wife. However, Fred did appear to have the potential for insight. His response to the therapist's question about patterns in his relationship was met positively, and seemed to get him thinking. The therapist was encouraged that this might be a fruitful area in which to continue.

Fred's in-session communication to the therapist, and the way in which he was forming a therapeutic relationship, was also informative. Although there were few overt signs of dependency, the therapist did note Fred's statement that, 'It would sure be helpful if you [the therapist] could see her so that you could talk some sense into her!' This struck the therapist as more information supporting the hypothesis that Fred had some dependent personality traits as well as some preoccupied attachment traits, and that these were being manifest in his attempts to get his wife (and the therapist) to 'care for him'.

When evaluating the ways feedback might most effectively be given to Fred, the therapist considered three options. First, he could give Fred direct feedback. This might be in the following form:

> It sounds from what you have told me that you and your wife are clearly having some trouble communicating, and that you don't feel that she is responding to you the way you would like. I wonder if some of the things you feel that you are communicating clearly might not be quite so clear to her. For instance, you seem to be assuming that she will know what you want, both in terms of emotional closeness and sexual response, but it doesn't sound as if that has been communicated to her clearly. She may be operating under a completely different set of assumptions than you have been. What are your thoughts about that?

This option is completely consistent with the spirit of IPT, and might be quite reasonable for a patient who was relatively securely attached, and who had already developed a solid alliance with the therapist. Both would be required for the patient to be able to tolerate this kind of direct feedback. If the patient were able to use it productively, it would be the most expedient and helpful way to work on the problem. In Fred's case, however, the therapist judged that Fred was neither able to tolerate such feedback at this point in therapy, nor would he be able to use it – he would likely experience it as critical and as a lack of empathy by the therapist.

Option number two, also consistent with the spirit of IPT, was to gently persist with similar questions about Fred's interactions with his wife, with the goal of helping him to appreciate how his communication style and expectations of his wife were leading to problems. The therapist would begin to move to questions that pushed Fred to think about things in more depth, and which would (hopefully) stimulate some insight. This might be in the following form:

> Fred, it is clear that you don't feel that your needs are being met by your wife, and that you have been trying to communicate this to her, but she doesn't seem to respond to you like you would like her too. I would like to try to understand better how this happens, and to figure out why this seems to keep happening. What are your thoughts about why the two of you aren't connecting on this?

Such an approach would likely be much more tolerable to Fred, as the therapist would carefully convey empathy rather than 'blame' Fred for the communication problems. Asking for Fred to take the lead, rather than giving him direct feedback to which he could respond, would also be more tolerable given his insecure attachment style. This process, however, would require much slower pacing than the direct feedback approach.

The therapist would also need to be particularly careful to word his statements as attempts to understand Fred. That frame – trying to understand the patient better – has to be genuine and real. Genuineness cannot be faked, and insecurely attached patients are experts at picking up insincerity. Virtuoso IPT therapists really do want to understand their patients better. It is no act. It is sincere, and requires being present with patients and listening well.

Option three, also consistent with IPT, was to have Fred invite his wife to therapy for a session. This is the course the therapist elected to follow. Despite Fred's initial protests to the contrary, when he directly asked his wife she came quite willingly to therapy. The therapist used this opportunity to collect information from her about Fred's style of communication, and to observe their communication directly. It quickly became clear that Fred's wife was invested in the relationship, but was beginning to get fed up with what she perceived to be his unreasonable demands. She felt that he was not at all clear about what he wanted, and tended to pout when he didn't get his way. The interaction in the session went as follows:

Therapist: *Thanks for coming in today.*

Sandra: *You're welcome. I told Fred that I'd be glad to come in for therapy – I even suggested that we see someone together, but he said he didn't want to do that.*

Fred: *I did not – I said that I wanted to work on my problems, but I never said that you couldn't come!*

Sandra: *Well, that's not what I remember.*

Therapist: *At any rate, now that you're here, I would like to do two things. First, I would like to get some feedback from you, Sandra, about your perception of the communication that's occurring between you and Fred. Second, it sounds like we need to do some planning about how to proceed with therapy after this session.*

Sandra: *My perception is that Fred and I have had a pretty good relationship for the most part, but that recently it has gotten worse. I can even put my finger on when I think that things started to go badly. I had a miscarriage about 6 months ago, and we haven't really been close since then. Fred just kind of stopped talking after that. I'm not even sure that he knows how I feel about it – he sure hasn't asked.*

Fred (to the therapist): *Oh, I forgot to tell you about that – that was really difficult for both of us.*

Therapist: *That does sound like a pretty important piece of information. What was that experience like for both of you?*

Both Fred and Sandra began to share their experiences with the therapist, and in the process of doing so, began to feel that they were finally in a situation where their partner had to listen. At the end of the session, the therapist raised the possibility that he could meet with Fred and Sandra for two or three more sessions before returning to individual work with Fred. Both agreed to this, and time was spent both on the grief issues surrounding the miscarriage as well as the communication difficulties the couple were having. Fred continued in individual therapy for several sessions thereafter, and at the conclusion of treatment felt that the conflict was largely resolved. He was also able to appreciate that he needed to be more active and clear in communicating with Sandra in the future.

In sum, the case is an illustration of the value in obtaining information about communication from a variety of sources. It also illustrates the classic IPT paradigm in which an acute psychosocial stressor leads to interpersonal problems in a vulnerable individual. In this case, Fred's insecure attachment traits and communication style led him, in the context of the acute stressor of the miscarriage, to express his needs for connection and support in a way that led to conflict in his marriage.

Conclusion

Communication analysis is an extremely important part of IPT because it is aimed directly at one of the root causes of a patient's distress – namely that her attachment needs are not being met sufficiently. Helping the patient to recognize patterns in communication and understand the ways her communication is not effective, and then helping her to change her communication is the essence of the technique.

References

1. Kiesler DJ and Watkins LM. Interpersonal complimentarity and the therapeutic alliance: a study of the relationship in psychotherapy. *Psychotherapy*, 1989, **26**: 183–194.

2. Rogers CR and Truaz CB. The therapeutic conditions antecedent to change: a theoretical view, in Rogers CR (ed.) *The Therapeutic Relationship and its Impact*. 1967, Madison: University of Wisconsin Press.

3. Stuart S and Noyes R Jr. Treating hypochondriasis with interpersonal psychotherapy. *Journal of Contemporary Psychotherapy*, 2005, **35**: 269–283.

4. Stuart S and Noyes R Jr. Interpersonal psychotherapy for somatizing patients. *Psychotherapy and Psychosomatics*, 2006, **75**: 209–219.

5. Stuart S, *et al.* An integrative approach to somatoform disorders combining interpersonal and cognitive-behavioral theory and techniques. *Journal of Contemporary Psychotherapy*, 2008, **38**: 45–53.

10

Problem Solving

Introduction

Problem solving is a fundamental intervention in IPT, and is a primary method for helping patients to bring about change in their interpersonal relationships. It is often utilized at the end of communication analysis, and is a way of helping the patient find ways to communicate differently, or to develop new social support. Problem solving is of help with all of the Problem Areas, but is particularly useful in dealing with Disputes and Role Transitions.

Problem solving, absent the technical jargon, is a directive technique in which the therapist attempts to help the patient develop solutions to a specific interpersonal problem and to implement the best of those solutions. It involves developing an accurate understanding of the problem, brainstorming with the patient to develop possible solutions, and motivating him to implement the solution that seems to be best suited to the situation. Between sessions the patient attempts to carry out the solution, and reports back to the therapist at the next session with the results of that trial.[a] The results are discussed in therapy, and if needed, modifications are made or new ideas are discussed.

Though the primary goal of problem solving is to relieve the patient's immediate stressors, a desirable side-effect is to teach the patient to apply problem solving techniques to other interpersonal situations that he might face. The old adage 'Give a man a fish and feed him for a day; teach a man to fish and feed him for a lifetime' is a wonderful analogy for problem solving in IPT. The idea is both to help solve the immediate problem and to teach the patient the process of problem solving so that he is better equipped to deal with future interpersonal problems (Figure 10.1).

The patient and therapist clarify a particular interpersonal problem. The patient then brainstorms with the therapist to generate solutions to the problem (1), attempts to implement one of them (2), and additional modifications are made if needed in the next session (3). The feedback process may lead to new problems which can be clarified, another round of brainstorming solutions (4), or to modifications of the solution that was implemented. This process enables the patient to develop a greater sense of mastery over interpersonal problems.

---

[a] This is, of course, an ideal situation; the use of homework and various directives as a means of influence and encouraging the patient to follow through with the proposed changes is the subject of subsequent chapters.

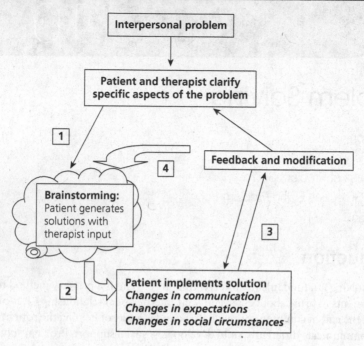

Figure 10.1 An overview of problem solving in IPT

An Overview of Problem Solving

Problem solving has five basic components:

1 Detailed examination of the problem
2 Generating (brainstorming) potential solutions
3 Selecting a course of action
4 Monitoring and refining the solution
5 Practicing

Detailed Examination of the Problem

The examination of the specific interpersonal problem should include all relevant historical aspects as well as the patient's attempts to resolve it. Approaches he has taken to similar problems in the past, successful or otherwise, should be explored. Throughout the process, the problem should be linked to the patient's symptoms and distress. The therapist should also help the patient to define the problem as specifically as possible. Attempting to address a general complaint that 'My marital relationship is going badly' is extremely difficult, as opposed to addressing a specific problem such as 'My spouse and I are having trouble talking about our finances'. The more specific the problem, the easier it is to address. It is the therapist's task while problem solving to help the patient break the problems down into manageable pieces. Consider the following situation in which the therapist is actively trying to narrow the focus of a marital dispute:

Patient: *My husband never seems to want to spend time with me – he's not interested at all in my day or what's happening with me.*

Therapist: *Sounds like the two of you don't talk much.*

Patient: *My whole life and schedule is totally messed up – he doesn't understand at all.*

Therapist: *I can imagine how difficult it must be to juggle all the responsibilities you have. Going back to the dispute with your husband, can you tell me how you have tried to approach your communication problem with your husband thus far?*

Patient: *Well, I have told him his work has to come second to his marriage!*

Therapist: *How has that worked thus far?*

Patient: *Not well – he just gets defensive.*

Therapist: *I think that if we concentrate on a specific communication problem the two of you are having the problem might be easier to address, and may also go a long way towards resolving the dispute with your husband. What seems to be the primary issue that leads the two of you to get into conflicts?*

Generating (Brainstorming) Potential Solutions

Solutions to interpersonal problems should be based on the patient's own ideas as far as possible, and the ownership of the process should remain with the patient. The therapist should try, wherever possible, to have the patient generate the ideas to be discussed, as the aim of the intervention is not merely to resolve the acute crisis, but also to help the patient develop problem solving skills.

Brainstorming solutions to interpersonal problems is basically a technique within the general rubric of problem solving. The patient should be encouraged to develop any and all ideas, even ones that at first may seem impractical. The goal at this stage is to develop a list of alternative solutions from which he can choose the one most likely to be effective. During this process, the therapist can also introduce new solutions to the patient without directly telling him what to do. For instance, the therapist may (maintaining confidentiality) share possible solutions developed by other patients with similar problems. The therapist could, if therapeutic judgment suggests it would be helpful, also offer suggestions which are framed as questions. Questions such as 'Have you considered...?' or, 'I wonder if this approach might be helpful?' are less direct than giving advice, or than statements that tell the patient what course to follow. Introducing suggestions at this point also allows the patient to consider them as one of many options, and allows the patient to retain a sense of autonomy when choosing the option he wishes to follow.

Selecting a Course of Action

The bottom line in IPT is that the patient must take action to resolve his interpersonal problems. This may take many forms – often a change in communication or an extension of social support – but action must occur. The process at this point involves evaluating the relative 'pros and cons' of the potential solutions, and then deciding upon a course of action. Unless there is a direct threat to the patient's well-being, it is nearly always best to encourage the patient to make an autonomous decision about which course to follow.

If it suits the individual patient, the discussion can be summarized in written form. Doing so may, with some patients, provide further impetus to complete the task. In some cases the therapist could even give the paper to the patient as a homework assignment.

Monitoring and Refining the Solution

At the beginning of the session after a solution is chosen and a course of action is agreed upon, the therapist should always ask the patient about the implementation of the solution. This reinforces the therapist's expectation that the patient will work on the problem between sessions, and that implementation of the specific solution is expected as well. This also implies to the patient that he has the capacity to make changes and to resolve his problems.

The patient should report back to the therapist with information about how he implemented the proposed solution. The patient may have enjoyed some degree of success, or he may have encountered some difficulties or unforeseen contingencies. The therapist should direct the patient to 'walk the therapist through' the application of the proposed solution, including the details of conversations and interpersonal interactions. Specific Interpersonal Incidents in which the patient has attempted to implement the solution are helpful to discuss. Throughout the entire process the therapist should positively reinforce the patient's attempts to implement solutions, emphasizing his strengths and minimizing or 'shoring up' the patient's relative weaknesses. For example, the therapist might start a subsequent session as follows.

Therapist: *Last week we developed a plan that you would talk to your wife about your desire to change jobs. How did it go?*

Patient: *Not too bad, but not so well either, I guess.*

Therapist: *I'd like to hear about all of it – can you walk me through the process from start to finish.*

Patient: *What, the whole thing?*

Therapist: *[directing the patient towards an Interpersonal Incident] Sure, the whole thing, step by step, from beginning to end. It would be good to start with how you brought the subject up with her.*

The Process of Problem Solving

The Spectrum of Interventions

There is a continuum of specific interventions that fall within the scope of problem solving. The spectrum extends from more directive interventions, such as the therapist offering direct advice, to interventions which encourage the patient to be autonomous in both developing and choosing the solutions to be implemented. Determining which level of intervention to use depends on a number of factors, including the point in time in the therapy, the patient's attachment style, the patient's ability to realistically develop solutions, and the degree the patient can tolerate directives from the therapist.

As with all therapeutic interventions, the therapist should be guided by the patient's attachment style when engaging in problem solving. When working with patients with more secure and flexible attachment styles, the therapist is likely to be able to operate along the entire range of the spectrum. A more securely attached patient is usually better able to use suggestions and directives from the therapist than a less securely attached individual, and ironically is also more likely to be able to function more independently and to more effectively generate his own solutions. As is the case with other techniques, security of attachment is a clear prognostic indicator.

Patients with less secure attachment styles often may have more difficulty with therapist directives that may be seen as non-empathic or authoritarian. A patient who has traits of preoccupied attachment may develop an excessive dependency or a passive hostility if a therapist is overly directive, and may not complete homework or initiate change as a result. The therapist should be mindful of the possibility of generating problematic transferential reactions if he uses explicitly directive interventions uninformed by clinical judgment. When working with less securely attached individuals, the therapist is usually best advised to use interventions which encourage the patient to be autonomous, doing so by providing lots of positive reinforcement and encouragement without offering direct advice.

The use of more directive problem solving interventions also raises the risk that the therapist's own personal feelings or judgments will unduly influence the patient's choices. This is a threat particularly when the patient's problem resonates with the therapist's own life experience and the therapist offers directives that are based on this, rather than attending to the patient's unique situation. As in any kind of therapy, the therapist is well-advised to be very aware of his personal reactions to the patient and the patient's story.

Developing New Solutions

Solutions to problems can be developed using many specific interventions. Various interventions which range from more directive to autonomous include:

- Therapist direct advice
- Therapist-directed brainstorm
- Therapist self-disclosure
- Patient-initiated brainstorm
- Drawing on the patient's past experiences.

Therapist direct advice

The therapist may choose to be explicitly instructive with some patients. Being more directive usually works best with more securely attached patients who are able to tolerate and use direct advice, but is sometimes necessary with patients who are simply unable to generate any solutions to their problems. The therapist should always be aware, however, that a patient who claims to be unable to generate any ideas may be setting a trap for the therapist similar to those that he has laid for unsuspecting significant others in his social relationships. Pushing the therapist to generate the 'answer' to the problem may allow the patient to be passive and may foster more dependency.

Some patients, however, because of state dependent factors such as a severe depression, are temporarily unable to generate enough momentum to brainstorm with the therapist. If this is the case, particularly early in therapy, the therapist may want to offer more behaviorally oriented suggestions or directives to the patient. This is completely compatible with IPT, and is reflected in a much greater emphasis on behavioral interventions and activity scheduling (activities with other people or in a social context to be consistent with the spirit of IPT) which are appropriately used with severely depressed inpatients, for example.

When being more directive and even when assigning specific tasks, the therapist should model the process of problem solving, explicitly using the process of listing options and evaluating the relative pros and cons of each. The therapist should frame this as a process to which the patient can contribute. Some useful statements and questions are:

> I'd like to offer you some suggestions as to how you might approach this problem – you can contribute your own as you feel you are able.

Which of the ideas that I mentioned seem plausible to you?

What ideas can you think of that I may have missed?

Therapist-directed brainstorm

Most patients have an intrinsic capacity to generate solutions to their problems. Their responses to queries about previous attempts to solve their problems is often a good indicator of how willing they are to exercise that capacity. The therapist should explicitly invite patients who are able to problem solve into the brainstorming process. Positive feedback and encouragement will further foster the patient's attempts to develop a solution and implement it. This should enhance the patient's sense of competence. Useful phrases include:

Why don't you run some ideas by me, and then we can try to find some solutions by looking at how each of them may affect your relationship problem.

The approach you used before sounds like it would work really well for you. What might be some of the advantages/disadvantages of trying something similar now?

For each idea generated by the patient, the therapist should lead the patient through the process of evaluating the option, and then decide together upon the most suitable approach. The therapist might also review with the patient the steps to take in the problem solving process:

- Specify the problem
- Break it down into smaller problems which can be addressed
- Brainstorm – list all the possible solutions, no matter how implausible
- Identify the pros and cons of each
- Decide on a solution that can be implemented
- Apply the solution
- Review what happens so that it can be fine-tuned if needed
- Practice.

Therapist self-disclosure

For patients who are less likely to develop problematic transference, and for situations that are not too personal, the therapist may elect to disclose some of his foibles as a way of suggesting solutions to the patient's problem. To be crystal clear, this is not a recommendation that the therapist self-disclose about any meaningful personal issues. However, comparatively neutral topics may be suitable pretexts for self-disclosure – if the therapist chooses to use this intervention – and may include things like minor household or workplace problems, common difficulties in child-rearing, or managing busy family schedules.

As an example, one of the self-disclosures I use quite commonly to emphasize the need for persistence and practice is my experience with flossing my teeth. Though I have the best of intentions, I often am too tired at night to take those few extra minutes to floss – it's just too easy to put it off. There's no immediate consequence, no one to scold me if I don't do it, and most importantly, it is not a well-developed habit. I haven't practiced it well. Of course when I have a dental appointment coming up in a few days, my guilt takes over and I'll floss vigorously for a day or two, and then be embarrassed when my dental hygienist asks whether I have been flossing regularly. The point? Making changes takes hard work and persistence – there's no easy or magical solution. Practice makes perfect.

With proper timing and judicious use, self-disclosures like this can enhance the therapeutic alliance and convey a sense of understanding and empathy; the risk is that poor timing and judgment about when to use disclosure, and especially what to disclose, can lead to disastrous consequences. Therapeutic judgment should rule the day, with non-disclosure being a very good default in nearly all cases. When it is not clear what to do, err on the side of not self-disclosing. But it is a good idea to have one or two good benign and humorous self-disclosures in your back pocket; just be prepared for the patient to ask you if you floss regularly now, or are still having trouble doing it every day.

Patient-initiated brainstorm

In many cases the patient will readily engage in the problem solving process, and will report progress to the therapist. In this situation the therapist should support and encourage the patient, reinforcing the gains made and the fact that the patient has been diligent in tackling the problem directly. The therapist can also review the process by which the patient came to a particular solution, further reinforcing it:

> That seems like a great idea. Could you walk me through the process you used to come to that decision?

Drawing on the patient's past experiences

One of the most useful and helpful ways to facilitate problem solving is to simply ask the patient questions such as:

> What have you done to resolve similar situations in the past?

> How could you apply this to your current problem?

These questions reinforce the idea that the patient is capable of solving his problems, support his strengths, and help him to develop solutions that enhance his sense of autonomy and competence. In circumstances in which the patient insists the problem is unique, the therapist may generate some response from a question like this:

> What usually works for you when you find yourself in other difficult situations?

Homework

All of these problem solving strategies can be coupled with a homework assignment as a way of increasing the likelihood that the patient will successfully follow through with the solution that is agreed upon. Homework is not necessary in IPT, but is often a great way to facilitate interpersonal change – the details of this technique are described in Chapter 13. The '*in vitro*' process of directed problem solving in therapy can be coupled to an '*in vivo*' homework component in which the patient applies the solution to the problem outside of therapy and monitors the results. This can literally be assigned as homework, or the directive given to the patient to attempt the solution between sessions can be implied. In either case, the patient should report the results to the therapist at the next session.

As therapy progresses, the patient may demonstrate increased competence in solving problems. If so, the therapist can give the patient a homework assignment to apply the method to other problems outside of the therapeutic relationship. This might be framed in the following way:

> You certainly have been able to approach problems and evaluate potential solutions here in our sessions. I would like to suggest a homework exercise that might help you consolidate this skill even further. You mentioned that there were

problems related to your mother-in-law, though we haven't had a chance to discuss them yet in therapy. Why don't you, between now and our next session, try to apply the problem solving techniques we have been discussing with respect to your wife to the problem with your mother-in-law. Then we can review how things went next week.

Potential Difficulties Using Problem Solving

The Patient Has Difficulty Engaging in the Problem Solving Process

To state the glaringly obvious, all of the IPT techniques work better when the patient is motivated and engaged. In our initial iteration of this guide, we wrote that 'excessive passivity by the patient should be discouraged'. That stunningly useless comment is problematic both because it lays the responsibility entirely on the patient (i.e. 'passivity by the patient') and gives absolutely no guidance to the therapist about how it should be discouraged even if that were a reasonable and desirable thing to do. Our experience since that initial iteration is that telling the patient directly to 'stop being passive!' is usually not very effective. A second and more subtle strategy employed by quite a few therapists, namely attempting to 'out-passive' the patient by being even more inert than he is, usually doesn't work well either.

This clinical experience (and common sense) has led to a major shift in the therapeutic approach to IPT.[b] Specifically, in IPT and other short-term therapies, it is now understood that the therapist also bears responsibility for the patient's engagement in therapy and motivation for change. To make the implicit explicit, this means that engagement problems are seen as a function of the therapeutic alliance – a dyadic relationship to which both participants contribute – rather than 'resistance' on the part of the patient.

Some of the reasons a patient's engagement and motivation to change may be poor are obvious and have nothing at all to do with the alliance. They may be due to the effects of depression or severe anxiety, or may reflect realistic fears about change. The patient's real-life experiences to date, reflected in his attachment style, may well be that change is risky, that support from others will not be there if needed, or that he is not capable of managing change.

The therapy process, particularly the pacing of IPT by the therapist, may also negatively influence engagement and motivation. Pushing change too quickly with an incomplete understanding of the patient's experience – not listening well before being directive – will impact engagement. That is why IPT is flexible – the therapist can take an extra session or two in the Assessment/Initial Phase, or add a session or two in the Middle Phase if more gradual change is needed. The therapist can also bolster the therapeutic alliance by providing support and positive reinforcement for the patient if his social support network is not yet able to do so. The therapist can focus early in therapy on more simple and concrete changes. The therapist can back up and encourage the patient to take smaller steps. These are just a few of many adjustments that may be helpful.

For instance, the therapist may choose to select an issue that is less difficult and encourage the patient to achieve mastery with that problem first, aiming to develop momentum for

[b] Yet again an example of the way that clinical science proceeds from clinical observations to more effective interventions.

more difficult problems or tasks later. It may be helpful for the therapist to be more directive and active in the problem solving process early in the therapy as a temporary measure in order to get some momentum going. When the therapist does need to artfully step in to be more directive early in therapy, he should ensure that additional instances of problem solving occur later in order to support the patient's autonomy and enhance his sense of competence. This can be a gradual shift which fosters the patient's growing sense of efficacy.

It is critical to note that efficacy and self-esteem are understood in IPT as both internally and externally derived constructs. They are understood as part of the patient's lived experience, and are influenced both by his internal working models and ongoing external relationships with others. Efficacy, self-esteem, and even autonomy are derived from lived social experience. They are derived from relationship.

Thus IPT recognizes that it is simply not possible for anyone (and certainly not a distressed patient who is feeling misunderstood, isolated, and insecure) to take a mental wrench and pry his sense of self from negative to positive. Our plumbing doesn't work that way: we are intimately connected to others, or at least wish to be, and our sense of self-esteem, self-value, and of being loved is developed and sustained within relationships. So instead of conceptualizing the patient's difficulties in engaging in problem solving as resistance, in IPT it is the therapist's task to step into the patient's attachment void for a while and to provide some support. This is what we do as real human beings in our role as therapists: we care for, support, empathize with, and even love our patients with all of the agape we can muster. And then we help them connect with others who can do the same, and with whom they can reciprocate that care and love.

There Do Not Appear to Be Any Solutions to the Problem

There are some circumstances in which the problem does not have a clear solution, or in which the patient is simply unable to generate a solution. In the first instance the patient and therapist should return to clarification of the problem and re-evaluate the patient's expectations for change. It may be that a minor alteration in the severity of the interpersonal problem, or a less substantial change in the way the patient deals with it, may be sufficient to bring about relief. At other times, appropriately implemented solutions may fail to bring about improvements in the patient's interpersonal problems, and the focus of intervention may need to shift to altering the patient's expectations about the situation or to looking for social support elsewhere.

The Implementation of the Solution Results in a Worsening of the Situation

Change may have an adverse effect rather than a beneficial one. Interventions in Interpersonal Problem Areas may intensify problems, lead to dissolution of relationships, or lead to an increase in distress. The 'pros and cons' of any potential solution require careful consideration. If the intervention has a risk of backfiring, then the patient and therapist should generate contingency plans for this possibility. If the adverse outcome was unexpected, the therapist should inquire about the details of the implementation of the solution, and also what transpired afterwards – another Interpersonal Incident regarding the attempted solution is often helpful. In all circumstances, the therapist should reinforce that the patient should persist with the problem solving approach, and that the setback is new information which can be used to understand the problem more fully and to develop modified and improved solutions.

Case example 10.1: Anne

Anne was a 46-year-old self-employed woman who had been referred for management of generalized anxiety in the context of significant conflict with her husband. Anne described her husband as having an 'awful temper', and as having a tendency to 'put her down' and 'speak badly to her'. She identified a number of supportive relationships and good social support outside of the relationship with her husband (Figure 10.2). At the end of the Assessment/Initial Phase, she clearly identified her problem as an Interpersonal Dispute with her husband (Figure 10.3).

Anne was quickly able to recognize that there was a clear pattern to her interactions with her husband. He would become angry and verbally hostile when he was frustrated, and this led to outbursts which caused Anne great anxiety. Anne described that her typical response to his rages was to feel intensely angry herself, but rather than express that anger to her husband, she would withdraw and try to pretend that nothing had happened. Not surprisingly, she noted that her own father had been controlling and verbally abusive with her mother, and that this had an influence on her reaction to conflict. The therapist and Anne discussed this in detail in the Middle Phase of IPT:

Therapist: *It seems the question is how you should respond to your husband's angry outbursts.*

Anne: *How to stop them?*

Therapist: *Well yes, but perhaps more how to respond to them.*

Anne: *Uh huh.....*

Therapist: *What have you tried to do in the past when he gets angry?*

Anne: *I usually run for cover and end up with a migraine.*

Therapist: *What has been the result?*

Anne: *Well, he quiets down, but we usually don't speak for days. I end up feeling worse because I know that it's just going to happen again – it's only a matter of time.*

After exploring the communication further by developing an Interpersonal Incident, the therapist suggested that they attempt to solve the communication problem together, and that the next step was to brainstorm about potential solutions. She first asked Anne how she had dealt successfully with similar problems in the past. Anne described how she

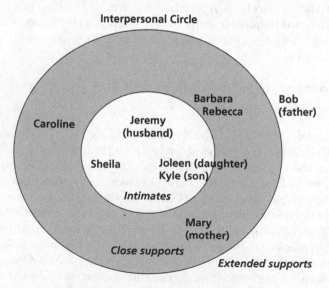

Figure 10.2 Interpersonal Circle – Anne

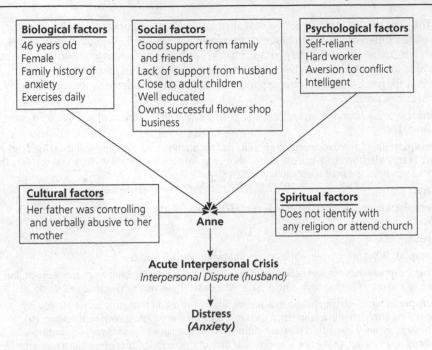

Biological factors

46 years old
Female
Family history of
 anxiety
Exercises daily

Social factors

Good support from family
 and friends
Lack of support from husband
Close to adult children
Well educated
Owns successful flower shop
 business

Psychological factors

Self-reliant
Hard worker
Aversion to conflict
Intelligent

Cultural factors

Her father was controlling
 and verbally abusive to her
 mother

Anne

Spiritual factors

Does not identify with
 any religion or attend church

Acute Interpersonal Crisis
Interpersonal Dispute (husband)

Distress
(Anxiety)

Figure 10.3 Interpersonal Formulation – Anne

often dealt with difficult and irate customers, which seemed to her to roughly parallel the problem with her husband. Anne generated her possible responses to an angry and hostile customer. She came up with the following options:

- Asking the customer to leave
- Ignoring the hostility and continuing as if there were no conflict
- Asking the customer to refrain from aggressiveness in her place of business
- Inquiring what the customer was angry about and offering a compromise.

The therapist then asked Anne how she might apply the same problem solving approach to her husband's hostility. Anne stated that she felt the best option with her husband was to simply ignore the hostility and continue as if nothing had happened. The therapist felt that this was a poor choice, as it seemed largely to be the same strategy that Anne had unsuccessfully used to that point. Noting that Anne had a long-term aversion to conflict, she recognized that giving Anne a concrete directive to follow a different course would likely provoke a superficial agreement from Anne without a real commitment to change. Therefore, she bit her tongue and encouraged Anne to try this the next time her husband became angry. The therapist was primarily concerned at this point with engaging Anne in the problem solving process, and in fostering her sense of ownership of the solution.

At the next session, Anne reported that ignoring the problem had not been helpful, and that her husband's outbursts seemed to have worsened. The therapist inquired about what had not worked, and Anne reported that she had not been able to 'ignore his temper long enough'. They worked through another Interpersonal Incident involving this specific interaction, and it appeared that as Anne ignored his anger, he had responded by becoming even more irate. Eventually she had, as in the past, left the room and gone to bed with a migraine. Despite further discussion about the available options, Anne insisted on persisting with the option of ignoring his anger. The therapist then chose to encourage Anne to refine the way in which she implemented the approach of ignoring her husband, again comparing it to the way Anne had customarily dealt with these types of problems at work.

At the next session, Anne reported that she had come to an important realization: there was a key difference between her customers and her husband. She didn't have to live with her customers, and if they got too unruly, she could ask them to leave. In contrast, she was literally 'stuck' with her husband, and the relationship problems were too important to ignore. It had become apparent to Anne that her approach was not bringing satisfactory results.

Anne: *I've tried ignoring him, but he is still getting angry all the time, and now I'm even more frustrated.*

Therapist: *Based on your description of your last interaction with him [Interpersonal Incident] I think I can understand why you are feeling that way. Perhaps we should go back and reassess the options you have to communicate to him differently.*

Anne: *OK.*

Therapist: *You recall the options we discussed? [Opens file and produces original paper with options].*

Anne: *Oh yes.*

Therapist: *What are your thoughts about what you would like to try?*

Anne: *I suppose that the best option would probably be to ask him what he is angry about, but when he's in one of his rages, he simply isn't reasonable. I just don't think that will work.*

Therapist: *I agree – trying to talk to someone when they are in that state won't get you anywhere. This brings to mind, however, a woman I was working with several months ago. Her circumstances were quite different from yours, but she did have problems communicating with her husband when he got angry. She landed on the idea of approaching him about the anger after he had cooled down, since he just wasn't reasonable when he was mad. I wonder if that might be of some help to you?*

Anne: *I am skeptical, but I simply can't ignore it any longer.*

Therapist: *How do you imagine you might do that with your husband?*

Anne reported at the next session that she had spoken with her husband about her response to his anger. He had been somewhat responsive, but had another 'episode' during the week, which left Anne feeling discouraged. However, she did note that though her husband was still 'rude', his anger was less intense. Although still unhappy with the situation, Anne did report feeling a bit more hopeful that things might change. Several sessions later, her expectations about the relationship were discussed.

Therapist: *It sounds like you have done a nice job of talking with your husband about your frustrations and your response to his anger outbursts.*

Anne: *I think so. He has listened, and it has gotten better. But I'm still not satisfied – he still gets angry, and every time he does, I keep getting frustrated.*

Therapist: *Realistically speaking, how much more do you think that his behavior will shift?*

Anne: *Probably not much more – it's hard to know – I suppose only time will tell.*

Therapist: *Well, perhaps we should shift the focus of our discussion a bit. What are your expectations about how he will behave?*

Anne: *I think originally I was expecting that he would stop altogether, and that there wouldn't be any more of the outbursts. He seems to be working on it, but I just don't know if he can completely contain them. He has always had a pretty quick temper. Maybe it's unrealistic to think that he can control them completely.*

Anne and the therapist focused on her explicit expectations of her husband and their relationship, and how these might be modified given that her husband was unlikely to change completely. As therapy continued, Anne was able to come to a more balanced view of her husband – as his outbursts diminished, she began to realize that there were many good things about their relationship. She ultimately elected to remain in the relationship, and though at the end of therapy she continued to express some dissatisfaction with his temper problems, she felt on balance that the relationship had improved and that she had the ability to address his temper directly when it flared.

Conclusion

Problem solving is a very effective way of generating productive change in the patient's interpersonal relationships. The therapist should ensure that the patient is active and contributes to the process as much as possible. A successful problem solving intervention usually helps the patient develop a sense of mastery over his problems, as it allows him to experience the benefits of his self-initiated efforts and fosters self-efficacy. It is also likely to lead to significant relief of symptoms and distress. The ultimate goal when using problem solving in IPT is to assist the patient to creatively solve his problem as well as to develop the skills to address other problems in the future.

Use of Affect

Introduction

The more affectively engaged the patient is, the more likely it is that change will occur. Drawing attention to the patient's affect, understanding it better, and helping the patient use it to graciously communicate more effectively, is critical in Interpersonal Psychotherapy (IPT).

In IPT, there are three goals regarding affect:

1. To assist the patient to recognize complicated affective and emotional reactions
2. To help the patient describe her affect and emotional state
3. To assist the patient to communicate her affect and emotions more effectively to others.

The therapist's tasks to accomplish these include:

1. Recognizing discrepancies between content and process affect
2. Identifying these differences for the patient
3. Facilitating discussion of affect and emotion and understanding them more completely.

Content and Process Affect

The most obvious technique that the therapist can use to reach these goals is to give direct feedback to the patient regarding the therapist's observation of the patient's affective state. This must be done, of course, in the context of a therapeutic relationship in which the patient can tolerate this feedback, and in which the patient can make use of it. This requires a high degree of inclusion in the treatment relationship – a strong therapeutic alliance. If these conditions are met, remarking to the patient that she appears sad, angry, pleased, or demonstrates other affective states may be of great help.

In IPT, the therapist should be aware of, and draw the patient's attention to, two kinds of affect: *process* affect and *content* affect. *Process affect* is the affect and emotions that the patient displays while talking about a particular issue during therapy, for instance, the death of a parent. *Content affect*, on the other hand, is the affect and emotions that the patient reports she experienced at the time of the event, say when she received news of her parent's death, or at the funeral. Process affect develops as the story is told in the therapeutic present; content affect is what was experienced as the event happened in the past.

These two types of affect may be congruent, or they may be dissimilar. For instance, when describing the death of a spouse a year previously, a patient may describe the following:

> When my husband died, I was an emotional wreck. I was really depressed, I couldn't eat for several days, and I slept terribly for a month.

The *content affect*, or the emotional state reported at the time of the death, was further described by the patient as sad, upset, and depressed.

When describing the experience in therapy, however, the same patient may display a *process affect* very different from the *content affect* that she described occurring at the time of the event. For instance, the therapist may note that as the patient describes the event in the therapy session, she speaks in a very flat or monotonous voice, or is telling the story as if she is reporting that it happened to someone else. In a case like this, the *process affect* would be described as neutral or flat. The converse might also occur. The patient might describe the death of her spouse in the following way:

> When my husband died, I was the one who kept the family together. I took care of all of the arrangements – I was so busy I never had the chance to cry. I mostly remember feeling numb.

The *content affect* in this case would be described as flat, neutral, or non-reactive. The therapist should elicit more description about it from the patient. When describing the experience in therapy, however, the patient might be upset, sad, or even tearful; the observed *process affect* might be sad or depressed.

When working with content and process affect, it is extremely important for the therapist to be aware of incongruities in the patient's presentation. When process and content affect are dissimilar, it signals to the therapist that the topic under discussion should be explored further. It also signals that the therapist, when the patient is able to tolerate the feedback, should point out the incongruity to her. This will assist the patient to become aware of emotions that she may be suppressing, or that she may be aware of but is finding difficult to experience or describe.

Case example 11.1: Joe

Joe was a 45-year-old man who came to therapy following the death of his father, which he identified as the primary issue leading to his depression. His father had died a year previously, and Joe had avoided coming to therapy until his wife had finally insisted that he do so. Though he reported being able to function both at home and work, he reluctantly admitted that his productivity had gone down, he was having trouble concentrating and sleeping, and his libido was greatly decreased. Though he was reluctant to come to treatment, he did admit that, 'my wife was right, I should have come to therapy a long time ago'.

After completing the Interpersonal Inventory (Figure 11.1) and Formulation (Figure 11.2), both Joe and his therapist agreed that the primary Problem Area was Grief and Loss, and that further discussion about the death of Joe's father would be helpful.

In the third session, the therapist asked Joe to describe in detail the circumstances surrounding his father's death, to which Joe replied:

> My father died quite suddenly of a heart attack…. he had been in good health, and no one expected it. My mother found him outside in the yard where he had been gardening, and he was already gone.

> My mother must have felt really guilty somehow, because she insisted that they do everything they could to save him, even though he had probably been dead for several hours. When they brought him to the hospital, they tried to do CPR [cardiopulmonary resuscitation] and stuck him full of tubes and lines … When I finally got to the hospital they wouldn't let me in to see him. It was several hours later that I got in, and by then, he had wires and tubes stuck everywhere – it didn't even look like my dad.

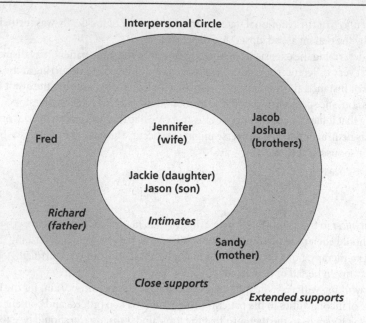

Figure 11.1 Interpersonal Circle – Joe

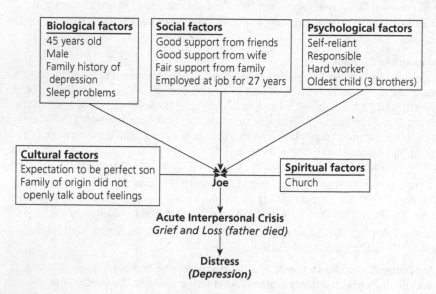

Figure 11.2 Interpersonal Formulation – Joe

I don't remember feeling anything when I saw him, just thinking, 'This isn't really him – I just need to get this mess cleaned up.' So I started throwing all the needles and tubes and stuff away until a nurse came in and told me to stop.

I didn't feel anything at the funeral either – I was too busy trying to help my mom, and I had to take care of all the funeral arrangements. I haven't even been to the cemetery since he was buried …

154

During this description, the therapist noted that Joe's affect when relating the story was extremely sad and tearful. His voice was quivering, and he clearly had a great deal of difficulty in telling the story without breaking down. Noting the discrepancy in process and content affect, the therapist remarked:

> As you're telling the story, I can really begin to understand what that must have been like for you. It's clearly difficult to talk about – you even look sad and tearful as you're speaking. There is clearly a lot of emotion you're experiencing now (process affect). At the time he died though, it sounded very different, almost as if you weren't feeling at all (content affect).
>
> *Help me to understand more about the difference* between the way you felt then, and the way you are feeling right now as you're telling me about your father's death.

The content and process affect incongruity was a clear signal to the therapist that the grief experience was at the core of Joe's difficulties. Further work needed to be done in helping Joe to express his emotional reaction to his father's death – both his reactions to the immediate circumstances surrounding it, and his current feelings. The therapist's open-ended directive to, '*Help me understand more about the difference ...*' was designed to get that process started. Simply pointing out the discrepancy also avoids any judgment – it is an opening of discussion, especially when coupled with the therapist's genuine desire to understand more.

Subsequent sessions, consistent with the IPT goals of helping patients to better communicate their needs and to build a more effective social support network, focused on a discussion about friends and family members Joe could talk to about his experience and his feelings about his father's death. He was very willing to share his feelings with his wife, who he found to be extremely supportive. He also approached a friend at work who had lost his own father recently, and felt very supported in that relationship as well. Towards the end of therapy, he made a decision to speak with his mother, whom he had largely avoided, about his anger that she had not let his father 'die in peace' in the hospital. Though this issue was not resolved when therapy was concluded, he did feel that he had made some progress with her, and had at least 'opened the door' to developing a better relationship with her.

In addition to being an extremely useful technique when dealing with Grief and Loss issues, the use of content and process affect is also very helpful in dealing with Interpersonal Disputes. The technique is particularly effective when combined with the use of Interpersonal Incidents.

Many patients who report Interpersonal Disputes will do so in a dispassionate way. A patient will 'present the case' to the therapist in a logical and unemotional way, largely because one of her motivations in relating the conflict to the therapist is to externalize the blame for the problem. The goal is to convince the therapist that she is not to blame – it is the fault of the 'other person' with whom she is in conflict. The story gets modified to convince the therapist that the patient's point of view is correct. In order to do this dispassionately, patients will often report the emotional content of an Interpersonal Incident with a neutral process affect, despite reporting a very angry or hostile content affect. Stories of conflicts with content affect such as anger expressed by yelling and screaming are often reported by the patient with neutral and unemotional process affect.

When there is a clear discrepancy between the reported content affect in a conflict-laden Interpersonal Incident and the process affect that is apparent in therapy (typically lack of strong affect), it is a signal to the therapist to delve more into the conflict – to have the patient describe it more. The discrepancy should also direct the therapist to reflect the difference in content and process affect to the patient. The purpose in doing this is twofold: (1) it leads the patient to become more affectively engaged in the process of therapy, and as a consequence more likely to be motivated to change; and (2) it gives the therapist a much more accurate report of the emotions that were expressed in the Interpersonal Incident, allowing both therapist and patient to more accurately understand her communication.

Case example 11.2: Debbie

Debbie was a 32-year-old woman who reported difficulty and distress in her relationship with her husband (Figures 11.3 and 11.4). Though she denied specific symptoms of depression and did not meet diagnostic criteria for any major psychiatric disorder, both she and her therapist felt that she would benefit a great deal from IPT with a focus on her relationship with her husband. While he was perfectly happy to have her come to therapy, she reported that he had no interest in attending sessions himself.

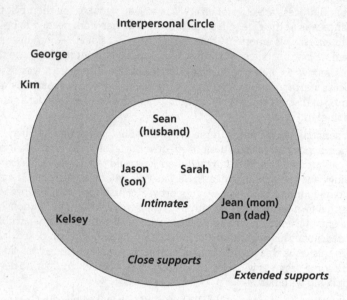

Figure 11.3 Interpersonal Circle – Debbie

Early in therapy, Debbie related an incident which she felt characterized the communication with her husband. The conflict involved the care of their 1-year-old son: several days before the session, her husband had called her at her workplace late in the afternoon to tell her that he had 'forgotten' he had a meeting that evening, and would be unable to pick up their son from daycare. After a brief phone call which concluded with her hanging up on him, she canceled her last meeting of the day in order to be able to pick up her son herself. She reported that she felt her meeting was at least as important as that of her husband's, and that she was furious about his refusal to keep his commitment to pick up their son. The following therapeutic dialog ensued:

Therapist: *Tell me more about the incident between yourself and your husband.*

Debbie: *I was in the midst of an important meeting when the secretary interrupted me to tell me I had an important call. At first, I was afraid that something serious might have happened to my son at daycare – calls like that always worry me. When I got on the line and found out it was my husband, I felt relieved at first.*

Then he told me that he had a late meeting that he had forgotten about, and wouldn't be able to pick up Jason from daycare. My first reaction, of course, was to make sure that Jason was alright – that someone would pick him up. Then I thought, 'My husband always does this – he never follows through on things or keeps his commitments.' I felt really angry at him (spoken with virtually no

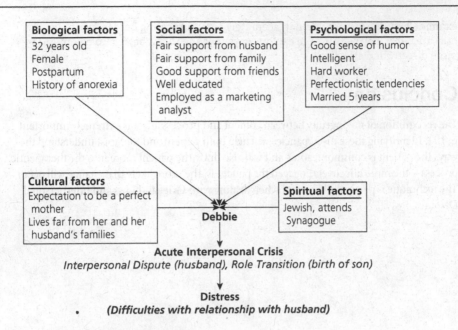

Figure 11.4 Interpersonal Formulation – Debbie

process emotion), but then I thought things through logically, and decided that if I didn't pick up Jason myself, no one would.

Therapist: *How did the phone call end?*

Debbie: *Oh – I hung up on him ... slammed down the phone I think. My husband is always doing things like that, you know. (Again spoken completely dispassionately, almost matter-of-factly.)*

It was clear to the therapist that there was much more to the story – Debbie's process affect was quite neutral and objective, and she was communicating to the therapist that she was behaving logically and rationally. The fault, as she presented it, was entirely with her husband. However, there was a clear discrepancy between Debbie's content and process affect, as the content of her story revealed a great deal of anger that Debbie was not displaying as she recounted the incident in therapy. Slamming down the phone, for instance, was likely a very forceful communication of anger or hurt, but that affect was not apparent as Debbie was describing the incident to the therapist. The therapist felt that helping Debbie to recognize the incongruity between her content and process affect would help her to better understand how she was communicating, and how her communications might be misunderstood by her husband. Further, the therapist believed that it would help her to become more engaged in therapy and increase her motivation to change. The therapist intervened in the following way:

Therapist: *It sounds like there was quite a bit of conflict between the two of you even during that brief phone call. I noticed, however, that as you were relating the story, it was almost as if you were telling the story about someone else. I didn't get much of an idea about how you were really feeling. It would **help me to understand better** what that was like for you if you could tell me more about how you are feeling about that incident right now as we're talking about it.*

Debbie: *Well ... actually I am pretty angry about it. I don't like to think about that though, because I'm afraid that if I think about how angry I am, I won't be able to control it. One time that actually happened ...*

Debbie went on to relate an incident during which she felt she had gotten really angry at her husband, and as she did so, became much more affectively engaged in telling the story. With an emerging recognition of her feelings, Debbie and the therapist were able to examine how she was (or was not) accurately communicating her feelings to her husband, and they were able to explore ways that she might be able to communicate more directly and effectively.

Conclusion

The recognition of incongruity between content and process affect is extremely important in IPT. Identifying these discrepancies will help both patient and therapist understand the ways the patient is communicating, and will also draw the patient more into the therapeutic process – the more affectively engaged the patient is, the more likely that change will occur. The technique is particularly helpful when dealing with Grief and Loss and Interpersonal Disputes.

Role Playing

Introduction

Role playing is a technique in which the patient and therapist create an '*in vitro*' interaction in therapy to reinforce behavioral change outside of therapy. While role playing, the patient's communication style and his mode of affective interaction can be examined in detail. In addition, the patient can often gain a better understanding of the experience of others involved in his social relationships.

Role playing is best used to model and practice past or future interactions between the patient and his significant others. Role playing allows more effective communications to be discussed, demonstrated, and practiced. Role playing doesn't have to be used in Interpersonal Psychotherapy (IPT); it is best used with selected patients and with selected problems. It tends to be most effective when the therapeutic relationship is good enough that the patient is feeling supported and can tolerate a degree of confrontation by the therapist. Patients with more secure styles of attachment are more likely to benefit from role playing, but it can be used with a wide variety of patients if done with a bit of curiosity, support, and humor.

The goals of role playing in IPT are:

1 To gather more information about the patient's style of communication
2 To help the patient develop new insights into his interpersonal behavior
3 To help the patient understand the reactions of others to his communications
4 To allow the therapist to model new modes of interpersonal behavior and communication
5 To allow the patient to practice new interpersonal communication skills.

Therapeutic Uses of Role Playing

Role playing is extremely helpful when used as a tool to gather information. The therapist, while observing the patient playing himself, can learn a great deal about the patient's style of communication, particularly the way affect and emotion are communicated. Problematic interactions can also be re-enacted and examined for specific instances of miscommunication.

It can also be used as a way to help the patient develop insight into his own interpersonal behavior. As he observes himself interacting in a role playing situation, he can reflect upon what is being communicated, what he really wants to communicate, and how clear the communication is. Role playing literally requires that the patient enlist his 'observing ego' as the communication occurs, and requires that he stop and think about what is being said.

159

Great insights can also be developed when the patient plays the significant other. It is an experience of 'being in the other person's shoes' for a while, and the patient can often much more fully appreciate how the other person is hearing communications, and what she may be wanting to communicate herself. The motives of the other person may become clearer as well.

Role playing can be used as a tool for implementing changes. In addition to modeling new ways to communicate, the therapist can give the patient direct constructive feedback about his communications which can then be incorporated into new ways to communicate more effectively. And of course role playing can be used as a means of practicing and reinforcing communication. New styles of communication can be practiced before extending them to the patient's social relationships. Practicing in session will increase the likelihood that the patient attempts new communication and communicates differently outside of therapy.

Conducting a Role Play

Role playing should almost always be structured with the therapist playing the role of the patient and the patient taking the role of the significant other first, especially early in therapy. There are several important reasons for this.

Having the therapist take the role of the patient first allows the therapist to demonstrate or model new ways of communication without being critical of the patient. He can demonstrate being more open, less defensive, and describing things more – any number of things can be modeled. If the patient plays himself first, the therapist is then left with having to correct or be critical of the patient if the communication is not going well. It is much better to have the therapist demonstrate, discuss the interaction, and then have the patient give it a try. A virtuoso therapist could even ask the patient to critique his role playing communication if he plays the patient first.

Having the patient play the significant other also promotes a different understanding by the patient. It is an experience similar in concept to gestalt techniques, in which the patient may get a different perspective about what the other is experiencing. The therapist can enhance this by stopping the role play at opportune times to ask the patient to reflect on the experience of playing the other. This is an extremely effective way to generate insight, and to get the patient to think about the impact his communication has on others.

It is critical that the therapist, when playing the patient, never acts out what the patient is doing wrong. This may come across as demeaning or humiliating, and will have enormous negative impact on the therapeutic alliance. Moreover, it is communicating in exactly the opposite way from what should be modeled, i.e. the therapist should always model graciousness and genuineness in all interactions, but especially when playing the role of the patient.

The Therapist as Patient

Playing the patient role affords the therapist the opportunity to demonstrate different styles of communication. The therapist may model communication techniques such as reflective listening by paraphrasing what was said by the other person. Techniques such as assertiveness, non-confrontational feedback and appropriate handling of aggression may also be modeled by the therapist, and then reinforced by switching the roles so that the patient plays himself and can practice the techniques that have been demonstrated.

A portrayal of the patient which emphasizes his relative strengths in interpersonal interactions may be greatly reassuring for the patient, particularly when the patient is insecurely attached. Positive reinforcement is nearly always therapeutic if honesty delivered.

The therapist should, however, generally avoid depicting negative aspects of a patient's behavior, such as poor communication or maladaptive non-verbal communication, because it risks appearing insensitive at best and derisive at worst.

There is certainly good reason, however, for the therapist to model new and more positive ways of communicating. This can be done either subtly without calling direct attention to the new communications, or can be done after bringing the patient's attention to the new communication that is being demonstrated. The therapist should use his judgment to determine which is most suitable at any given moment in therapy.

The Patient as Other

Having the patient depict a significant other while role playing can provide the patient with a unique window into the experience of that person and the interpersonal problem in which he is engaged. Patients frequently become more affectively charged as they engage in role playing and more accurately convey the types of behavior exhibited by others – this is often quite enlightening for the therapist. As noted, the therapist can break the role play at times and ask the patient about his experience of playing the other person.

The patient may also alter his impressions of the significant other when depicting that person during a role playing exercise. For instance, a patient may describe the other person to the therapist as unreasonable, but when depicting the other in the context of a role play, may recognize that some of the other person's responses may be provoked by his own communication.

There is risk in having some patients play a significant other. If the patient is somewhat passive-aggressive, he may be bent on 'proving' to the therapist that the other person, not the patient, is completely to blame for the interpersonal problem. The patient may then portray the other as completely unreasonable in an attempt to convince the therapist that this is the case. The patient may, by dramatically portraying a hostile significant other, make it nearly impossible for the therapist (playing the role of the patient) to respond. Therapeutic judgment should rule the day – if an aggressive, hostile, or histrionic patient is bent on proving to the therapist that the other is at fault, the therapist should beat a hasty retreat and move on to other techniques.

The Patient as Self

Having the patient play himself while role playing is useful in two ways. During the initial phases of IPT, when the goal is to better understand the nature of the patient's interpersonal problems, role playing can provide very useful information about the way the patient really communicates, as opposed to simply relying on the patient's self-report. The patient's particular style of communicating with, interacting with, and approaching others is often readily apparent during role playing. Affect is often more apparent as well. Role playing often reveals discrepancies between a patient's report of his communications and what is actually occurring.

In later sessions, role playing may be an ideal medium for the rehearsal of new communication skills. Behavioral changes such as anger or anxiety management can be practiced. Specific situations, such as confrontations or interviews, can also be practiced. Role playing is enhanced if the therapist is able to give the patient direct feedback about his specific communications. Doing so requires a solid therapeutic alliance, as this feedback can be threatening to some patients, particularly those with less secure attachment styles. Nonetheless, in such instances where the therapist judges that it will be helpful, interrupting the role play periodically to give direct feedback can be quite helpful.

An example in which direct feedback can be productively used is a role play of a job interview. As the patient plays himself, the therapist can intermittently step out of the interviewer role to give direct feedback to the patient about verbal communication, such as being too soft-spoken or too digressive. Non-verbal communication can also be addressed, and is often even more important in such situations. The therapist might reflect, for instance, that maintaining more direct eye contact or giving a firmer handshake might better impress prospective employers.

This feedback need not be given harshly. The therapist can give it directly if the patient can utilize the feedback well, but could also be framed more gently. For instance, the therapist might say, 'I wonder what would happen if you really focused on being concise?' or 'What do you think about keeping more eye contact?' Or the therapist can simply reflect his experience and ask the patient to brainstorm ways to improve communication further, for example saying, 'As you are talking, I find myself getting a bit confused about where you are heading. Could you help me to stay on track a bit more? Let's try that last interaction again.'

The Therapist as Other

In this mode, the therapist depicts one of the patient's significant others. In the early stages of IPT this may be useful to gain insight into the patient's typical style of communication beyond what is obtainable through the patient's self-report; later in therapy it is useful as a means of having the patient practice new communication skills. New situations which the patient might encounter can also be enacted. In all of these situations, the therapist can intermittently stop the role play to give direct feedback to the patient about his specific communications.

Potential Difficulties Using Role Playing

The Patient is Reluctant or Unwilling to Role Play

As role playing is an active and potentially anxiety-provoking process, some patients may be reluctant to participate in it, or may find it difficult. In these circumstances the therapist may choose to postpone the role play and move to a less confrontational intervention. The therapist should also consider that the therapeutic alliance may not be sufficiently strong for the patient to feel comfortable role playing, and if that is the case, he should delay the intervention and work on fostering the alliance.

The therapist may also explore the possibility that the patient's reluctance to participate in role playing is a manifestation of his interpersonal difficulties, and that these should be further explored in therapy. Among other possibilities, he may be anxious about meeting the therapist's expectations, fearful of negative evaluation by the therapist, or anxious about 'performing'. If so, the therapist can gently discuss with the patient the factors that seem to make engaging in role playing difficult, work to understand what the experience is like for the patient, and take care not to blame the patient nor frame the difficulty as a therapeutic failure. The therapist can then question how such factors affect the patient's relationships outside of therapy.

As with all interventions, the therapist can anticipate problems in advance by considering the patient's attachment style. Those patients who tend to be insecurely attached may find role playing distressing or anxiety provoking. In these cases the therapist may opt to postpone the role play or consider a shorter role play about a less critical issue. In some situations the therapist might opt to use a one-sided form of role play, such as asking the patient to imagine his or her spouse was present and could be directly addressed. Such a modification, however, will nearly always lose some of the affective impact of a true role playing intervention, as the patient will often be looking to the therapist for the 'right' way of saying things rather than being more spontaneous and engaged in his part. While an option, this modification should be used sparingly.

Nearly all patients are a bit reluctant to engage in role playing initially (so, for that matter, are therapists who have little experience with it). Leavened with a bit of humor, and supported by a strong alliance, patients usually warm up to it quite quickly. Repeat performances are usually well met. Keep in mind that the role play need not be long – 8–9 minutes of interaction is quite sufficient, and even that should be split up into 2–3 minute increments of role playing with discussion in between. Going longer than 2–3 minutes without breaking will diminish the immediate impact of the feedback; most patients (and therapists) have trouble sustaining attention for more than 2–3 minutes without a break in any case.

The Therapist Cannot Accurately Depict the Significant Other

The therapist can only base his rendition of the significant other upon the account the patient offers; although if structured correctly, the therapist will have already seen the patient play the significant other in the first part of the role play while the therapist was playing the patient. If the therapist depicts the patient's significant other in a way the patient deems inaccurate, the therapist can use the opportunity to explore the basis of the inaccuracy. This can often lead naturally into asking the patient about how his partner behaves and communicates, followed by an invitation to the patient to play the role of the other to demonstrate. It may also be an opportunity to ask the patient, once he describes the partner in more accurate terms, to describe how he responds to the difficulties presented by her.

For instance, if the patient tells the therapist that he is not accurately portraying the anger that his wife usually displays, the therapist can ask the patient for more details about how that anger is expressed. This can be followed with queries about how the patient deals with the anger:

What does he do when confronted by his wife?

How does the anger affect the relationship?

How does the patient feel in response, and how is that communicated?

In sum, though the therapist should certainly attempt to get it right the first time, there is a great deal of material that can be gleaned from unintentional poor acting.

The Therapist Depicts the Patient in a Manner that the Patient Perceives as Critical

When role playing, an ounce of prevention is worth a pound of cure. This situation should be avoided at all costs, and can best be averted by keeping to the rule that the therapist's task in playing the patient's role is to reinforce the patient's strengths and to model new communication techniques. In IPT, the therapist should never portray the patient in a negative fashion, nor use the patient role to point out the patient's faults. There is simply no justification for doing so, as it will invariably come across to the patient as demeaning. Further, this type of indirect and critical communication is a very poor example for the therapist to set. In cases in which feedback to the patient about his communication style would be helpful, the therapist can provide this directly and constructively while the patient is playing himself, rather than when the therapist is playing the patient.

Case example 12.1: Sarah

Sarah was a 34-year-old woman who had been referred for IPT for marital problems. She complained that after the birth of her daughter Jenny, her husband James had failed to contribute to the care of their baby as he had agreed to do. While Sarah initially reported in the first session and Interpersonal Inventory that this had been the first major dispute during their relationship, there were, after a careful history was taken, several other conflicts which became apparent. In each, Sarah's typical style was to attempt to avoid the conflict by ignoring it, and she was rarely able to communicate her anger to James. The couple had been able to 'bypass' the specific postpartum conflict with Sarah avoiding the issue, although it left her with all the work as well as feeling misunderstood and without support (Figure 12.1).

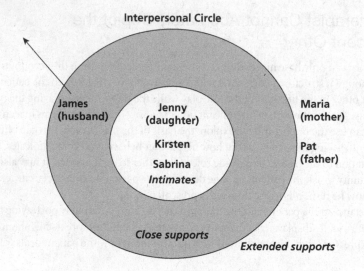

Figure 12.1 Interpersonal Circle – Sarah

In contrast to previous situations, however, her anger about the lack of help with childcare, though not expressed to James, had gotten to the point that she was considering leaving the relationship. She had yet to express this to James, who had apparently only noticed that she was much more sullen and withdrawn than usual (Figure 12.2).

In her accounts of her interactions with James, Sarah had found it difficult to describe in detail the character of James's interactions with her. More importantly, she had trouble identifying the specific aspects that distressed and angered her. In order to further clarify this, the therapist proposed a role playing exercise in which Sarah depicted her husband. The following exchange took place during the role play:

Therapist (as Sarah): *James, I want to talk about Jenny.*

Sarah (as James): *[Sarah pretends to pick up a newspaper and is holding it to obscure her face] Hmmm?*

Therapist: *Can we talk about Jenny?*

Sarah: *Um hm.*

Therapist: *Does that mean yes?*

Sarah: *What?*

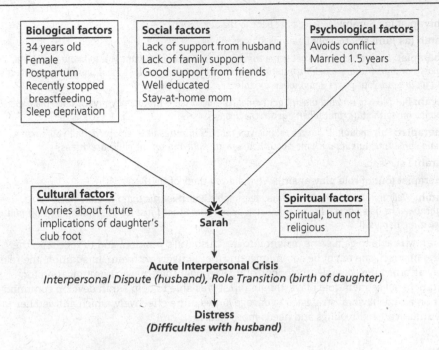

Figure 12.2 Interpersonal Formulation – Sarah

Therapist: *Does that mean yes we can talk?*

Sarah: *[still buried in the newspaper] About what?*

Therapist: *Jenny.*

Sarah: *[Still behind newspaper] Our daughter Jenny.*

Therapist: *YES!!!!*

Sarah: *Mmm hmm.*

Therapist: *[secretly wishing that a projectile was close at hand] I would appreciate it if you would stop reading the paper for a minute and participate in the discussion. When I feel that you aren't paying attention to me when I'm trying to talk to you, it makes me feel very angry.*

Sarah: *No, I'm listening.*

The therapist then suggested they stop the role play.

Therapist: *Is that how it really is?*

Sarah: *(with satisfaction) Oh yes.*

Therapist: *If he truly communicates like that, I can understand why you must feel so frustrated.*

Sarah: *Anyone who had to live with that guy would be frustrated, believe me!*

Therapist: *When he behaves like that, how does it make you feel?*

Sarah: *Incredibly angry!!! I feel ignored and unimportant, as if I don't matter at all.*

Therapist: *So what do you do?*

Sarah: *I usually just walk away – there's no point in talking to him.*

Therapist: *How well do you think that he understands how angry you are?*

Sarah: *Probably not at all – he doesn't seem to notice when I leave, or at least it doesn't seem to bother him.*

Therapist: *I wonder if there might be another way of communicating how you're feeling – let's try the role play again. By the way, you made it pretty tough on me when you were playing your husband – if you could help me out just a bit I think we could get a little farther.*

Therapist (as Sarah): *OK – let's get back to the discussion.*

Sarah (as James): *I thought I was discussing things.*

Therapist: *I think we need to get some things out on the table. I want you to know that I feel ignored and very angry when I try to talk to you and you don't look at me. I would appreciate it if you would put your paper down when we talk.*

Sarah: *But I like to unwind when I get home! All I need is 15 minutes by myself with the paper. You hit me with stuff right when I get in the door.*

Therapist: *Fair enough. If I agree to give you that 15 minutes uninterrupted, will you agree to spend some time talking with me about how we are splitting up the childcare duties?*

Sarah: *I guess so.*

Therapist (out of role play again): *What did you think of that?*

Sarah: *Well first, I don't think he'd be so reasonable. But it is true that I usually try to corner him right when he gets home – I'm so exhausted by that time that I just want to hand Jenny off and take a break myself.*

Sarah was able to gain some insight into her husband's position, and to reflect on the ways in which she might be communicating ineffectively with him. In addition, the role play afforded the therapist the opportunity to model some new communication for Sarah. In subsequent role plays, the therapist was able to help Sarah develop communication and behavioral strategies to engage James more effectively, which allowed her to communicate her feelings and needs more clearly to him.

Conclusion

Role playing is one of the most demanding techniques in IPT, as well as being one of the most rewarding. It is invaluable as a tool for gathering information, particularly about the patient's communication and style of interpersonal interaction. As a tool for creating change, it provides a supportive '*in vitro*' environment for the therapist to model new ways to communicate, and for the patient to modify and practice them. Role playing will work well as a tool to help the patient resolve his interpersonal problems as long as it is used with a good measure of clinical judgment.

13

Homework and Other Directives

Introduction

The term homework has many connotations, conjuring up for some unpleasant reminders of tests and papers, often put off until the last minute. Psychotherapeutically, homework has a long but mixed history, and its use has ranged from the 'requirement' that it be applied in behaviorally oriented therapies to a complete exclusion in psychoanalytic treatments.

Homework is but one of many variants we refer to as directives. Used as an adjective, 'directive' refers to 'a type of psychotherapy in which the therapist actively offers advice and information rather than dealing only with information supplied by the patient'. By that definition, every single therapy that exists is directive. Granted, some are more so than others, but in every therapy that exists, the therapist actively offers information, if only to tell the patient that the hour is up and it is time to finish.

The structure of Interpersonal Psychotherapy (IPT) is directive, just like the structures of all other therapies. The clearly stated goals of IPT – to reduce distress, improve interpersonal functioning, and increase social support – are directive. So are the goals articulated in other psychotherapies such as changing cognitions, discussing values, or talking about dreams: they imply at the very least that the patient should have cognitions and values and dreams, not to mention that they should be discussed in therapy. It is a simple and undeniable fact that all therapies are directive and that all are laden with implicit or explicit expectations about what the patient should be doing. So let's call a spade a spade: in IPT the therapy is generally directed towards change in communication and social support, and it is generally expected that the patient will participate in that process.

A directive as a noun can be defined as any intervention by the therapist that increases the likelihood that the patient will engage in behavioral change. Understood broadly, there is a spectrum of interventions which are more or less overt or directive. For example, as the patient is talking about interesting or pertinent material, the therapist might nod encouragingly: a subtle but effective directive to continue to produce more of the same. At the other end of the spectrum, the therapist might explicitly tell the patient to do something, for instance, to pay her bill, take her medication, or stop whining.

Understood in this way, the use of directives in therapy is a direct extension of the Interpersonal Theory described in Chapter 2. Everything – literally everything – the therapist does elicits a response from the patient. The key in IPT (and of course other therapies as well) is that the therapist should think about what she is saying and be constantly aware of the responses it may be eliciting. The use of homework and other more overt directives in IPT follows directly from its undergirding theory and interpersonal orientation. In essence, more overt directives such as homework or advice giving should be utilized when, in the therapist's judgment, it increases the likelihood that the patient will make productive changes in her interpersonal functioning and communication. The time-limited nature of IPT makes the logic of homework obvious – if it can facilitate more rapid improvement, then it should be used.

Since brief psychotherapies are inevitably more directive, particularly a therapy such as IPT which is explicitly directed towards improvement in current functioning, the therapist's job is to persuade or influence the patient to make changes to bring this about as quickly as she is able. This includes enlisting the patient as a cooperative participant in the process, and in many cases involves helping the patient become the primary agent of change. Nevertheless, this cooperative endeavor always includes directive interventions by the therapist – it is simply a matter of degree whether this takes the form of more subtle techniques within the therapy session or takes the form of overt homework assignments. Homework is a natural extension of the therapeutic process used in IPT.

Homework in IPT: What Is It?

Homework is nothing more than a task that the patient is expected to do in the interval between sessions. The goal of homework assignments in IPT is to increase the likelihood that the patient will engage in constructive communication change, that her symptoms will be decreased, and that her interpersonal functioning will be improved.

This broad definition leaves open a multitude of possibilities, all of which may be used as long as they adhere to the basic tenets of IPT. Homework assignments and other directives are congruent with the spirit of IPT as long as they are interpersonal in nature. A variety of techniques consistent with these principles might be used in IPT. For instance, an intervention in which the patient is asked to schedule pleasurable activities would be outside of the scope of IPT, but an assignment in which the patient is to schedule pleasurable activities *with a significant other* is well within the scope of IPT. Requesting that the patient engage in a relaxation procedure as a stand-alone intervention would be outside of the scope of IPT, but asking the patient to *explain to a significant other* why time alone and meditation are important to the patient is completely consistent with IPT.

It is critical to clarify at this point what is, and what is not, within the realm of IPT, and to clarify what is consistent with the spirit of IPT and its interpersonal focus. This is not to say that other interventions may not be helpful as an adjunct or addition to IPT, but rather to say that they are not within the IPT circle of interventions. Our intent is simply to be precise in how IPT is defined and described, and to be precise in describing other interventions that a therapist may choose to use with IPT. For the purpose of describing exactly what is being done in therapy or in research, this precision is necessary.

One can well imagine that using motivational interviewing[1] techniques during the course of IPT would be extremely useful in some cases.[2] So would discussing the patient's cognitions or values, and so would some relaxation or exposure work. But it would be disingenuous to suggest that all of these things are IPT, just as it would be disingenuous to suggest that IPT is really just a subset of some of the other approaches to therapy. The differences in foci, targets, and tactics are readily apparent. We simply encourage therapists (and advocates of particular psychotherapies, including IPT) to be fair and clear and honest in their descriptions of the therapy they are conducting.[a]

The general guideline is that tasks which involve communication and interaction with other people are within the scope of IPT. These homework assignments can be categorized as:

- Direct communication assignments
- Appraisal assignments
- Activity and behavioral assignments.

Direct Communication Assignments

These are perhaps the most obvious of all of the homework assignments, and simply involve having the patient engage in direct communication with others. A patient with a dispute about finances, for example, might be given the assignment to have a conversation with his partner about his concerns at 7 pm on Wednesday evening. A patient with social phobia might be given the assignment to go to a social engagement and to attempt to speak to at least one other person while there. The essence is that the assignment is directed towards a specific direct communication.

Appraisal Assignments

Rather than assigning a direct communication, the patient may be asked instead to monitor and record her communications. The purpose of this is twofold. First, it provides important information about the patient's interactions and communication patterns to both the patient and therapist. Second, it has the effect of raising the patient's awareness of her communication. Asking the patient to record her conversations draws attention to her communication, and makes her more aware of what she is saying, how well she feels understood, and the responses of others. In essence, it enlists the patient's observing ego. This is a very effective way of helping the patient develop some insight into her communication patterns, and the self-monitoring which occurs may also be a very effective mechanism for change.

Activity and Behavioral Assignments

Having the patient engage in specific activities, such as exercise, is by itself outside of the scope of IPT. This is not to say that it ought not to be done, but rather that it is better conceptualized as an adjunct to IPT. There is no doubt that such activities may be very helpful for selected patients. If the therapist's judgment is that activity scheduling would be of help to the patient, then it can certainly be added to IPT. In addition, assignments like these can be brought within the scope of IPT by focusing the primary point of the intervention on improving communication and building social support.

Practically speaking, this means that giving a narrow assignment to practice relaxation techniques is not, precisely speaking, consistent with IPT, while requesting that the patient

[a] Unfortunately, parochialism and universalism have been a great hindrance to progress in psychotherapy research and dissemination of effective treatments. Parochialism has been a problem because many devout adherents to a particular therapy, including IPT, have insisted that their therapy be delivered precisely as specified, and that no other contaminants be included. Universalism has been a problem because some adherents to particular schools of therapy insist that their therapy really encompasses all the others, for instance, that all therapies are really behavioral therapies. Open-mindedness and flexibility are called for in religion, politics, and psychotherapy: after all, in each, the common goal is to serve the wonderful and complex array of people we are fortunate enough to develop relationships with, a goal not well met with arguments placing purity above practicality.

ask someone else to participate with her in relaxation does address the goal of increasing social contact and support. Similarly, asking the patient to exercise alone would be outside of the spirit of IPT, while assigning a patient the task of finding someone to exercise with, or of joining a health club with the goal of meeting other people as well as exercising, would be well within the realm of IPT.

'Paradoxical' Assignments

These types of assignments, though they have been widely used in strategic therapies to great effect, are not within the realm of IPT. Though they may be directed at relationship change and communication specifically, they should not be utilized in IPT because they do not allow the therapist to model direct communication. In IPT, the therapist should constantly and consistently model effective communication for the patient – a paradoxical directive does not do this, and therefore undermines one of the basic principles of IPT.

Homework in IPT: Patient Selection

The obvious criterion for homework is to consider it for anyone whom the therapist believes will benefit from a specific assignment. Several additional guidelines are useful in IPT.

The primary consideration in IPT is to assign homework to patients who are likely to complete it. While this seems obvious for all therapies, it is extremely crucial in IPT and other short-term therapies. This is because if the homework assignment is not completed, non-compliance is likely to become the dominant issue in the therapy. Not only does this shift the focus to the patient–therapist relationship, as the non-completion of the homework assignment must be discussed within the therapeutic relationship, it also detracts from the focus on immediate symptom resolution and improvement in interpersonal functioning.

Directives such as the assignment of homework subtly shift the therapeutic relationship. As understood from the perspective of Interpersonal Theory, giving a directive is a communication which shifts the therapist to a more powerful or a higher status in which she is telling the patient what to do, with the expectation that the patient will complete the task assigned. While this shift is quite tolerable to some patients, some will withdraw, and others will be provoked by the challenge for higher status and contend with the therapist. The latter responses change the therapeutic relationship in ways that make the alliance more difficult to manage.

With more passive-aggressive patients, for example, the assignment of homework is likely to elicit passive-aggressive behavior towards the therapist. Not only is it unlikely that the homework will be completed, but the assignment itself – putting the therapist in a more dominant position – is likely to cause problems in the therapeutic relationship.

Assigning homework to some preoccupied patients may also cause problems in the therapeutic relationship. If the therapist takes on a more dominant role, she may elicit even more dependent behavior from the patient. As opposed to the passive-aggressive patient, who often will not even attempt the assignment or complain that 'the dog ate it', dependent patients will often complain that the assignment is too difficult, and use the failure as a means of reinforcing their dependency on the therapist.

There are many patients, however, who benefit a great deal from homework and other overt directives such as advice giving. In general they tend to be quite motivated, relatively securely attached, and may even ask the therapist for additional work between sessions. In the best of circumstances, the patient will even go beyond the assignment, or modify it in creative ways that bring about even more positive change.

By way of analogy, imagine that the therapist is a University Department Chair who is able to influence her faculty, but unlike a real Chair, is unable to enforce direct orders by cutting salaries, assigning faculty to broom closet offices, or denying tenure. Thus the therapist/Chair can rely only on personal persuasion, charisma, and charm (as well as therapeutic techniques) to get patients/faculty members to leave their offices and generate more clinical income. For more courageous patients/faculty members (i.e. those more securely attached), giving a direct command to see more patients is sufficient, and is the best and most direct way to bring about change. For other faculty/patients, a direct order will increase anxiety and fear, and result in the patient digging in even more deeply to seek protection. Dependency will be exacerbated. For some faculty/patients, the therapist/Chair's command to leave the relative security of their offices will be met with disdain, with the patient saying in a passive-aggressive way, 'I'll show the arrogant dag who's boss.'

While the analogy may be a bit too far-fetched for some, it nonetheless illustrates the principle that the therapist should assign homework that is likely to be completed, and homework that is in the patient's interest. The therapist should also very carefully select those patients to whom she assigns homework. To do otherwise is to risk iatrogenically causing more transferential difficulties in a therapeutic context in which examination of the transference is not only outside of the scope of the treatment, but detracts from the aims of the therapy. There is no reason to do this in IPT. As a general rule, patients who are more securely attached are more likely to benefit from directives, while those who are less securely attached should be approached with caution.

The Process of Assigning Homework in IPT

There are a number of ways homework can be assigned, but they all ultimately depend upon the therapist persuading the patient to undertake the task. The difference is simply a matter of degree, with the spectrum running from therapist-generated to patient-generated tasks. The point at which the therapist intervenes along that spectrum, however, has great impact on the likelihood that the homework will be completed; great care should be taken to ensure that the level of intervention matches the individual patient.

The best assignment is one which is initiated by the patient. An astute and motivated patient, for example, might remark to the therapist that it would be helpful if she initiated a conversation with her partner to resolve a conflict. The therapist need only concur and encourage the patient. Patients like this are, unfortunately, few and far between, though they are much sought after by therapists. Nonetheless, the more the homework is generated by the patient, the more likely it is to be accomplished. The therapist can encourage this kind of patient-initiated problem solving by using non-specific directives with the patient. For example, the therapist might ask questions such as:

What do you think would be helpful to accomplish between sessions?

How do you think you can best initiate the communication changes we've been working on?

How do you think this problem might best be addressed between now and next week?

This type of implicit directive accomplishes two things. First, it clearly implies to the patient that she is expected to work between sessions. While doing so, however, it also gives the patient a great deal of autonomy in developing solutions. Gentle guidance by the therapist, or collaborative work to refine the homework following the patient's suggestion, can be used.

Special care should be taken to ensure that the patient's assignment is not overly ambitious – homework should always be within the ability of the patient. The goal of homework in IPT is not to frustrate the patient but to maximize productive change.

Further along the spectrum towards specific therapist-generated directives are those such as psychoeducation. For instance, the therapist might tell the patient that increasing activity and decreasing isolation is helpful to most depressed patients. Acknowledging the fact that it is difficult to do some of these when depressed, the therapist might then ask the patient for ideas about how these general goals could be accomplished between sessions. The therapist is, with intent, influencing the patient to begin to generate specific solutions which can be collaboratively refined. Giving the patient ownership and working collaboratively will increase the likelihood of completion.

More specific directives can be given by the therapist using examples gleaned from other patients. Maintaining confidentiality, the therapist might find it useful to mention strategies that other patients have used to deal with similar problems. A postpartum woman who is dealing with a conflict with her partner, for instance, might be influenced to address the conflict with her partner more directly if the therapist describes a situation in which a similar problem was successfully addressed by another patient. The use of details which are like those of the patient will enhance the power of the intervention, as the patient recognizes similarities with her own situation.

As with all interventions, care must be taken with such approaches. The more overtly directive the therapist, the greater the risk of rupturing the therapeutic alliance. Though the specific interventions noted above may be quite beneficial and help some patients feel better understood, others may feel alienated, thinking that the therapist is not understanding them as individuals.

The most overtly directive intervention is simply for the therapist to tell the patient exactly what to do between sessions. While some patients will benefit a great deal from this, and a few will even honestly ask for homework to do, the therapist must take great care to ensure that taking a more dominant role does not precipitate transference problems.

In sum, the therapist is generally best served by using the least directive approach that is feasible and effective. Allowing the patient to take the lead encourages her to take responsibility for the task, and increases her sense of ownership. Moreover, it keeps the therapist from assuming that she ultimately knows what is best for the patient instead of listening well to the patient for her ideas about solving the problem.

Case example 13.1: Tom

Tom was a 40-year-old business executive who had come to therapy for help with marital problems. His wife of 15 years was threatening to leave him, stating that he was too invested in his work and didn't prioritize her or the family. Tom had a very high-powered job with a legal firm, and though he claimed he 'intellectually recognized' that his wife had a good point, he also felt that she didn't understand how stressful his job was.

In the Interpersonal Inventory (Figures 13.1 and 13.2) the therapist learned that Tom had a number of social relationships, mostly at work, and mostly with men. Like Tom, most of them were also devoted to their work, and expected everyone else to be equally obsessed. The culture was that men were not supposed to show weaknesses; any discussion of emotion was taboo. Tom described himself as having difficulty with emotional expression outside of this setting as well – though very articulate, he described never having had close relationships in which he could discuss his feelings.

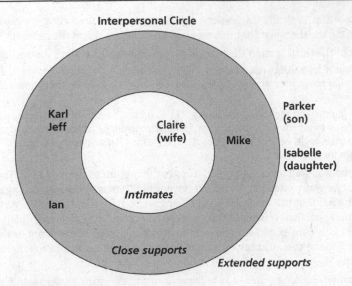

Figure 13.1 Interpersonal Circle – Tom

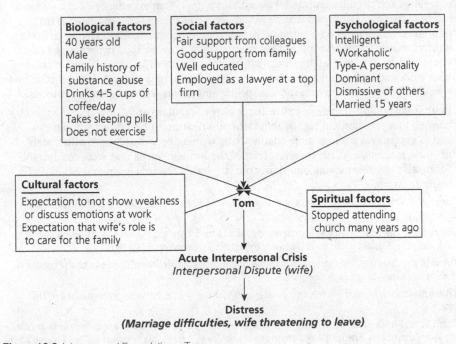

Figure 13.2 Interpersonal Formulation – Tom

The therapist noted that Tom was very goal-oriented, and that he tended to be fairly dominant. This was apparent in both subtle and direct ways within the therapy itself. Near the end of the first session, for instance, Tom rather adamantly told the therapist that they 'needed to meet again the next week', before the therapist had the chance to bring up the topic of future appointments. Tom always had a particular agenda to discuss, and always brought in a written list of materials to cover, somewhat like a business meeting. Typically the sessions would begin with Tom setting out his agenda and informing the therapist that this was how they would spend the session.

At the end of the third session the topic of homework arose at Tom's instigation.

Tom: *We've met for 3 weeks now, and you still haven't given me any assignments to do. That would never happen in my company – if you were working for me, I'd be giving you a lot of stuff to take home!*

Therapist: *[fighting off the temptation to say, 'I'm glad I don't work for you!'] Many people I work with do find that having something specific to accomplish between sessions is very helpful in achieving their goals. Before thinking about a specific task, let's think those through. What are your goals for the next week?*

The therapist was well aware of several things at this point in therapy. First, Tom's attachment style was somewhat dismissive; given this, Tom was likely to disengage from therapy if he felt that the therapist wasn't being responsive to his requests. At the same time, the therapist also recognized that giving a direct and specific assignment to Tom was fraught with danger, as Tom was used to being in charge and was not likely to respond well to the therapist taking a more dominant position within the therapeutic relationship.

The therapeutic challenge, then, was to assist Tom to develop an assignment for himself that both maintained a productive therapeutic alliance and helped Tom to discuss his feelings and to communicate better with his wife. If Tom experienced some success with this, the therapist hoped that he would begin to develop some insight into his communication style as well, ultimately leading to a more permanent change in his communication and a deepening of his relationships. The therapist hypothesized that Tom would benefit from talking directly to his wife about his feelings of conflict and stress about work and their relationship, but he realized that simply giving Tom a directive to do so would likely be disruptive to the therapeutic alliance as well as unlikely to succeed.

The therapist chose, therefore, to use Tom's own vocabulary at this point in the therapy, choosing to more subtly influence Tom rather than confront him directly about the need to express his feelings more openly. Using words like 'people I work with', 'goals', and 'tasks to accomplish', the therapist framed the issue in terms that were comfortable to Tom, all the while moving him slowly but inevitably towards improving his communication.

Tom: *Well, my main goal is to save my marriage. And my wife has made it pretty clear that she isn't happy.*

Therapist: *The goal to save your marriage sounds like a very good general goal – kind of like a business plan, I guess. How do you usually approach a general goal like that?*

Tom: *In my business, we start by breaking it down into smaller steps. Then you can set some specific deadlines to get each one done.*

Therapist: *Sounds good – what specific steps do you see that need to be accomplished in this case?*

Tom: *First, I need to set up some time to talk with her – I still don't quite know what she sees as the specific problem. She just keeps saying that she doesn't feel 'close' anymore. Then I guess I better communicate what I'm thinking more clearly to her.*

Therapist: *Sounds good so far – what is it that you'd like to tell her, exactly?*

Tom: *The main thing is that I don't feel like she understands all the stress that I'm under. Work is difficult enough, but now to have to deal with this kind of dissatisfaction at home too ... and I want her to know that even though she may not think so, I do still love her very much.*

Therapist: *It seems to be helpful to you to have a kind of written agenda to get things done – I noticed that you have used that for our sessions. Would it be helpful to write down what you want to tell your wife?*

Tom: *Great idea doc! [takes out a sheet of paper from his briefcase and proceeds to write several notes].*

Therapist: *Now that you've got a good idea of where you're heading, what's the next step?*

Tom: *Setting some specific deadlines. Why don't we say that I should have a good conversation with her by this time next week?*

Therapist: *Sounds ambitious, but you seem like the kind of guy who gets things done when he sets his mind to it. Do you think figuring out a specific time would be of help?*

Tom: *Now I know why they pay you the big bucks, doc. Yeah, Thursday night is usually fairly free – no meetings or any activities with the kids. I'll talk to her after we get the kids to bed.*

Therapist: *Sounds like a plan. I'll look forward to hearing how it turns out.*

Tom approached his wife the next Thursday. He reported in the next session that the attempt wasn't very successful – his wife had been put off by his 'demand' that they talk, and more so by the fact that he had a written agenda for the conversation. According to Tom, she said that having an agenda made her feel like he wasn't listening to her. Though the attempt was not as successful as it might have been, the therapist pointed out that Tom had made a strong effort. Further, Tom was now more open to other suggestions about how he might approach his wife differently.

Conclusion

The intent of homework and other directives is to increase the likelihood that the patient will engage in communication or social activity that will lead to improved functioning and symptom resolution. Though homework is not required in IPT, it is extremely helpful for many patients. The therapist should tailor the tasks in the directive, and the way it is delivered, in order to maximize the likelihood that the assignment is carried out. Refusal of homework or a passive-aggressive response to it will shift the focus of IPT away from improvement in external relationships to a focus on transferential issues. When used, homework in IPT should be interpersonal in nature, and ideally should be generated by the patient.

References

1. Miller WR and Rollnick S. *Motivational Interviewing: Preparing People for Change*, 2nd edn. 2002, New York: Guilford Publications.

2. Swartz HA, *et al.* Engaging depressed patients in psychotherapy: integrating techniques from motivational interviewing and ethnographic interviewing to improve treatment participation. *Professional Psychology: Research and Practice*, 2007, **38**(4): 430–439.

Section 4

Problem Areas

Interpersonal Disputes

Introduction

Disputes, arguments, disagreements, and differences of opinion are intrinsic to all human relationships – the 'seasoning', so to speak, of human life. At times, more piquant life-seasonings may lead to problems. Interpersonal Disputes may be utilized as a Problem Area in Interpersonal Psychotherapy (IPT) when they are relevant to the patient's acute distress. They should first be identified in the Assessment/Initial sessions, then collaboratively determined to be a focus of treatment during the Interpersonal Formulation. As with all of the Problem Areas, 'Interpersonal Dispute' is not a diagnosis. It is simply a shorthand way of describing the interpersonal issues involved in the patient's acute distress, and a way of maintaining focus over the course of treatment.

The Interpersonal Dispute that is identified is understood as one leg of the Interpersonal Triad; namely the acute crisis that has precipitated the patient's distress. The patient's response to this crisis – divorce, family conflict, conflict at work or school, or any other specific problem – is influenced by the other two legs of the triad. Biopsychosocial/Cultural/Spiritual vulnerabilities, including the patient's attachment style among many others, are the diathesis or predisposition to respond with distress. The context for the Interpersonal Dispute is the patient's social support, which often is lacking and therefore exacerbates the distress.

The general approach to Interpersonal Disputes, moving from identification to exploration to acute resolution, is displayed in Figure 14.1.

During the Assessment/Initial Phase, and particularly during the Interpersonal Inventory, the therapist should explore the possibility that an Interpersonal Dispute is the acute crisis that brings the patient to treatment. This can be collaboratively agreed upon as a focus of treatment when constructing the Interpersonal Formulation. To further assess the Interpersonal Dispute, the therapist can use the Conflict Graph to help the patient describe the conflict and clarify communication. Communication styles are analyzed to identify problems. Problem solving then follows to help the patient determine a course of action. Modification of communication or expectations about the dispute can be achieved using role playing or problem solving.

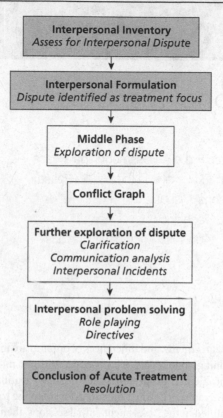

Figure 14.1 Interpersonal Disputes

IPT is designed to assist the patient to resolve the acute Interpersonal Dispute crisis. There are three specific goals:

1 To help the patient understand the dispute more fully
2 To work towards resolution by improving interpersonal communication
3 To enlist any social support that is needed.

The IPT therapist should not enter into therapy with a prejudice about the outcome of the relationship. There is a spectrum of outcomes for any given relationship which will differ depending on the individual and his circumstances. These can be roughly categorized as: (1) the patient may elect to end the relationship and move to other social supports and relationships; (2) the patient may decide to maintain the relationship with a change in expectations and an increase in social support external to the relationship; (3) the patient may elect to maintain the relationship after making positive changes in it. In each case, the goal in IPT is for the patient to make an objective, well-considered decision about how to manage the relationship, as opposed to an uninformed, impulsive one.

Interpersonal Disputes can be overt and obviously related to the onset of distress, or may be subtle and not immediately apparent in the compilation of the Interpersonal Inventory. Overtly hostile conflicts such as abusive or violent relationships are usually obvious in the early stages of history gathering, but may not be disclosed by the patient. In some cases, the dispute is in the form of a 'betrayal' of trust; in the case of intimate relationships, for instance, this might be a sexual affair. 'Disappointments' may occur at any stage of a relationship and are often more subtle, particularly when expectations are not clearly communicated. In some cases factors peculiar to the patient, such as personality or cultural context, or specific to the dispute, such as physical or psychiatric illness in a partner, may preclude it becoming overt. Some disputes are subtle and may only become apparent incidentally; for instance, a patient may inadvertently disclose a conversation or Interpersonal Incident that uncovers the dispute.

Interpersonal Disputes may also be developmentally determined. In many of these cases, the disputes arise as part of the lifecycle and the therapist should aim to help the patient place the dispute within this context. Role Transitions may also be considered as a Problem Area in such cases. Box 14.1 lists some examples of common disputes.

Box 14.1 Examples of Interpersonal Disputes

- *Overtly hostile conflict*: domestic violence, verbal abuse
- *Betrayals*: infidelity, impropriety, conflicting loyalties within a family
- *Disappointments*: unmet expectations at work or school
- *Inhibited conflicts*: anger at partner's illness or disability
- *Subtle mistreatment*: verbal abuse, denial of intimacy
- *Developmental conflict*: separation-individuation issues

Identification of Disputes in the Assessment/Initial Phase

Interpersonal Disputes often become evident while the initial history is being taken, and may well be the presenting problem. Some disputes may only emerge during the construction of the Interpersonal Inventory. Box 14.2 lists some specific questions that can be used during history taking or the Interpersonal Inventory to identify a dispute.

Box 14.2 Questions for eliciting Interpersonal Disputes as a treatment focus

- How have things been with your spouse/partner?
- How have you been getting along with your family?
- How are things going with colleagues at work?
- Are you having difficulty communicating with people around you? Anyone in particular?
- Have you found yourself unhappy or disappointed with anybody around you?
- Are you finding yourself in more arguments with people than usual?
- How do you express anger to others?
- Are you happy with the way people treat you? Anyone in particular?
- How well do you think that others understand you?

The therapist should *never* rigidly impose a Problem Area as a treatment focus upon the patient at the expense of the therapeutic alliance, particularly given the overlap of the areas. The goal when working with the Problem Areas is not to be dogmatic nor to make a correct 'diagnosis' but rather to maintain the therapeutic focus on interpersonal problems. The specific Problem Area is less important that maintaining a general interpersonal focus.

So if a patient conceptualizes his problem as a Role Transition while the therapist thinks it is better understood as a dispute, it should be dealt with under the rubric of a transition. Conversely, the therapist may view the patient's problem as a Role Transition while the patient describes the issue as an Interpersonal Dispute; the experienced therapist will go with the patient's conceptualization. After all, one of the primary goals in

IPT is to understand the patient better; that can hardly be done well if the therapist begins rigidly imposing his terminology upon the patient.

Interpersonal Disputes: Exploration in the Middle Phase

Once a dispute is identified and agreed upon as a Problem Area, the therapist should begin to collect information regarding the following questions during the Middle Phase of IPT.

When did the patient first become aware of the dispute?
> The therapist should explore how the patient recognized that there was a dispute, as well as whether the patient has been able to link the dispute and the onset of psychological distress.

What are the patient's expectations of the other person or situation and how did these change over time?
> The therapist should establish whether the patient's expectations are unrealistic in the context of the relationship. He should clarify the ways any changes in expectations have resulted in improvement or worsening of psychological symptoms and distress.

What attempts has the patient made to try to resolve the dispute, and what has kept a resolution from occurring?
> The therapist should explore the ways the patient has attempted to resolve the dispute prior to therapy. On occasion, the patient's attempts will have exacerbated the problem. Exploring these is a good way to further establish the patient's style of communication and motivation for change.

How does the patient communicate his needs in the relationship, and how has this changed over the course of the dispute?
> The therapist should establish how the patient's communication style has contributed to the development of the dispute. Information gathered using communication analysis will help to establish how dysfunctional communication has contributed to the development and persistence of the dispute. This should also provide guidance regarding which specific interventions, aimed at improving the patient's communication, may help bring about a resolution.

What is the patient's attachment style, and how has it contributed to the development of distress in the context of the dispute?
> The Assessment/Initial Phase of IPT should clarify the patient's basic attachment style, but it can be clarified further when discussing disputes. This style – a diathesis for the distress – should inform the therapist about the way the patient's distress and problems in communication have developed. The patient's attachment style should influence the interventions chosen by the therapist; it also has implications regarding the development of the therapeutic relationship.

What does the dispute suggest about how the patient will function within the therapeutic relationship?
> The therapeutic relationship will be influenced by the same factors that operate in the patient's other relationships. The therapist should take care to note the style

of communication the patient uses in therapy, the patient's expectations of relationships in general, and how these expectations are communicated, in order to anticipate and deal with parallel problems which may develop in the therapeutic relationship.

Graphing the Interpersonal Dispute

The initial iteration of IPT in 1984[1] and our first edition of *Interpersonal Psychotherapy: A Clinician's Guide*[2] both described a process of 'staging the dispute' as a required step in characterizing it. Disputes were staged as either in negotiation, impasse, or dissolution. Clinical experience and more recent research have led to an important shift in the therapeutic approach to disputes, which has discarded the staging process.

The shift is due largely to the theoretical and clinical emphasis in IPT on listening well to the patient. Categories, such as the dispute 'stages', have the effect of constricting further communication rather than expanding it. The goal in IPT is to have the patient more fully describe his experience, not place it in an arbitrarily defined category. As this description and expansion occurs, the therapist can better understand the patient's relationship problems, and the patient can also develop more insights into his contribution to it, and to solutions for the problem. Moreover, the process of expanding and describing more to the therapist can be carried over to the patient's relationships outside of therapy, helping others to understand him better and to respond to him differently.

Reliability may come from categorization, but validity and meaning come from detailed description and stories. It is far better to start working with Interpersonal Disputes by asking the patient to describe the dispute in his own words, and in terms that have meaning for him, than to require him to fit it into a category. It is far better to have him describe more, to elaborate on what he is thinking and why, and to have him give details about his experience and perspective. That is communicating well, and the therapist should encourage it at every possible opportunity in IPT. The key in IPT is to provide structure that facilitates more description and listening well.

The method used in IPT to more completely understand disputes and listen well while providing structure is to graphically diagram them. Figure 14.2 illustrates the Conflict Graph, the clinical tool that has been developed to facilitate this. It is designed to be very intuitive and easy to use, particularly for patients. It is also designed, unlike the old staging method, to open the conversation, to invite the patient to describe more, to explain more fully, and to help the therapist understand the patient's problem and perspective more completely. It is a structured way to obtain more information efficiently while listening well.

When an Interpersonal Dispute is identified, the therapist can use the Conflict Graph to help the patient visualize and describe the conflict. The first step in the graphing process is to introduce the Conflict Graph to the patient as a way of more fully understanding the conflict. The x-axis represents the importance of the relationship, while the y-axis represents the severity of the conflict. The therapist can then hand the graph to the patient, and ask him to plot the dispute on the graph, using a single point to note his perspective regarding the severity of the dispute and the importance of the relationship. After further exploration, the patient is then asked to plot the perspective of the significant other – i.e. how the other person in the conflict perceives the dispute severity and relationship importance. Further clarification can help to understand the differences in perspective and suggest how communication can be changed.

A critical part of the graph is that there is *no scaling or numbers*. That is because the goal is to help the patient to *describe the conflict in words*, not to categorize it or to use an arbitrary rating scale. As an IPT therapist I want to know what the conflict is like; I am not interested in knowing that the patient rates the severity of the problem a 7 or an 8 or any other number. I am listening for words and descriptions, not ratings. Numerical ratings have no point of reference,

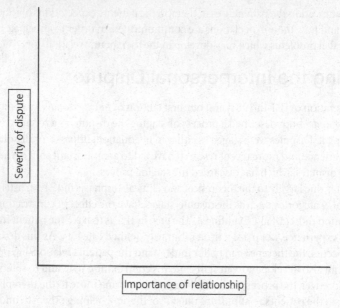

Figure 14.2 The Conflict Graph

no anchor. There is no shared meaning for a rating of '8'. Similarly, using staging categories has little shared meaning: what does a conflict in the now discarded category of 'impasse' really mean? The therapeutic goal in IPT is to have the patient describe, not to categorize.

The eventual goal of describing the patient's experience – communicating more effectively – with his significant other makes this opening up and sharing of individual experience even more critical. A patient telling his significant other that there is a problem because the severity of their conflict is an '8' is not helpful – there is no shared meaning. A rating won't allow the patient to be better understood; instead, it will actually hinder communication. The dispute won't change or shift without words and descriptions and communication. In contrast, having the patient describe in detail why the conflict is so important to him, the nuances of how he is feeling about it, the impact it is having on him – these are the seedlings of new and different communication that will grow into more complete understanding. That is how social support is enlisted.

Plotting the conflict also facilitates two other aspects of change. First, it forces the patient to think about the dispute differently. Not in a confrontational way, but in an open and inquisitive way. It forces the patient to struggle with questions such as: 'What makes the dispute so severe?' 'What makes the relationship important?' 'Why have I plotted the conflict here?' The process literally enlists the patient's observing ego, and should lead the patient to 'look over his own shoulder' at how he is perceiving the relationship and the conflict. It gently forces an internal shift from a fixed understanding of the relationship to an open examination of it. The second aspect of change is that the graphing process – with no scales – shifts the perspective on resolution from 'all or nothing' or a categorical outcome to one of degree. Rather than all or nothing, perhaps a moderate shift might be sufficient. Rather than a categorical change, perhaps there is room for compromise. Perhaps it is possible to be met halfway. Perhaps it is possible simply to understand more fully.

Both of these aspects of change are enhanced even more when adding the second step of the graphing process, which is to ask the patient to plot on the same graph the perspective of the other person in the dispute. Again this forces the patient to confront questions such as: 'Where would she plot the dispute?' 'How severe is it for her?' 'How important is the relationship to her?' 'Why would she plot it there?' 'Why are our perspectives different?'

Both after the patient plots his own perspective, and after he plots the perspective of the significant other in the dispute, there should be an opening of discussion facilitated by lots of clarifying questions. Questions like these are often helpful as a start:

What has changed?

Where would the dispute have been plotted a month ago? A year ago?

Has anyone's perspective shifted?

Why is the relationship so important, and why is the conflict so important?

The plotting of the other person's perspective gently encourages yet a third element of change: it requires the patient to step out of his own shoes for at least a few moments and imagine what others might be thinking and feeling. It requires the patient to take a different perspective and observe from that perspective. It is literally a technique to help the patient think about the thoughts, emotions, wishes, desires, and needs that he has as well as those of the significant other. When there is a discrepancy between the points plotted for each individual, it should lead directly to the therapist asking the question:

What does the other person need to know to understand your perspective?

And these secondary questions:

What do you need to know to understand the other person's perspective better?

What is leading to the gap in understanding?

These questions are critical in IPT, because they all lead to change in insight and communication. Asking what the other person needs to know to understand the patient leads straight to directives to the patient to describe his experience to his partner. Asking what the patient needs to know to understand his partner leads straight to directives to have him ask her about her perspective. And asking what is causing the gap in understanding leads straight to directives to discuss the conflict and introduces the possibility of compromise. All foster change in insight and communication.

Further exploration of the communication problems in the relationship can be examined using techniques such as Interpersonal Incidents and communication analysis. The patient and therapist should clarify all aspects of the dispute as well as the affect which is generated by it. This should include both the content affect which the patient reports when describing various conflicts, as well as the process affect observed by the therapist as the patient discusses the dispute in therapy. The therapist should also address the patient's communication style to help identify the ways in which the patient's communications are contributing to the dispute. Modification of communication or expectations about the dispute can be achieved using role playing or problem solving.

Utilizing techniques which help the patient generate solutions to his relationship disputes enables the patient to improve his ability to deal not only with the 'acute' aspects of the specific relationship dispute, but also to develop skills to deal with problems which may develop in the future. This will ultimately help to prevent the relationship from deteriorating after treatment has ended. It should help with new relationships as well. Even in those cases in which the patient is in a relationship which he ultimately chooses to end, the goal in IPT is to help him to better understand how he has contributed to the conflict. If this is accomplished, the patient will be better positioned to enter into new relationships without making the same mistakes. This is particularly crucial, given that patients tend to manifest the same attachment styles, and develop relationships in the same way, across time. If insight is not forthcoming, the patient is likely to step from the frying pan of one bad relationship into the fire of another just like it.

Interpersonal Disputes: Techniques

After establishing that a dispute exists, graphing it, and exploring it in detail, the therapist and patient should work to resolve the acute crisis which has led to the dispute (Figure 14.3). There are a number of techniques that can be used in the Middle Phase of IPT to collect information and to help resolve the dispute.

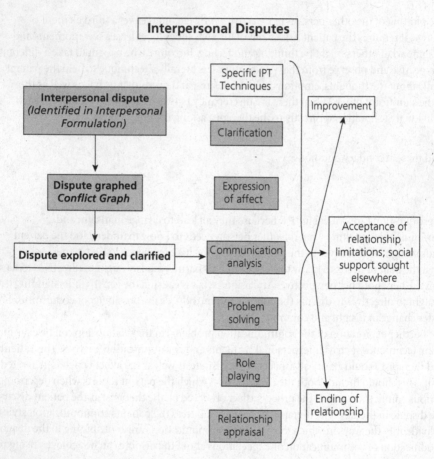

Figure 14.3 Therapeutic interventions in Interpersonal Disputes

The dispute is identified in the Assessment/Initial Phase and included in the Interpersonal Formulation. After graphing the dispute, it is explored in detail during the middle sessions. The therapist helps to bring about change by altering the patient's communication patterns (using communication analysis and Interpersonal Incidents), using problem solving, or helping the patient modify his expectations about the relationship. The dispute either begins to improve, or the patient may decide to end it or invest less in the relationship. Regardless of the outcome of the dispute, a primary goal of IPT is to help the patient emerge from it with increased social support.

Clarification

The use of open-ended questions and empathic listening will help build a therapeutic alliance with a patient who is experiencing Interpersonal Disputes. This is the foundation of all interventions in IPT, but is particularly important when dealing with disputes. This is in large part because a patient in a dispute often comes to therapy feeling frustrated and misunderstood, an experience which is likely to be imposed upon a therapist who neglects to establish a good alliance and doesn't listen well.

Clarification will help identify specific aspects of the patient's dispute, which is crucial given that the patient's report to the therapist is likely to be biased. The reports of less insightful patients will often convey an implicit message that the other person is to blame, and at least part of the communication to the therapist about the dispute is an unspoken invitation to the therapist to side with the patient against the 'oppressive other'. The therapist should therefore take care to expand on these areas further, as 'what is not said' is often extremely important in determining the nature of the dispute.

Clarification is also helpful as a way of practicing different ways to communicate with a significant other. The simple principle is to describe and clarify to the therapist first, and then to share the more complete and detailed description of the patient's unique story with significant others.

Expression of Affect

When relating the history of the dispute the patient may begin to experience emotions such as sadness or anger. It is vital for the therapist to help the patient recognize these – this can often be accomplished by exploring both process and content affect as the history unfolds. The affect can best be elicited simply by having the patient discuss the relationship – in particular, focusing on specific Interpersonal Incidents in which conflict has occurred will often help the patient to recognize and express emotional reactions. Once identified, these emotions can be used to motivate change in the conflicted relationship.

Communication Analysis

Disputes may arise out of poor or maladaptive communication, or they may lead to ineffective communication in a situation in which the communication was once much better. The therapist should direct the patient to report verbatim conversations and Interpersonal Incidents that he has had with others. This will provide material so that the patient's communication style can be examined, and hypotheses can be drawn about the ways the patient's communication is contributing to the perpetuation of the problem.

Problem Solving

Once the history of the patient's relationship problem is well understood and the therapist has a good understanding of the patient's communication style, the therapist and patient can collaborate on generating potential solutions. Both old strategies for dealing with similar problems as well as new approaches should be discussed. It is important for the patient to be as active as possible in this process in order to increase his sense of mastery. This should also help the patient to develop the skills to address other problems in the future.

Role Playing

Role playing can be a valuable intervention when dealing with Interpersonal Disputes. The patient can first play the role of the significant other, which is a helpful strategy for the patient to gain insight into the other's experience. The therapist can demonstrate new ways of communicating when playing the patient. The therapist can then play the role of the significant other to gain further insight into the patient's communication style, and can give feedback to the patient so that his communication can be discussed. Role playing may also be used to help the patient develop assertiveness or communication skills, providing an 'in vitro' environment in which to practice them.

Relationship Appraisal

Disputes are often based on expectations about the relationship that are non-reciprocal. Unrequited love, unrealistic expectations, or conflicts about the role that each person is to assume lead to conflict because of differences in expectations. In addition, conflicts can be exacerbated because the patient's expectation of the other exceeds what she is capable of doing, or exceeds what is possible to do in the particular situation.

For instance, a woman having postpartum difficulties may expect her husband to take over the childcare responsibilities when she returns to work. If he is working as well, this may simply prove to be unrealistic, as it is literally not possible for him to fulfill her expectations. A patient with a spouse who is relatively detached and who may have avoidant traits may expect her spouse to be able to communicate deep emotional feelings – this too may be an unrealistic expectation given the limitations inherent in the spouse. Conversely, the husband's expectations that his wife will only need the amount of communication that he is comfortable with may also be unrealistic. In these situations, the therapist should examine the expectations of the patient in detail, and help to determine whether they are realistic. If they are not, then the patient is bound to be disappointed no matter how much her communication improves. The therapist can give direct feedback to the patient about the expectations in some circumstances, or in others may want to let the patient take the lead. In either case, the goal is to help the patient realistically appraise her situation.

This particular technique bears many similarities to approaches taken in cognitive therapy. *Technically* speaking, IPT and cognitive behavioral therapy (CBT) utilize a similar technique: the therapist is challenging the patient's expectations. *Tactically* speaking, however, IPT and CBT are very different. In IPT:

- The primary goal is change in communication and increase in social support and not challenging the patient's underlying cognitions or maladaptive schemas.
- The therapist helps the patient to examine his expectation about a specific relationship to effect interpersonal change and is always concerned with expectations about relationships.

Interpersonal Disputes: Additional Therapeutic Tactics

The Patient Reports an Absence of Disputes

During the Assessment/Initial Phase of IPT, a patient may fail to acknowledge the presence of significant Interpersonal Disputes, despite the fact that elements of the history strongly suggest a serious conflict is present. Possible reasons for this may include the patient's attachment style (often preoccupied if he over-idealizes and is reticent to criticize significant others), his personality, psychological defenses, cultural factors, or a reluctance to self-disclose during the early stages of the therapeutic relationship.

In these circumstances, the therapist should retain a high degree of curiosity about the presence of a dispute without 'pathologizing' the situation and potentially damaging the therapeutic alliance. In other words, the therapist should continue to listen well. Disputes should be reframed as common and reasonable parts of relationships; moreover, their presence should not imply that the relationship is doomed or dysfunctional. The therapist should look for inconsistencies reported by the patient, as well as examining the patient's communication and problem solving styles. If an interpersonal conflict becomes apparent, the therapist can suggest to the patient that working on the dispute can improve the relationship and help relieve symptoms.

The Patient Who Appears Unmotivated for Change

Needless to say, a patient who is unmotivated can be very difficult to work with in IPT. Such patients are, of course, not highly sought after by therapists who use other modalities either. Lack of motivation can be a significant phenomenological feature of a mood disorder, or may be a reflection of the characterological qualities of some individuals, such as those with avoidant or dependent personalities.

If the therapist and patient recognize amotivation as a feature of the patient's illness, the initial stages of therapy should focus on achieving more limited goals or achieving change in smaller, more manageable aspects of the patient's interpersonal problem. As the patient experiences success, his motivation may well improve in tandem with mood. The therapist should continually emphasize the patient's gains, and use this to reinforce motivation over time. If the amotivation is related to attachment style, the therapist should adapt his own style to accommodate it. This means setting more realistic goals for treatment, slowing the pace to focus on the therapeutic alliance if needed, and engaging the patient collaboratively to solve problems.

An important distinction is the patient's motivation to *engage* in therapy and his motivation to *work* in therapy. Dependent patients, for example, are often quite willing to seek help (i.e. to engage in treatment) but may not be motivated to change once some of their dependency needs are met by entering a therapeutic relationship. Fortunately, with therapeutic effort such patients can usually be influenced to work once they are engaged in therapy. While threatening termination of therapy with a rigid time limit is a tempting way for the therapist to make the patient change, the damage done to the therapeutic alliance, the anxiety produced in the patient, and the empathic misfire all suggest that threatening or imposing termination is a very poor tactic indeed. In contrast, persistence and the techniques described in previous chapters can be much more helpful in increasing motivation in these situations.

Put simply, patients who are able to walk through the door for the first appointment and return for subsequent sessions are at least motivated to engage in therapy, and therefore have the opportunity to benefit from it. Those who do not seek treatment, who are not able to tolerate therapy, or who are sporadic in their attendance and commitment to therapy usually don't do well. There is simply no therapeutic technique that is effective if the patient is not present.

The Patient with Overwhelming Social Adversity

The presence of overwhelming social adversity, such as financial deprivation or poor social support, coupled with chronic and seemingly intractable Interpersonal Disputes may precipitate a sense of hopelessness for both the patient and therapist. That ought not, however, limit the implementation of IPT. Despite apparently overwhelming social problems, such patients are often motivated for change, often have a specific interpersonal focus, and often have the capacity to work towards realistic goals. Our experience with indigent patients and others with difficult social circumstances suggests that there is no reason to assume that these factors alone will adversely affect outcome.

In such cases, the therapist should avoid suggesting that all of the patient's problems will be addressed and can instead work collaboratively to set modest and achievable goals. Working towards outcomes such as developing attachments and social supports outside of the problematic relationship, or improving assertiveness and problem solving skills, is appropriate. The therapist should also provide the patient with a warm and collaborative relationship which supports the patient in his efforts to deal with these difficult situations. The combination of empathy and an interpersonal problem focus may well contribute to improving psychiatric symptoms in illnesses previously regarded as 'chronic' or 'treatment resistant'.

The Patient Who Has Difficulty Communicating Well

Difficulties in communicating often reflect both the patient's attachment style and his dysfunctional way of communicating attachment needs. The silver lining to these behaviors is that they can, when they occur in therapy, be a veritable gold mine of information, as the patient's interactions with the therapist will reflect his interactions with others. If the therapist can identify these behaviors in a constructive and non-critical way in the patient's interactions outside of therapy, he can then help the patient to alter problematic interactions in communication or interpersonal behavior in these relationships.

In IPT, difficulty in communicating within the therapeutic relationship should be promptly extrapolated to real relationships in the patient's life to avoid shifting to a transference-based treatment. If the patient's behavior in relationships outside of therapy remains the focus of treatment, significant progress can be made in helping the patient understand his contribution to the interpersonal problem.

Case example 14.1: Donna

Donna was a 41-year-old woman who sought counseling for a marital conflict. During the Interpersonal Inventory, Donna reported that she felt a profound lack of intimacy in her relationship with her husband, Blake (Figure 14.4). Donna reported that their communication was quite limited, that they didn't seem to have much in common any more, and that their sexual relationship was very poor. Donna reported that she had attempted to talk to Blake about this, but reported that the conversation 'just didn't get anywhere'. During the Interpersonal Formulation (Figure 14.5), Interpersonal Disputes was chosen as a Problem Area.

In the next session, Donna and the therapist graphed the interpersonal conflict (Figure 14.6). She reported that she was far more invested in the relationship than Blake was, and that the problem was much greater for her as a result. She had quite a bit of difficulty articulating why that was the case, and when asked about what Blake needed to know to understand her perspective better, was unable to provide much information. Instead, she seemed to think the problem was intractable, and that he would never really understand her.

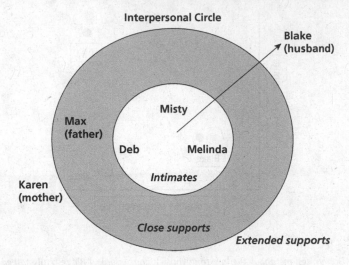

Figure 14.4 Interpersonal Circle – Donna

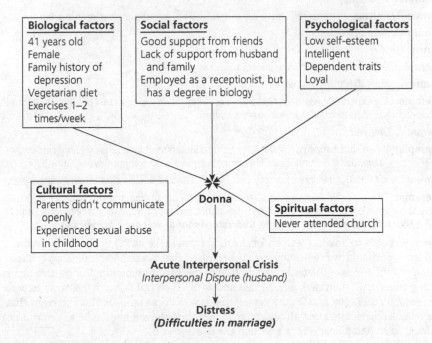

Figure 14.5 Interpersonal Formulation – Donna

During both this exercise and the Assessment/Initial Phase of IPT, the therapist had difficulty getting Donna to engage in the therapeutic process. The therapist found herself frustrated and at times irritated with Donna, as she typically answered queries with only brief or incomplete responses. The therapist began to work on the hypothesis that this same style of communication was impairing Donna's relationship with her husband, and decided to get more information by reflecting briefly on the in-therapy communication, and extending it to her relationship and communication with Blake.

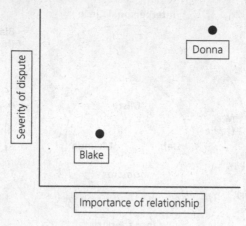

Figure 14.6 Conflict Graph – Donna

Therapist: *Donna, tell me about the last time you felt that you and Blake really talked.*

Donna: *[Long pause, then softly] A few weeks ago.*

Therapist: *What happened?*

Donna: *[Long pause, then softly] Um ... we ... um ... talked about our relationship a bit.*

Therapist: *Was it like this?*

Donna: *Hmm?*

Therapist: *Was it like you and I are talking now?*

Donna: *[softly] I don't understand.*

Therapist: *My experience has been that there are times when we talk together that there is a lot of non-verbal communication, but not much is spoken.*

Donna: *... Um, yes.*

Therapist: *When that happens, I find it very hard to understand well what you are thinking or experiencing. I wonder if that might be happening when you are communicating with Blake?*

Donna: *I don't know ... he does often say that he is frustrated when I shut down I guess ...*

Therapist: *I wonder if Blake really understands how you are feeling and thinking. It's difficult at times to communicate in words, and to provide details, but that is how we come to understand others better.* **How well do you think he understands what you are experiencing?**

Donna was able to link her feelings of isolation from Blake with her communication problems, particularly identifying with the thought that Blake had no idea what she was feeling. As the focus of the treatment shifted to her communication, Donna also reported feeling angry and frustrated with herself and with Blake, but felt at a loss as to how to proceed. The therapist and Donna agreed that it was important for Blake to know that she was feeling isolated and alone, and that this had affected her desire to communicate, which in turn had a deleterious effect on the relationship.

A conversation was enacted using a role play. First, the therapist played Donna, and modeled some different and more direct ways of communicating. Next, the therapist played Blake. During the process the therapist became even more aware of how Donna's communication elicited a frustrating response from others. She commented on this experience while role playing, and asked Donna how Blake typically responded to her communication. The therapist and Donna continued to rehearse her communication over the next few sessions, using the role playing technique to improve her ability to describe how she was feeling.

Towards the end of the therapy, Donna described a number of conversations in which significant improvements in her communication style were evident. She reported an improvement in her dispute with Blake and also a significant improvement in her sense of isolation. The therapist encouraged Donna to begin to utilize other social supports during this time, including several friends who were receptive to providing her with support.

The Patient with an Impaired Significant Other

There are often instances in which the IPT therapist will encounter a patient with a significant other who may have psychological difficulties – adversity affects families as well as individuals. The burden of caring for or interacting with an impaired partner or family member can often lead to interpersonal problems for the caregiver. Family therapists often use the term 'identified patient' to describe a particular family member who presents or is brought for treatment for a problem that has complex origins in a dysfunctional family. These kinds of systemic problems are often encountered in IPT.

The clinician has a number of options in such cases, including inviting the impaired partner to a session, conducting couples therapy, seeing the partner separately, or providing a referral for the partner if warranted. When the significant other is reluctant to address her psychological problems, the therapist may have to help the patient reframe the behavior or responses of the significant other as maladaptive communications, and encourage the patient to find out what they are intended to convey. In cases in which the significant other refuses treatment, changes made by the individual seeking treatment will hopefully affect both parties in the relationship, and may have benefits for the significant other as well. Even in the most difficult cases in which the significant other is impaired and not willing to seek treatment, the therapist should never withhold treatment from the individual who is seeking it simply because the significant other will not attend.

Case example 14.2: Peter

Peter was a 44-year-old man who presented to a psychologist with a history of feeling excessively sad and hopeless over the previous few months. He told the therapist that this had developed as a result of an argument he had with his 19-year-old daughter, Cassandra. He described his symptoms as fluctuating with the vicissitudes of the problems with Cassandra. Though Peter's symptoms were not intense enough to constitute a depressive episode, his distress was marked, and as a result he was highly motivated for treatment. Peter's previous physical and mental health had been good.

The problem between Peter and Cassandra appeared to be related to the breakdown of Peter's marriage to Cassandra's mother 3 years earlier. Since that time Cassandra had spent most of her time with her mother, who had apparently depicted Peter's contribution to the failure of the marriage in a one-sided manner. Cassandra herself had experienced difficulties with her health (complaining of chronic fatigue) and had also engaged in a number of problematic behaviors including several self-harm incidents, substance abuse, and suicidal ideations. Despite the seriousness of her distress, Cassandra had not sought help. Peter had encouraged Cassandra to get some treatment, but had received an indifferent and at times a hostile response from her.

Peter also complained that he felt stressed because of demands being placed upon him by his partner, Jane. Peter and Jane had been together for 12 months and Jane had been offered a job in another city. As a consequence, Jane had been pressuring Peter to marry her in order to 'cement their relationship' and to 'let us get on with our lives'.

After completing the Interpersonal Inventory (Figure 14.7), Peter and the psychologist agreed that the difficulties he was currently experiencing with Cassandra and Jane were best conceptualized in the Interpersonal Formulation as Interpersonal Disputes (Figure 14.8). Peter was most concerned with his difficulties with Cassandra, and opted to focus

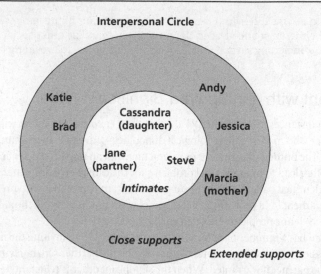

Figure 14.7 Interpersonal Circle – Peter

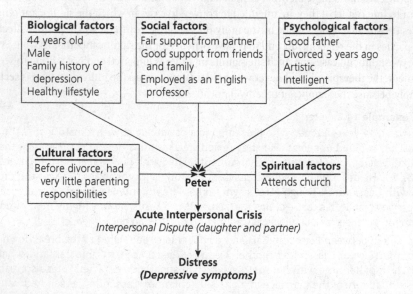

Figure 14.8 Interpersonal Formulation – Peter

on these first. A Conflict Graph was constructed, and clarification of the problem started (Figure 14.9).

Peter and the therapist were able to clarify the nature of the dispute with Cassandra in detail. Peter felt that Cassandra was nearly equally invested in the relationship, and that she also saw the disruption in their relationship as very serious and distressing. Despite having plotted both of them quite close, Peter was still able to describe a lot of misunderstanding and communication problems. He reported that the visual picture of their relationship highlighted the problems – Cassandra had largely shut down her communication, which he saw as a signal of her distress. He also believed this to be the case with her self-injurious behavior. He was convinced, however, that she would be able to change

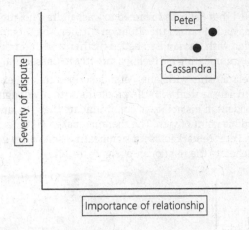

Figure 14.9 Conflict Graph – Peter and Cassandra

if he could convince her that he really cared about her. He also realized that he would have to initiate the process of opening communication again.

Peter described that his expectations of Cassandra were that she should 'try and hear my side of the story' and also 'look after herself more effectively'. He also felt she should realize that his suggestion that she seek treatment was well intended, and was a reflection of his concern for her. He felt that he had great difficulty communicating this to Cassandra. As Peter described the situation in detail, the therapist noted that he became quite tearful and agitated. The therapist called attention to Peter's process affect, noting the discrepancy in his rather factual presentation of the story in the presence of obvious sad affect. Recognizing and admitting to his sadness helped motivate Peter to further address the dispute.

In the Middle Phase, the therapist and Peter discussed an Interpersonal Incident with Cassandra that had taken place prior to the session.

Therapist: *Can you tell me about the last time you and Cassandra spoke?*

Peter: Yes – it was a disaster.

Therapist: *That's an interesting word to describe it. Perhaps we could consider that interaction in detail, so that we can better understand the problems with communication and how you might resolve them.*

Peter: OK. I'll try to remember what happened.

Therapist: *Fine. Can you describe the context of the conversation?*

Peter: Yes. I rang Cassandra.

Therapist: *What did you say exactly when you spoke to her?*

Peter: What I said? 'Cassandra, it's Dad'.

Therapist: *And what did Cassandra say then?*

Peter: She said, 'What do you want?'

Therapist: *How did you respond to that?*

Peter: I think I said, 'What do you mean, what do I want?'

Therapist: *Was that how you sounded?*

Peter: [confused] What do you mean?

Therapist: *As you're relating it to me, it sounds very neutral and without emotion. What was the emotion that was communicated?*

Peter: Well, now that you mention it, I was pretty hot. I think I was shouting.

Therapist: *OK. Can you tell me how Cassandra responded to you after that?*

195

The discussion revealed that Peter had reacted to Cassandra's hostile responses in kind, and that his responses had inflamed the situation further. The therapist and Peter agreed that his communication with Cassandra needed further work, and the next few sessions focused on clearly communicating his feelings directly to Cassandra.

When exploring his relationship with Jane, Peter described that he expected Jane to 'give me some space' and to 'let me deal with the problems with my daughter first'. Peter felt slightly more confident in his ability to communicate these to Jane, but felt that she still didn't understand his point of view. The therapist asked Peter to construct another Conflict Graph, which Peter remarked had a significant discrepancy in the respective importance they attached to the relationship (Figure 14.10).

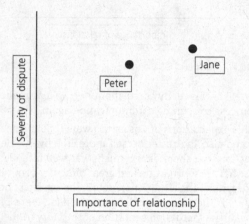

Figure 14.10 Conflict Graph – Peter and Jane

Peter and the therapist opted to work on clarifying his expectations of Jane and on rehearsing his communication to her. The therapist and Peter agreed that the particular problem was how to reconcile Jane's wish to move interstate without the need to force the issue of her wish to marry Peter, who stated, 'I am still getting over my last marriage.' The therapist and Peter discussed a number of potential solutions including a trial period of living apart with arrangements to meet every weekend, Jane looking for similar employment close to home, and Peter relocating to another city with or without getting married.

Peter rejected the last option given it would further distance him from Cassandra and make the resolution of that dispute more difficult. Peter then communicated this to Jane and a decision was reached to temporarily live apart. He then applied similar problem solving strategies to his conflict with Cassandra, in particular brainstorming about how to approach her most effectively, and how to communicate his desire that she seek help for her problems. Peter was able to communicate with Cassandra in a way that acknowledged her anger but also conveyed his message clearly. Cassandra then agreed to see a psychologist. With the resolution of both disputes, Peter felt a significant improvement in his functioning.

When working with Interpersonal Disputes it is important for the patient and therapist to clarify as explicitly as possible the core expectations of the other person in the dispute. This should be coupled with an exploration regarding the way the patient communicates his expectations and attachment needs to the other person. Once this is done, problem solving work can commence with the goal of improving communication.

Case example 14.3: Gerry

Gerry was a 45-year-old single man who lived alone and worked as a costume designer for a large theater company. He was referred by his local medical officer for worsening depression and anxiety. Gerry stated that he had been quite successful working as a costume designer, and that his work had been much appreciated by those working with him. However, a new director for the company had recently been hired, and Gerry described her as demanding and emotional. She was, according to his report, 'micromanaging everything and getting into my business. Nothing I do is ever good enough.'

Gerry described a long-standing pattern of social anxiety to the therapist. He described that literally any form of intimate social contact was anxiety provoking, and stated that at times he would have quite severe panic episodes in response to perceived negative evaluation by others. He found that while he was quite comfortable working on his own in the costume department, the new director had caused him serious problems, as it placed him outside of his 'comfort zone'. His mood had deteriorated, he had developed a great deal of anxiety, and he reported that he had been drinking more in order to cope.

Gerry had no psychiatric history. His local medical officer had prescribed an antidepressant medication which had been of some benefit in reducing his symptoms of depression, although he still remained depressed and anxious about his work in particular. Gerry was the only child in his family, and spent his formative years growing up in a communist country in Europe. He described his father, a local communist party official, as a 'harsh and distant man'. His recollections of his mother throughout his childhood and early adulthood were of a long-suffering, sad woman who was unhappy in her marriage. He had immigrated to Australia as a young adult.

Gerry had no intimate relationships apart from a platonic relationship with a woman at work who worked on scenery projects (Figure 14.11). He was also very clear that he had no particular desire for more relationships, and that he was quite happy with his solitary life. He enjoyed his designing work, and found meaning in his hobbies of reading and cinema. He was very clear that it was the conflict with the new director that was the problem (Figure 14.12).

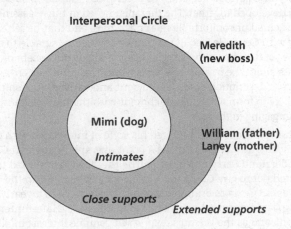

Figure 14.11 Interpersonal Circle – Gerry

At the end of the Assessment/Initial Phase, the therapist and Gerry discussed options for treatment. Though the therapist was aware that one option was cognitive therapy, which was clearly indicated for social phobia, social anxiety was not Gerry's complaint nor his conceptualization of the problem. Further, Gerry had made clear that he was not

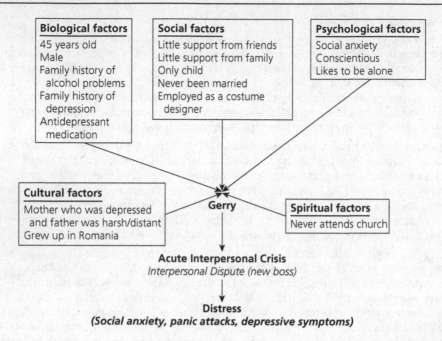

Figure 14.12 Interpersonal Formulation – Gerry

interested in or motivated to develop more social relationships. The therapist suggested that the immediate crisis – the dispute with the new director – would be a good focus for treatment. Gerry agreed to IPT with the goal of resolving the immediate job crisis, and also agreed to continue with antidepressant medication and cut down on his drinking.

The therapist made a mental note to add Gerry's fearful attachment style to the Interpersonal Formulation. They had used Gerry's description that he 'liked to be alone' in the formulation they developed together. The therapist noted in the Assessment/Initial sessions that Gerry seemed uncomfortable relating to him, and that he felt somewhat bored when interacting with Gerry. He also noted that Gerry seemed unable to accept positive comments, such as statements expressing optimism about the benefit of treatment or positive comments about the quality of Gerry's work. This information, along with data gleaned from Gerry's description of his few current and early relationships, made it clear that Gerry was likely to form a fearful attachment with the therapist and was likely to have difficulties engaging in therapy.

As a result, the therapist consciously altered his style of interaction with Gerry. He used primarily open-ended questions, and made a point of emphasizing that Gerry's responses helped him to understand Gerry much better. The therapist also slowed the pace of therapy, and elected not to give Gerry any homework assignments in the early sessions of treatment. He asked Gerry to bring some of his design work to an early session, and spent time having Gerry explain the work he did in detail. The latter intervention was particularly helpful, and as the therapist expressed genuine interest in his work, Gerry began to engage more in the relationship and in therapy.

Gerry's description of his relationships prior to the onset of his symptoms highlighted his avoidance of intimacy. Gerry found initiating and maintaining relationships difficult, and had not found any of his previous relationships particularly gratifying. The therapist asked Gerry about his current relationship with his parents who had remained in Europe; Gerry stated that he had little or no contact with them as he had feared his father's disapproval of his leaving his homeland. There simply did not appear to be much in the way of meaningful relationships, and Gerry did not appear interested in developing any.

The Conflict Graph (Figure 14.13) was interesting because Gerry placed the importance of the relationship with his new director at the very bottom of the scale, commenting, that 'if he didn't have to put up with her because of work, he'd be rid of her entirely'. The importance of the conflict was very high, however, as he recognized that it was not only causing him distress, but that his job might be at risk if he did not come to an accommodation with her.

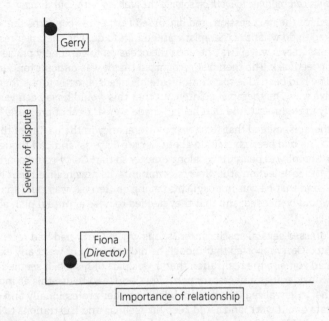

Figure 14.13 Conflict Graph – Gerry

In session 6 the therapist suggested that they address the dispute with his supervisor head on. After brainstorming ways that he might initiate a discussion with her and address his sense that she was interfering with his work, they engaged in some role playing. The therapist took Gerry's role first, and demonstrated some pleasant and graceful ways of asking the director to allow him more autonomy. Gerry was able to utilize some of these when he played himself in the role play.

The day before the next session, Gerry called the therapist and left a message that he was canceling all further appointments. The therapist noted the obvious: the cancellation followed a session in which a role play was used, and that the implication at the end of the session was that Gerry would follow-through and initiate a conversation with the director about his dissatisfaction. The therapist telephoned Gerry at his home and the following conversation took place:

Therapist: *Gerry, I got the message that you wanted to cancel our appointments – is everything OK?*

Gerry: *[long pause] Well, I went home after our last session and was very upset and started to drink again. I … I didn't want to tell you. I just don't know if I can do what you want me to do and talk directly to that woman. I find this really hard.*

Therapist: *Gerry, I really appreciate that feedback from you. In retrospect I think I may have been pushing too hard – I was paying more attention to my agenda for treatment rather than yours. I was very impressed with the way you were able to handle the role play that we did, but I don't think I realized how difficult it is for you to do that with other people.*

Gerry: *You must be really disappointed with me – I know that you were expecting me to talk to her, and I just can't do it.*

Therapist: *I think I understand much better how hard it is for you to talk to her right now. I think I can also understand now how concerned you must be about my reaction to all of this, but I missed recognizing that at our last session. Again, I appreciate your feedback – had you not said something, it would have left me wondering what had happened. Now I think I understand much better where you're coming from, and also understand that I need to slow down and listen more carefully to what you want to accomplish in therapy. As far as I am concerned we still have work to do, and I would very much like to meet with you. Why don't we plan to meet at our regular time next week and we can continue to work on solving the problem with your director.*

Gerry returned for the next session, and discussed further his concerns that he was being pressured to do what the therapist wanted him to do. The therapist responded to these comments in two ways. First, he used the occasion to genuinely praise Gerry for giving him the feedback. The therapist recognized that it was difficult for Gerry to do this, but that he had been able to communicate his needs directly to the therapist in a very productive way. The therapist pointed out that this would have been very difficult for Gerry early in treatment, and that he had made a great deal of progress.

Second, the therapist agreed that there was a discrepancy in the pacing of the therapy. He related that he had been concerned about Gerry's distress, and had thought that it would be most helpful to push things along quickly so that Gerry could confront the director. On further reflection after Gerry's comments, he now realized that he was not listening well, and that he was imposing his pacing on Gerry. It was clear that more preparation would be needed, and that they needed to have a mutual plan about how fast to go.

They then addressed several specific interactions which Gerry had had recently at work with his director. Gerry reported that though he did not enjoy or want any extra contact with her, he had come to the realization that it was part of his job. It seemed to be helpful to him to consider it as a necessary part of his work and to use this as motivation to 'put up with her'. He realized that he could deal with her professionally and only had to communicate about work, and could keep his feelings and frustrations to himself. Gerry did not feel obligated to talk about anything personal, nor to develop any personal relationship with her.

At the next session, Gerry reported that he seemed to be able to get along a bit better using this style of interaction. He suspected that she saw him as a 'bit of an ass' but he felt the same about her, and she had begun to realize that his work was good and to accommodate him. As he began to see this as a viable solution to his work problem, he had begun to feel somewhat hopeful that things would 'return to normal' and that he could get back to the solitary work and pursuits he enjoyed. The therapist went over several of these interactions with Gerry in detail, and highlighted how he had used his interpersonal strengths. As the Acute Phase of Treatment approached its conclusion, the therapist had the following interaction with Gerry.

Therapist: *Gerry we are coming to the end of the time we had agreed to meet. It seems to me that you are much less anxious and depressed since you started coming here.*

Gerry: *Well … work is much more tolerable at least.*

Therapist: *I think you have managed to adapt to the change at work quite well. I also appreciate the direct feedback you were able to give to me about feeling pushed to do something you didn't want to – slowing down the pace was clearly the right thing to do. I appreciate the effort you made to communicate that to me.*

Gerry: *It was really unusual for me to be able to talk that way. I'm still not sure how other people might take comments like that, but I appreciate you sticking with me.*

Therapist: *Before we conclude, I wanted you to know that I would be glad to meet with you again if you would like. Things seem to be going quite well now, but I can imagine other circumstances that might be a problem – another director for instance?*

Gerry: *I'll call you if I need to. This was helpful – not that I want to continue mind you, but I'll probably give you a call if something comes up in the future.*

Conclusion

Interpersonal Disputes are frequently encountered in IPT, and are the bread and butter of therapy, as nearly all interpersonal relationships engender conflict at some point. The goals in IPT are to identify the dispute, assess it fully using the Conflict Graph as a visual aid, and then to help the patient move to resolve the dispute, modify communication, and increase social support. The therapist should pay particular attention to the patient's style of communication and his expectations about the relationship; both are frequent contributors to the problem as well as factors that maintain the dispute.

References

1. Klerman GL, *et al. Interpersonal Psychotherapy of Depression.* 1984, New York: Basic Books.
2. Stuart S and Robertson M. *Interpersonal Psychotherapy: A Clinician's Guide.* 2003, London: Edward Arnold Ltd.

15

Role Transitions

Introduction

Change happens. It is inevitable. In many ways adaptation to change both determines and is determined by one's physical and mental health. In most circumstances change is dealt with successfully, and individuals adapt to their new conditions without developing psychological problems. In others, individuals with poor interpersonal resources or who are faced with overwhelming change become distressed.

All interpersonal relationships occur in complex psychosocial contexts. When the context changes, as in a Role Transition, relationships change. An example of this process is the Role Transition faced by a young adult who graduates from high school and leaves home to go to college. While there may be no major intrapsychic changes in the person or in those around her, the context of relationships with parents, siblings, and others changes, and the transition leads to dynamic changes in those relationships. The young adult becomes less dependent upon her family, moves towards more adult responsibilities, and begins to relate differently to her parents in her new role. In other circumstances lifecycle transitions or deterioration in health may be significant contextual changes which also affect relationships. In interpersonal psychotherapy (IPT) the process of change within relationships which occurs as a consequence of contextual changes in the patient's life is conceptualized as a Role Transition.

Though some transitions, such as loss of health, may be seen as wholly negative by the patient, most change involves both good and bad elements. When working with a patient who is experiencing a Role Transition, the therapist should first work to understand what the transition has been like for the patient – to listen well. The Life Events Timeline is a tool developed specifically for this purpose; it is designed, like all of the tools in IPT, to provide structure which facilitates listening well. While constructing the timeline, the goals are:

- To help organize the patient's narrative about the transition in a balanced and realistic way
- To help the patient tell her story more effectively to others
- To enlist social support that is needed to manage the transition well.

The discussion of the transition should certainly include a review of all of the good, bad, and indifferent feelings the patient may be having as she goes through it, but there is no presupposition that the transition is problematic because of some sophisticated intrapsychic processes. Having difficulty with a transition to poor health following a heart attack, for instance, doesn't involve repression or undoing or any unconscious mechanisms, nor does it involve difficulty resolving ambivalent feelings about the change. No one wants to have a heart attack or the resulting physical disabilities. In IPT, it is understood simply that the transition – the deterioration in health status – is an acute crisis which has led a vulnerable patient to become psychologically distressed, and that improving her interpersonal functioning and social support as she manages the transition will be of help.

Role Transitions can be developmental life events, such as adolescence, pregnancy, or aging, or situational changes such as unemployment or divorce (Box 15.1). As in all life events, Role Transitions should be viewed in the context of the person's interpersonal and socio-cultural environment, and in light of psychological factors such as personality and attachment style. Seemingly minor Role Transitions can be experienced as major crises by a patient who has poor social support or attachment vulnerabilities. In other situations such as forced immigration, the loss of a known old role and the advent of a formidable new role literally force the patient to move from conditions in which she felt comfortable and able to function into a new environment which is perceived as overwhelming.

Box 15.1 Examples of Role Transitions

- *Life stage Role Transitions*: adolescence, parenthood, aging, retirement
- *Situational Role Transitions*: job loss, promotion, graduation, migration
- *Acquisitive Role Transitions*: career advancement, new house, financial windfall
- *Relationship Role Transitions*: marriage, divorce, step-parenthood
- *Illness-related Role Transitions*: diagnosis of chronic illness, adaptation to pain or physical limitations

Role Transitions: Identification in the Assessment/Initial Phase

Role Transitions may be apparent during the initial history or may only emerge after careful exploration of an event or aspect of the patient's life and its significance to the patient. The therapist can ask questions like those in Box 15.2 to elicit information about potential transitions. This is typically done in the Assessment/Initial sessions of IPT, and may be developed further during the Interpersonal Inventory.

Box 15.2 Questions to elicit Role Transitions as a treatment focus

- What changes have occurred recently in your life?
- What changes have there been in your home, work, or social life?
- Have you recently passed any milestones in your life?
- Have you recently started (or talked about starting) a family?
- Are you expecting any major changes in your life over the next few months?
- Have there been any changes in your physical health?

Occasionally, Role Transitions may not become apparent until well into the course of therapy. As the patient and therapist clarify and develop a better understanding of the patient's interpersonal problems, or as interpersonal work proceeds and changes to relationships occur, the use of the Role Transition Problem Area may become more appropriate. Examples of this include the reformulation of a relationship dispute which is culminating in the ending of the relationship as a Role Transition, or the acceptance of a diagnosis of depression as a chronic recurrent illness requiring a Role Transition in the patient's thinking about her physical or mental health.

Role Transitions: Exploration in the Middle Phase

Once a Role Transition is identified and agreed upon as a Problem Area, the therapist should begin to collect information regarding the following during the Middle Phase of IPT.

When did the patient first become aware of the transition?
Though many transition points, such as moving to a different city, are obvious markers, there are often many others along the way that the patient may not recognize. For example, moving to a new city involves a point at which the possibility of moving arises. Then there is the process of making a decision to move, the preparation of finding a new place to live and making arrangements to move, the actual event, and then lots of adjustments afterward. What are the relevant transition points for the patient? Has she been able to link the transition and the onset of psychological distress?

What are the patient's expectations of other people or situations and how did these change over time?
The therapist should establish whether the patient's expectations are unrealistic. This includes both expectations of self and others in the context of the transition. He should clarify the ways any changes in expectations have resulted in improvement or worsening of psychological symptoms and distress.

What attempts has the patient made to try to adjust to the transition, and what has kept a productive adjustment from occurring?
The therapist should discuss the ways the patient has attempted to adjust to the transition prior to therapy, including their effects. Exploring these is a good way to further establish the patient's internal working model of self, and her sense of self-efficacy.

How does the patient communicate her needs during the transition, and how has this changed over time?
The therapist should establish how the patient's communication style has contributed to the difficulty with the transition. Information gathered using communication analysis will help to establish how the patient has solicited support and how effective she has been in eliciting it. This should also provide guidance regarding which specific interventions, aimed at improving the patient's communication, may help garner additional support.

What is the patient's attachment style, and how has it contributed to the development of distress during the transition?
The Assessment/Initial Phase of IPT should clarify the patient's basic attachment style, but it can be clarified further when discussing transitions. This style – a diathesis for the distress – should inform the therapist about the way the patient's distress and problems in communication have developed. The patient's attachment style should influence the interventions chosen by the therapist; it also has implications regarding the development of the therapeutic relationship.

204

What does the transition suggest about how the patient will function within the therapeutic relationship?

The therapeutic relationship will be influenced by the same factors that operate in the patient's other relationships. With respect to transitions, this should give the therapist information about how the patient is likely to handle the transition that will occur at the Conclusion of Acute Treatment. Are there indications that the patient will have difficulty with that conclusion? If so, the therapist can adjust the structure of IPT so that sessions are tapered in frequency as conclusion nears, and can include Maintenance Treatment as needed.

Constructing the Life Events Timeline

The Life Events Timeline is a simple but powerful tool (Figure 15.1). This tool, and the other simple tools that are used in IPT, have proven to be great ways to elicit information in an open and non-judgmental way while helping to open the conversation and get more information. They also facilitate more insight. By insight, we do not mean any sophisticated intrapsychic process, but simply a realization that the transition is more complex and more nuanced than the patient originally thought it was.

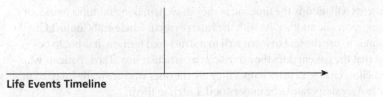

Life Events Timeline

Figure 15.1 Life Events Timeline

As with all of the tools in IPT, the Life Events Timeline can be drawn very informally on a piece of blank paper. The therapist simply draws a horizontal line with an arrow, and then draws a vertical line to intersect it. The vertical line is the identified Role Transition. The therapist then instructs the patient to use the timeline to note the events that proceeded, and followed, the acute transition, hands the paper over to the patient, and settles in to listen well.

There are two critical elements of the Life Events Timeline. The first is that there is no scaling on the horizontal line. There is no demarcation of weeks, years, etc.; the instructions are simply for the patient to note relevant events leading up to and following the transition. It is up to the patient to think about and determine what should go on the timeline. Second, the arrow to the right is critical. Many times transitions are difficult because the patient experiences them as endpoints. In fact, there is always more to the story. A divorce might seem like an endpoint, but life continues beyond that transition. The arrow implies that there will be more to the story, and the therapist can draw the patient's attention to that graphically. Even in the most desperate situations, such as a terminal diagnosis of medical illness, there is still more of the story to be written. A transition point – the diagnosis – is apparent, but what will the days left be like? What will happen after the patient has died? There is always more to the story, always the possibility of hope, and always the opportunity to transcend whatever transitions are occurring.

The idea is to get the patient to use the graph to more fully describe her experience, in part for the benefit of the therapist, but also for the benefit of the patient herself. It is a structured way of listening well. The benefit to the patient is the opportunity to work to tell her story in detail to the therapist first, and then to tell it to others who can understand and respond to the patient's needs as the transition is occurring. In addition, the reconstruction of her story allows the patient to bring more coherence to it, and to infuse it with meaning. This meaning is not a sense of cosmic or spiritual explanation; it is meaning in the sense of a cause and effect timeline or chain of events.

A good example of this is the Role Transition that women and men go through as they have a baby. Often the Role Transition is framed initially as a simple event: the birth of the baby. This single event is quite obvious – either you have a baby or you do not. But there are many events leading up to that transition point. Deciding (if such was the case) to try to become pregnant. Finding out that the pregnancy is underway. Telling others about it. Doctor's appointments, sonograms, decisions about testing. Planning for the baby, labor, and delivery. Holding the baby for the first time. Being in the hospital. Maternity or paternity leave. What seems an endless stream of sleepless days and nights. Grandparent visits (and interference).

Even in the most obvious transitions there are many, many additional events that lead to the identified transition and follow it. The timeline requires the patient put the transition into some kind of historical context, to give it coherency, and to understand why the transition stressor has arisen.

An additional note: the Life Events Timeline can also be modified and adapted to particular patients or cultures. For example, some therapists working with adolescents like to draw the timeline around the edge of a round table, and then physically walk around the table with the adolescent as she describes her experience, stopping at the various time points along the way. Some patients will modify the timeline as they draw it, making multiple marks, or stacking transitions upon one another. As with the Interpersonal Circle and Conflict Graph, the important point is to use the tool to listen well in a structured fashion. It is not to be rigid and insistent that the patient does the exercise in a particular way. Those patients who scribble on the timeline, change it, mark it up – they are the ones who are really invested in telling their story and are desperate to be understood. Listen to them.

Case example 15.1: Maria

Maria was a 27-year-old woman presenting for help at 2 months postpartum. She described feeling overwhelmed and completely exhausted. She noted that she wasn't enjoying anything; though she could identify a few times in the quiet of the night when she was breastfeeding her newborn daughter that were meaningful to her, nothing else seemed to feel right. It was, in her words, 'all gray'.

She quickly identified her husband of 4 years as being responsible for many of her problems. She noted that he had 'made a commitment' to do half of the childcare, but was instead working more. She did not feel that he was invested or contributing. She felt that he not only did not understand what she was going through, but that he was actively avoiding her and intentionally making things worse. Maria and the therapist completed the Interpersonal Inventory (Figure 15.2) and Formulation (Figure 15.3) and identified the birth of her child as a Role Transition and a focus of treatment.

In the Middle Phase of IPT, Maria and the therapist began discussing the transition in detail. As a way of organizing the narrative and obtaining more information, the therapist introduced the Life Events Timeline. Maria had a bit of trouble getting started, so the therapist suggested that she might think about other events surrounding the identified transition such as the decision to try to get pregnant and note them on the timeline. After a brief pause, Maria drew several points on the timeline (Figure 15.4). These included the discussion of becoming pregnant, the discovery of the pregnancy (it was planned for her, but not for her husband), telling her parents, and the time in hospital before and after delivery. The therapist asked her about any significant points after delivery. Again, after some thought, she identified a visit from her parents as an important point.

After Maria noted the specific points on the timeline, the therapist proceeded to ask her about the details of each, starting with the first (far left) and moving chronologically.

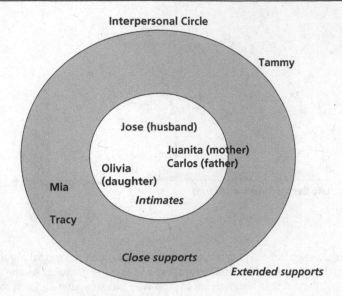

Figure 15.2 Interpersonal Circle – Maria

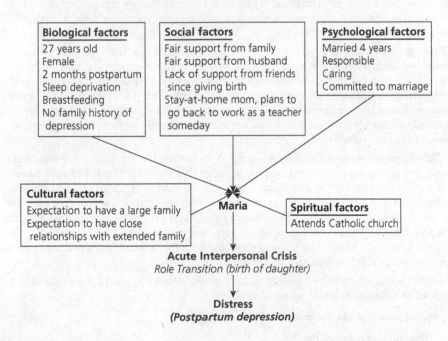

Figure 15.3 Interpersonal Formulation – Maria

The therapist planned on devoting at least an entire session to developing the timeline with her, and on utilizing it as a reference as they moved forward. Maria described that several months before she became pregnant, she and her husband had a long discussion about having children. Her husband, who was early in his professional career, was reluctant to start a family, and had suggested that they wait several years before trying. Though Maria was working at the time as a teacher, her long-term goal was to have a big family, and she was eager to get started. They ended the discussion without coming to a compromise.

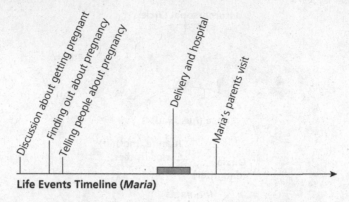

Figure 15.4 Life Events Timeline – Maria

It was about a week after that discussion that Maria decided to stop taking her birth control pills, though she did not tell her husband about her decision. As she described it, she had told herself that her decision to stop was not an active decision to get pregnant, but a decision to simply 'let things be in God's hands: if He wants us to have children then I'll get pregnant, and if not, then I won't'. Three months later she missed her menstrual period, and 2 weeks after that she discovered, to her delight, that she was pregnant.

The second transition point on the timeline was a huge disappointment for her. She described herself as being ecstatic that she was pregnant, but when she told her husband, he responded with great anger when she confessed to him that she had stopped her birth control. There was never any consideration that they would not continue with the pregnancy, but her experience of his reaction devastated her: she was happy and wanted to have a 'big happy family' but her husband's anger overwhelmed her experience of the excitement of the pregnancy.

Telling other people was another critical point: in contrast to her husband, her parents were also extremely excited, particularly because this was their first grandchild. They were quite critical of her husband's reaction, and frequently told Maria that it was 'too bad that he is ruining the experience for you'. A bit more history revealed that they had 'never really approved of him' as he was from a different religious background, and that they saw this as yet another failing on his part. She increased her contact with them during the pregnancy, planning and going shopping with her mother for baby things because her husband's reaction was 'so disappointing'.

As the story developed, the therapist artfully guided Maria to provide more information about her experience, asking questions such as:

What was that like for you?

How did you manage that?

How did you communicate that to your husband?

Gradually she also began to ask Maria to think about how her husband was reacting, and what he might have been thinking and feeling. The goal was to foster a different perspective for Maria: though her original conceptualization had been a very simple statement that her husband was not helping, there was clearly much more to the story, and a history that influenced everyone's reactions. Helping Maria to understand first that the story was more complex, and second to understand how her husband (and others) might have been reacting, was the goal.

Maria finished the timeline by talking about how her husband had 'really pulled things together' at the delivery and in the hospital, and how she had felt that he was very supportive in being with her and coaching her. The day after the delivery, however, her parents had arrived with the intention of staying for a month to help care for their new grandchild. Her mother 'swooped in and took things over'. While she appreciated this initially, as the story unfolded Maria began to describe that she resented her mother 'telling her how to do everything' and that her mother did all of the fun things like holding and playing with the baby, but was not helping out at all at night.

As the discussion unfolded further, Maria stated that she could understand a bit more about how her husband might have felt displaced by her parents, though 'he still should be helping more'. The therapist asked her *how well she felt her husband understood her experience*, to which Maria replied that he clearly did not understand what it was like to be a mother nor what it was like to be responsible for all of the childcare. The therapist also asked her *how well she understood her husband's point of view*. After a pause, she responded that she really hadn't thought much about how her husband might be reacting to things until the discussion in therapy.

The obvious point of intervention was to ask Maria what she thought might be helpful to deal with the transition and to foster better understanding with her husband. Appearing somewhat reluctant once again, she responded that perhaps it might be helpful to have another discussion with him about their experiences through the pregnancy and postpartum. The therapist considered giving Maria a homework assignment, but given her reticence about wanting to talk to her husband, elected to simply make a suggestion. Specifically, she suggested that Maria might want to take the Life Events Timeline with her to use as a way of introducing the topic with her husband; other patients, said the therapist, had found it quite useful as a start to discussions, and some had even asked their partners to mark up the timeline with points that they thought were important.

One of the critical things increasing the likelihood that she would open the discussion with him was that Maria now had practice in telling the story and relating her experience in a different way. Working through the timeline with the therapist had literally given her practice in presenting things in a more introspective way, and in a way that was not confrontational. Constructing and discussing the Life Events Timeline was practice in putting the transition into context and describing its complexities and nuances. Consistent with all of IPT, one of the goals was to have her tell that story – to describe her experiences – to her husband, and to help him understand what her experience and thoughts and emotions were like, and to ask him to help her understand his experiences as well.

A very wise patient once described the transition she was going through with her husband as a dance. Prior to the transition – in this case having a baby – she and her husband had a very good relationship. They were both dancing the tango, had learned to adapt to one another, and knew each other's moves. It was effortless and beautiful. Once the baby came, it was as if a third partner entered the dance. The couple was disrupted, and in order to try to accommodate the change, her husband had started dancing the waltz while she had been dancing the foxtrot. They were struggling because they were stepping on each other's feet, and needed to learn to dance together, and as a threesome, once again.

This magnificent metaphor was from a patient who was gracious and insightful; who saw the problem not as one that she was going through alone, but one that she and her partner were experiencing in different ways. Her partner was in session to hear it, and to appreciate her desire to understand him as well as to tell him her story. Needless to say, they did very well in therapy.

Role Transitions: Techniques

Clarification

The process of more fully understanding the patient's experience relies heavily upon the technique of clarification. The therapist should generally maintain the focus of discussion upon the transition, and explore details about the specific aspects of the patient's roles both before and after the transition and associated points on the Life Events Timeline. The therapist should also ask questions which clarify how the patient has come to see things as they have historically. When clarifying the transition, the therapist's tasks are to:

- Understand the patient, and to help the patient better understand the details of the circumstances and transition
- Engage the patient's affect so that change is facilitated
- Help the patient recognize and describe any sense of loss and subsequent ambivalence or anxiety about her transition
- Help the patient to conceptualize the transition in a more balanced, realistic, and meaningful way
- Help the patient develop new social supports.

To an untrained observer (including many in the patient's social network), a Role Transition might not appear to be a loss experience at all, and in some cases it may be seen by others as an overall positive change. In contrast, the therapist must work to understand the nature of the Role Transition from the patient's perspective, and to understand its meaning in the patient's life. As the therapist does so, not only will the patient's perspective become clearer to the therapist, but the patient should also come to understand her circumstances more fully. The Life Events Timeline is a tool to facilitate this: a structured way to listen well.

As an understanding of the patient's perspective develops, the therapist is more able to empathize with the patient's experience in the change of roles. As empathy develops, it can be communicated to the patient and can validate her sense of loss and her anxiety or ambivalence about undertaking the new role. The communication of empathy will foster the therapeutic alliance, and the recognition and management of anxiety about the future is also greatly therapeutic.

Engage the Patient's Affect so that Change Is Facilitated

The patient's emotional reactions in all of their detail should be discussed and described. Among many may be the patient's sadness at the loss of the old role and anxiety about the new role. There are likely many others, all of which are important to elucidate so that the therapist can understand the patient better, help her to understand her own experience better, and help her to tell the story to others and to communicate her need for support and understanding to them. All of the complex and conflicting thoughts and feelings should be acknowledged and explored by the therapist and used as motivating factors to help the patient manage the role transition.

Recognize and Describe Any Sense of Loss and Subsequent Ambivalence or Anxiety About the Transition

Even in the best of circumstances, change is stressful. Patients nearly always have a sense of loss or ambivalence about the old role, though social pressure or relationship factors may lead the patient to feel that her mixed or negative feelings are difficult or impossible to discuss with others. Creating a therapeutic space to talk about these feelings and providing a listening ear is always helpful. As in other areas of IPT, the therapist should help the patient organize her narrative, and then encourage her to share it with others in her social support network.

Help the Patient to Conceptualize the Transition in a More Balanced, Realistic, and Meaningful Way

The therapist should attempt to clarify the patient's perceptions of the positive and negative aspects of the old and new roles in order to help the patient develop a more balanced and realistic view of the transition. 'Realistic' refers to an understanding of the complexities of the change: rather than a simple single transition point, nearly all transitions include multiple meaningful events both prior to and after the identified transition. In this way the patient may come to see that the loss of the old role is a complex experience that may have its advantages as well as its disadvantages. The same is true for the new role – the patient should be encouraged to explore and articulate the positive and negative aspects of the new role. Helping the patient to recognize her ambivalence and to develop a balanced and meaningful view of both roles is the goal.

As described above, a classic Role Transition is childbirth. A new mother may see that her life before having a child had the advantages of freedom, career progression, and ample leisure time. Intrinsic to the old role is a comfortable and familiar social support system which may be dramatically affected by change in child status. She may also feel that parenthood leaves her tired, with little freedom, and with less time to spend with her partner. After conceptualizing the passage into parenthood as a Role Transition, the patient and her therapist review and clarify the positive and negative aspects of both the old and new roles. While doing so, the woman may recognize that, from a different perspective, she greatly enjoys being a mother, and in her old role had lost touch with friends who had entered parenthood. Despite the loss of some social support, she may recognize that having a child leads to new social connections as she spends more time with friends who have children (Figure 15.5). Insightful patients will also recognize that their partners also undergo major Role Transitions, though the experiences of those transitions vary greatly.

The patient and therapist should review the details of the Life Events Timeline, and can also develop a list of the positive and negative aspects of the old and new roles to develop a more balanced and realistic view of the transition. By doing so, the therapist can be most effective in helping the patient come to a resolution in the transition by helping her describe her transition experience. Becoming a parent is a profound transition, and one which is often difficult to describe. A therapist who is genuinely interested in the patient's unique experience can bring about tremendous change simply by encouraging the patient to talk about what having a baby is like – the therapist's empathy, warmth, interest, and caring go a long way. Asking questions such as 'What is it like to be a new parent?' 'What is it like to hold your child?' 'What about parenthood is different than you expected?' 'What does it feel like to care

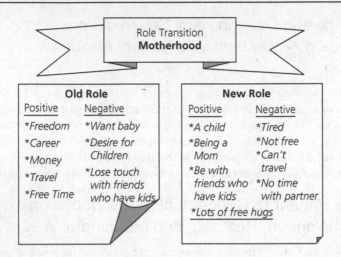

Figure 15.5 Role Transition of motherhood

for your baby?' and especially, 'What is it like to love someone like you do your child?' are literally life-changing ways to get the patient to think and talk about her experience.

Help the Patient Develop New Social Supports

The transition to parenthood is also an excellent example of the need to address social support in the new role. In addition to coming to a more balanced view of the transition, the patient should be encouraged to develop new social supports – people who can connect with her experience and whom she feels understand it better. New relationships provide both emotional support and help to meet the patient's attachment needs in the new setting.

Describing the Patient's Experience After the Transition

Patients who present for treatment tend to view their new roles as difficult and laden with challenges that they may feel incapable of meeting. Patients with less secure attachment styles may overestimate the scope of their challenges and underestimate their capacity to meet them. New roles become stressors for these patients as they attempt to cope with challenges they feel that they are not able to overcome. The therapist must help such patients to reappraise the challenges of the new roles and their ability to deal with the transitions, and should also help them develop new social supports. Consider as an example a patient who has developed depression in the context of being diagnosed with adult-onset diabetes mellitus. His appraisal of the new role he has been forced to assume – 'a diabetic'– may be that it is a process of increasing ill health and disability, full of difficulties such as the need to adhere to demanding lifestyle modifications, to take medications, and to make multiple visits to doctors, podiatrists, and dieticians. Many people would see this new role as an overwhelming challenge they felt poorly equipped to meet.

In cases like this, the therapist should first help the patient to develop a Life Events Timeline, which likely includes onset of symptoms, health concerns, diagnosis of diabetes, and other significant events before and after the actual diagnosis. As with all transitions, the timeline arrow pointing to the future is critical, because it allows the therapist to ask questions about what lies ahead, as well as to make explicit that the future is not yet written in stone – there are choices still to be made and hope on the horizon.

The therapist should then work back through the timeline and elicit descriptions from the patient about his old 'healthy' role, encouraging him to describe the experience of loss of the healthy old role, and to discuss how the change has affected his sense of self and his relationships with others. The therapist should also help the patient to develop a more balanced view of the new role. While this may be difficult in a situation in which the patient's appraisal that the new situation is mostly negative is accurate, the therapist can often discuss the life change as a point at which the patient can reassess his priorities and make a conscious decision about how to structure relationships and life in the future. Many patients are able, after working through the loss of health, to use the change as a point of transformation – a 'wake-up call' – and to use it to reassess their life goals and priorities.

The therapist should help the patient to consider some of the other potential positive aspects of the new role and future transition points, such as the opportunity to adopt a healthier lifestyle, and the recognition of a potentially fatal medical condition which had previously been unrecognized and can now be safely treated. The therapist should also help the patient to reassess the challenges of the new role, such as adherence to lifestyle adjustments such as dietary requirements, and should help the patient develop the interpersonal support needed to put these into practice. For instance, the patient may want to enlist his wife for both interpersonal support and practical support with his new dietary requirements. Other friends may be enlisted for help with exercise and other lifestyle changes.

The therapist can also help the patient to begin to communicate his experience of illness. In addition to enlisting social support, the patient can also begin to more fully meet his attachment needs by communicating his experience in a way that others can understand and can respond to. As a therapist, asking questions such as, 'How well do you think others understand your experience?' and 'What can you do to help others to understand your experience more fully?' are of great benefit.

Role Transitions: Additional Therapeutic Tactics

Patient Does Not Conceptualize the Problem as a Role Transition

As with all IPT Problem Areas, the patient's perceptions and expectations of particular events in her life may be vastly different from the inference drawn by others. It is the task of the therapist to help the patient recognize that her distress is temporally related to a particular acute event or change in circumstances, and to help the patient conceptualize this connection as a Role Transition. The Life Events Timeline is an obvious concrete way to do this. However, as with other Problem Areas, it is not necessary to 'diagnose' a Role Transition – it is vastly better to allow the patient to use terms which are meaningful for her. The interpersonal areas should be used flexibly with the primary goal of maintaining an interpersonal focus. For example, a woman who has become depressed in the context of her daughter leaving home for college may not choose to conceptualize this as a Role Transition, but see it instead as a Grief and Loss issue or perhaps an Interpersonal Dispute with her daughter who is attempting to establish herself as an adult in a context outside of the family. The therapist should acknowledge the patient's view of the problem, and work with the patient collaboratively rather than attempting to diagnose or impose the term Role Transition at the risk of damaging the therapeutic relationship.

There is a great deal of overlap between all of the Problem Areas in IPT. For instance, a divorce could be considered a Grief and Loss issue, a Role Transition, or an Interpersonal Dispute. All of these may be complicated further by being intertwined with fearful or dismissive attachment styles. Similarly, the death of a significant other may involve Grief and Loss issues, or involve transition issues as new responsibilities are assumed and new social supports are needed. The primary purpose of the Problem Areas in IPT is to focus both the patient and clinician on specific interpersonal problems and to maintain the interpersonal focus of treatment. For the clinician to insist on diagnostic specificity is simply to assume that the clinician is more familiar with the patient's problems than the patient is, an assumption which keeps the clinician from truly listening to the patient. The therapeutic alliance should never be sacrificed in order to force a patient into a particular conceptualization of her problem.

An astute therapist can use the discussion about how to conceptualize the patient's interpersonal problem as a means of enhancing the alliance by further clarifying the issue with the patient. For example, rather than rigidly interpreting for the patient that her problem must be a Role Transition, the therapist can 'offer' a tentative view which the patient can then accept or reject. This has the benefit of conveying to the patient a desire to understand her perspective more fully, and will go a long way towards enhancing the alliance. Further, this also allows the patient a more collaborative role in the therapy, and encourages her to offer the therapist important clarifications or additional information about how she perceives the problem.

The therapist might say to the preceding patient, for example:

We have approached the problem with your daughter as a 'dispute', and your communication and problem solving skills have really improved. I think I sense that there are still some things distressing you about the change – you've said on a few occasions that 'Maybe she needs to get on with her own life'. Perhaps it would be helpful to think about how the change in your relationship with your daughter has affected you and how you might be feeling about being the mother of a college student. What are your thoughts about looking at some parts of your experience as a Role Transition in addition to a dispute?

The Patient Does Not Recognize the Complexity of the Role Transition

Patients may have difficulty in understanding the transition as complex as opposed to seeing it as a single transition point. The use of the Life Events Timeline will help to deal with this, as it implies that there is a chronological flow to events, and that preceding events influence those that come after. Patients may also over- or underemphasize the positive or negative aspects of the transition. The effects of the patient's mood upon her thinking patterns may be particularly significant in influencing this assessment. In these circumstances the therapist can:

- Review and further clarify the aspects of the transition
- Highlight the likely effect of depression or anxiety on the patient's view of the role
- Empathically and gently note that despite her feelings about the lost or gained role, the transition has occurred, and the goal is to help the patient cope as well as possible with a difficult change.

The last point is particularly salient in IPT. The bottom line is action – the therapy is designed to help the patient cope and function maximally given the change.

The Patient Describes or Displays Little Affect when Describing the Transition

Some patients have difficulty experiencing or expressing emotion within the therapy sessions or in their life in general. This may be addressed by examining Interpersonal Incidents in which the patient may have experienced distress or other relevant affect. The patient will likely exhibit some degree of affective shift using this technique. The therapist can also use the technique of highlighting content and process affect. The question 'What are you experiencing as you are describing your experience right now?' is often very helpful. If the patient continues to have problems despite these techniques, the therapist can focus upon the more practical aspects of helping the patient to adapt to the transition, in the expectation that this, even in the absence of affective involvement, will aid in the reduction of symptom severity.

As a general rule in all therapy, and in IPT in particular, the more affect that is experienced by the patient, the more likely change is to occur. Therefore asking questions, with genuine interest, about how the patient feels or reacts emotionally to situations should be a focal and frequent intervention.

Case example 15.2: Terry

Terry was a 49-year-old married business executive who had been admitted to a general hospital with severe chest pains. Investigations demonstrated Terry had suffered a significant anterior myocardial infarction. Terry was also found to have elevated blood glucose and to be moderately hypertensive. After 3 days in the hospital's coronary care unit, Terry was seen by an endocrinologist, who diagnosed type 2 diabetes mellitus and instituted management with diet and oral hypoglycemic medication. After being examined by his cardiologist, Terry was also started on antihypertensive medication.

After being visited by his cardiologist, Terry complained to the nursing staff that he was unhappy with the consultation and wanted a second opinion. This was arranged, and another cardiologist confirmed the diagnosis of hypertension and also concurred with the recommended treatment. Terry became angry with the second cardiologist, and attempted to discharge himself against medical advice. A psychiatrist was called to see Terry in the coronary care unit. She gave Terry an opportunity to ventilate his frustrations and discuss his feelings about the situation. He reluctantly agreed to remain in the hospital, and she left Terry her details should he wish to contact her again.

Several days later, Terry was discharged and referred to a cardiac rehabilitation facility. After about 3 weeks, the psychiatrist received a phone call from the cardiac rehabilitation nurse, who had observed deterioration in Terry's mood. The therapist arranged for an outpatient appointment with Terry. At the conclusion of the evaluation, the therapist noted that Terry now endorsed numerous symptoms consistent with a depressive disorder. Terry told the therapist that he had not had any previous difficulties with his mental health, and that he had been physically well prior to his heart attack. Terry felt that he was unable to deal with the 'triple whammy' of ischemic heart disease, hypertension, and diabetes, as well as the fact that he was now taking so many medications that he 'rattled'.

After further discussion with the therapist it became apparent that Terry was quite driven in his work – he had been a highly successful businessman running his own chain of electronic stores for 20 years prior to his illness. Terry spent a great deal of time during the Assessment/Initial sessions (Figure 15.6) discussing how he had built up his business from 'small beginnings' and how it had become a successful chain of stores. Terry described himself as a 'hard-nosed professional' who had no time to be ill. To illustrate this, Terry stated to the therapist, 'in small business the weak are killed and eaten by their competitors'.

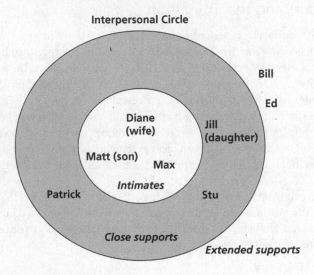

Figure 15.6. Interpersonal Circle – Terry

When the therapist inquired about Terry's feelings about being diagnosed with heart disease and with diabetes, she noted a marked shift in Terry's affect. Terry became tearful and dysphoric when discussing the impact of the event on his life. The therapist reflected the following to him as they were developing an Interpersonal Formulation:

> Terry, it seems that you have developed a number of symptoms that I think indicate you have developed a clinical depression. You have obviously been a strong and capable man throughout your life, and this catastrophic development in your physical health seems to have really overwhelmed you. I can certainly understand that this is your first experience with ill health, and it is a massive one at that. There are many reasons why people become depressed, but it seems that for you – quite understandably – that this particular event has been the main cause.

> I think that you would benefit from some counseling that focuses on how you can best adjust to your new health circumstances, and the impact that your health problems are having on your life. I think that there is also good reason to consider trying an antidepressant medication, and I think this would be of benefit to you. However, I also understand that you are reluctant to take yet another pill. I think that if we were to meet for about 12–14 sessions of interpersonal psychotherapy we would be able to address this issue in a more structured way, which would be of great benefit to you.

> What are your reactions to that?

The therapist's presentation captured many of the elements of a good formulation, and highlighted the importance of the delivery. First, she allowed Terry to respond to her tentative hypothesis regarding his Role Transition. This was particularly important given the fact that Terry described himself as fiercely independent. The therapist realized that she needed to give Terry even more of a sense of control than many other patients might need. Second, there was a clear sense of developing a collaborative relationship. The therapist was able, however, to maintain her role as a 'benevolent expert', setting up a positive transference relationship which could be maintained through the brief course of therapy.

As they further discussed the Interpersonal Formulation (Figure 15.7), Terry stated that he felt a strong sense of grief and loss at the change from his previous 'perfect physical health'. The therapist agreed that there were certainly significant Grief and Loss issues present, and she agreed that would be a reasonable way of conceptualizing the problem. The therapist also suggested the possibility that viewing the loss of health as a Role Transition would also be helpful, as it offered a way Terry could talk about the loss of his 'healthy self' while helping him to acknowledge the need to adjust to his new circumstances.

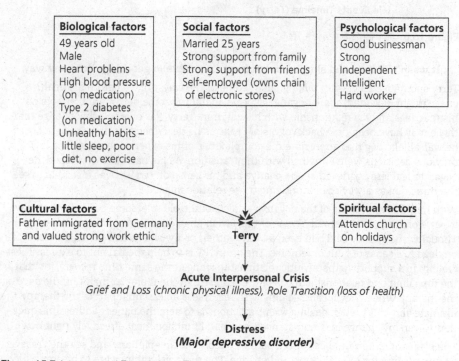

Figure 15.7 Interpersonal Formulation – Terry

Terry initially described his old role as being one of 'strength and invulnerability'. Terry recalled being able to work 16-hour days, 7 days a week:

> **I could get by on almost no sleep – I vowed that no one would every outwork me.**

Initially, Terry's Life Events Timeline (Figure 15.8) was minimal: he identified only the acute medical symptoms and time in the hospital as additional significant time points, and had also drawn a very large and dark mark in the future. The mark was labeled 'BACK TO WORK!!!' which he had underlined several times as well. Terry further underscored it by loudly proclaiming 'That's my only goal'.

The therapist thought about asking Terry directly whether he had any reservations about how his life was before the heart attack, and what might have changed, but on reflection, she realized that this was likely to be too confrontational given Terry's investment in his work and his attachment style. Instead, she simply asked him to describe in more detail what things were like prior to his heart attack. She also directed him to describe more about all of his roles: businessman, husband, and father. Terry responded that

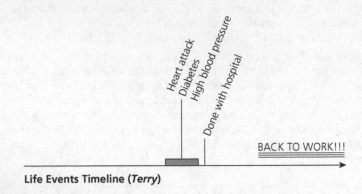

Life Events Timeline (*Terry*)

Figure 15.8 Life Events Timeline – Terry

It wasn't all beer and skittles, but at least I was able to get things done my way.

Terry spontaneously began talking about some of the ways things before his health crisis 'might have had' some negative aspects, including some detrimental effects on his marriage and his relationship with his children. Terry was able to acknowledge that these may have been drawbacks of his old role; as he described this in more detail, he was able to begin to appreciate the complexities of his experience, as well as how previous decisions were entwined with the transition. As his narrative developed, he began to feel less aggrieved by the change and his sense of loss. He was also able to see the transition as a way of reprioritizing these relationships.

With recognition of some of the negative aspects of the old role, some patients often have a sense of grief or loss as well. This is of the 'I wish I had done things differently' type. Thoughts such as, 'I wish I had been a better father' or 'I wish I hadn't gotten divorced' often lead to a sense of guilt or remorse. The art in IPT is to help the patient to express these feelings in a supportive therapeutic relationship while at the same time recognizing that the time limit and relationship focus of IPT require that the therapist maintain the pace of the therapy. While grieving and dealing with remorse is an essential part of the therapy, the ultimate aim of IPT when dealing with transitions is to help the patient address the question: 'Given my change in circumstances, how can I function most effectively right now?'

The ideal outcome would be for the patient to come to an epiphany and see the crisis as an opportunity for re-evaluation and change. The therapist, taking care to be empathic, can often reflect this directly to the patient. For instance, the therapist might say:

> **Despite the loss of health you have experienced, the 'silver lining' is that it has now forced you to think about what you want to do with your life. It has taken you off the 'fast track', and you can now spend some time thinking about how you want your relationships to be. That's what we should focus on in therapy, so that I can help you to follow through with the changes you would like to make.**

The therapist and Terry also discussed his new role. Terry acknowledged that his cardiac rehabilitation specialist had strongly urged him to limit the number of hours he worked, improve his sleep, allow time for exercise, and modify his diet. This would require that he work more routine hours and be home for meals rather than eating restaurant and take-out food. These lifestyle modifications were seen by Terry as important to his health. Terry also felt 'washed out' by his medication. The therapist and Terry engaged in a role play regarding how he might approach his cardiologist (with whom he had the initial disagreement) about changing his antihypertensive medication or looking at alternative interventions without getting angry or appearing demanding.

The focus of discussion then shifted to Terry's business and the need for him to modify his hours. The therapist suggested that Terry might benefit from a problem solving approach:

Therapist: *Perhaps we could brainstorm a few solutions to the problem.*

Terry: *Guess so, wouldn't hurt.*

Therapist: *OK. You've said that the problem is basically the business needs to be manned at least 12 hours a day to maintain the edge over your competitors.*

Terry: *That's right.*

Therapist: *And that you really need to limit your working to six to eight hours per day as well as taking time out to eat a healthy lunch and make sure that you're home in time to do some exercise.*

Terry: *That's right.*

Therapist: *OK. Well, what do you see as potential solutions to this?*

Terry: *Well, I guess one might be to hire some help.*

Therapist: *What would that involve?*

The therapist and Terry then developed four or five potential solutions to the problem. In each instance they evaluated the positives and negatives of the particular option, and Terry chose the one he thought most reasonable. Terry went about implementing this and reported back to the therapist. As Terry was able to make the appropriate lifestyle modifications needed for his health without compromising his business, he described his mood as improving. Terry stated that he still felt a great sense of loss when he reflected on his previous physical health status, but he was able to state that, 'at least I know I'm human'.

IPT offered Terry a way of concretely understanding the change in his life occasioned by his physical health problems. Terry had been provided with an opportunity to reflect on his old physically healthy role and describe in detail to the therapist and others what the loss was like, and also came to realize that his old role was 'not as mentally and relationship healthy as I thought it was'. He had also been provided with a collaborative working relationship which helped him formulate strategies to deal with his new role, which he felt poorly equipped to deal with. The therapist was able to help Terry regain a sense of control over his situation, which was a core loss for him.

Therapy was concluded after 12 sessions. The last two were held biweekly; given his experience in therapy Terry was quite willing to meet with the therapist in 3 months to 'check in' for a maintenance session, with the plan to re-evaluate the need for ongoing maintenance at that time.

Case example 15.3: Bob

Bob was a 40-year-old accountant who was referred by his local doctor for chronic symptoms of low mood. He was amenable to treatment with IPT as well as antidepressant medication. He had difficulty in describing a primary problem, stating that he had felt depressed for a long time and had simply decided that he should come in for treatment. His Interpersonal Circle had a paucity of relationships (Figure 15.9), and included only his parents and an older brother whom he placed in the middle circle and a few friends at work that he placed in the outer circle. Among the interpersonal issues identified during the Interpersonal Inventory were problems he had experienced forming intimate relationships with women. Bob had no current intimate romantic relationships, and was only moderately interested in developing new ones. He also described frustration at work, saying that he felt that he was in a dead end job he'd be doing for the rest of his life, and that he was 'doomed to boredom and a mundane life'.

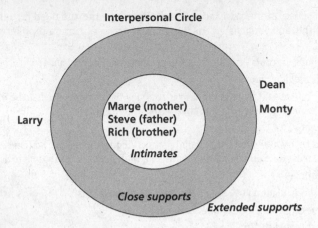

Figure 15.9 Interpersonal Circle – Bob

The therapist was tempted to move into Bob's intimate relationships (or lack thereof), but recognized that it was not likely to be very productive given Bob's apparent lack of motivation and his very clear fearful attachment style. Instead, he worked with Bob to pinpoint *what it was that led Bob to come to therapy at this particular time – the acute crisis*; after all, Bob had been depressed for a long time according to his report, but had never sought treatment until now. What specifically was different? What had changed acutely?

As they talked more, Bob began to describe that things had begun to be more distressing as he was nearing his fortieth birthday. He recounted the day of his birthday: he had received a call from his mother and a note from his brother, and his father had signed the card his mother had picked out. No friends had called, and he had spent the day at home reading a book he had read before and having a TV dinner while watching reruns. It dawned on him that day that this was his life, and even worse, that it was likely to be his life forever. He called in sick the next day and spent the day in bed feeling lonely; although he had 'pulled it together and been responsible' and had only missed one day of work, he had continued to feel dejected and demoralized since.

The fortieth birthday was also significant because his brother at age 40 had already been married for 12 years, had a great job and two kids, and Bob felt by comparison that he simply had not accomplished much. The therapist was tempted to move to a more cognitive approach to address what appeared to be the distorted comparison that Bob was making between himself and his brother. He also found it tempting to use this approach so he would have something or some kind of procedure he could *do to* Bob to make him feel better. Going through specific tasks and assigning homework would be active, and would help avoid the awkward silences that were occurring in therapy as Bob struggled for words. It would be much easier to '*do to*' Bob rather than to '*be with*' him. He was concerned, however, that such an approach, while intellectually appealing, would leave Bob with the same sense of isolation and hopelessness that he brought to therapy. He also felt that using a more cognitive approach would make it difficult to listen to Bob and to really understand what his sense of isolation was like.

Once the time frame of the symptoms were clearer, the therapist suggested as they were developing the Interpersonal Formulation (Figure 15.10) that they think about Bob's experience as a Role Transition. The transition, turning 40, was an acute crisis that had led a smoldering distress to flare up. Turning 40 had provided a different context for Bob, and the realization he had on his birthday was a new and much more dismaying way of thinking about and feeling about his life.

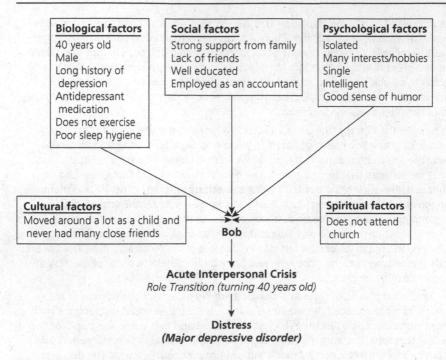

Figure 15.10 Interpersonal Formulation – Bob

They agreed to meet for about 20 sessions of Acute Treatment, with the plan of tapering sessions about halfway through the course. The therapist, slowing the pace, made great use of the techniques of clarification and empathic listening. He encouraged Bob to explain and describe what his situation was like. They developed a Life Events Timeline (Figure 15.11) which was at first quite cursory, but continued to work on it and elaborate it through several sessions. Bob gradually became more comfortable with the therapist, and began to disclose his feelings of isolation and loneliness. He described coping with them largely by convincing himself that he didn't care and wasn't invested in relationships, but that this covered a great deal of pain. The boredom the therapist had once felt, and the long uncomfortable silences, were gradually replaced with a deep sense of caring for Bob as he began to understand his distress.

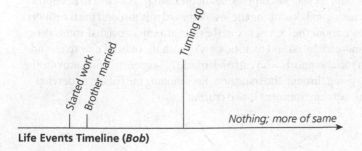

Life Events Timeline (*Bob*)

Figure 15.11 Life Events Timeline – Bob

The therapist made use of the developing therapeutic alliance to suggest to Bob that he still had much of his future ahead of him. The arrow, so to metaphorically speak, was headed into the future. What did Bob want to do? What were his goals? Bob related that he was interested in making some new friends; perhaps a few to go out to dinner with every once in a while, or to talk about books or movies with. Taking care not to assign any overt homework or be too directive, the therapist asked Bob to help him brainstorm some small steps that might get him started in that direction. Bob came up with several: going to a book discussion at the local library, joining a movie group, and asking a woman he knew at work to dinner. The latter two seemed far too difficult to Bob, but he agreed to consider the book discussion.

At this point in the therapy (the latter 10 sessions) Bob and the therapist were meeting every 2 weeks, giving Bob plenty of time to try some social interactions, and gradually lessening the attachment support the therapist was providing. Bob reported in the next session, 2 weeks later, that he had gone to the book discussion, and though he had not spoken much, did enjoy being out and having something different to do. He was planning on going to another one the next week. The next two weeks he set the goal of joining a movie group; this was more serious as it required a commitment to attend regularly rather than simply showing up as Bob was able to do with the book discussion. As therapy moved along, Bob continued to make slow but steady changes in his social activities. The 2-week intervals seemed to match his pace well, and helped him develop a sense of mastery and independence more easily.

At the Conclusion of Acute Treatment, Bob had not yet asked out the woman at his work, but was more confident he would be able to do so. Other social interactions had increased, but most importantly he felt less distressed and that there was hope for the future. The therapist, knowing that his support was still crucial to Bob, suggested that they plan on meeting once every 2 months for Maintenance Treatment. The decision was based on Bob's risk for relapse, an accommodation to Bob's fearful attachment style, and the therapist's recognition that an abrupt termination would be extremely difficult and unnecessary for Bob. In fact, given his chronic depression, all of the empirical evidence pointed towards Maintenance Treatment. Bob readily agreed, saying that he didn't think he needed to come in often, but that he was glad that he could stay in contact with the therapist.

Conclusion

Role Transitions are frequently presenting problems in IPT. Patients are usually able to make connections with the life events which have led to their distress. The strategy in dealing with Role Transitions is to utilize the Life Events Timeline to assist the patient to describe his experience and to begin to appreciate the complexities of the change, as well as to develop a hope for the future. Discussing and describing the loss of the old role through the transition is helpful, as are discussions about the experience of the new and any associated ambivalence. The goal is to develop a more balanced and realistic view of both the old and new roles, and to connect the patient to social supports who can understand his experience and provide the support he needs as he is going through the transition. Encouraging the patient to develop new social supports in his new environment is also crucial.

16

Grief and Loss

Introduction

Loss is a fundamental part of human experience. We live, we die. Those close to us die. And in a myriad of other ways we experience loss: loss of relationships, loss of health, expectations of loss and death of ourselves and others to name just a few. Grief and loss is encountered throughout life.

Human beings who suffer loss endure despair, separation, and a profound sense of isolation, not only from the loss itself, but from a deeply rooted sense that no one else understands them. It is the experience of being alone, of not being connected to others, that makes grief unbearable. A patient described the depth of her isolation after the death of her husband when she told a story of a beautiful sunset. As she sat watching the sun go down and the sky turn a beautiful rainbow of red, orange, and purple against a cloud-filled sky, she had a moment of respite, of wonder, a sense of connectedness to God and humanity that transcended her loss. She turned to her right before she even noticed she was doing so to grasp her husband's hand so that she could share the moment with him, only to have the moment crash into despair as she remembered he was no longer there.

Many theorists and academicians speak of the resolution of grief and loss, as if there were a specific process or set of steps that people should follow. Many, as specified in the *Diagnostic and Statistical Manual of Mental Disorders* (DSM)-IV, use a time frame to determine if the grieving has been too long, terming it 'pathological' if it goes beyond some arbitrary time limit. And many who do not sit with and listen to those who grieve and mourn imply, or even impose, the notion that there is an end to grief, or that there is a way to 'process' it or 'work through it.'

What does this 'working through' really mean? In Interpersonal Psychotherapy (IPT), there is no imposition; no specific way or process that people must follow. Each loss is understood as unique – it is the individual's experience that is important. The therapeutic task is to help the patient develop and, utilizing social support, to communicate his experience of loss, to find connection, and diminish isolation. In the beginning of the process, the therapist steps into the attachment void, providing a human connection with whom to share the suffering. A listening pair of ears, a caring and compassionate soul. Therapist warmth and empathy are crucial to this process.

As the patient tells his story, and his emotions are described and experienced in therapy, the therapist works to help him extend the expression of his loss experience to social supports outside of therapy. The goal is to help the patient understand the loss, to bring coherence to the story, and then to share that story with others. The process of sharing with others will begin to engage social support, diminish the patient's sense of isolation, and begin to help him connect once again – to be in community. While describing, discussing, and sharing the loss in therapy is extremely helpful and is a necessary part of IPT, it is the communication of the experience to others and the development of social support surrounding the loss which characterizes IPT.

IPT is designed to assist the patient to resolve the acute Grief and Loss crisis. There are four specific goals:

1 Facilitate the patient's grief and loss process by listening well
2 Help the patient describe his loss experience
3 Assist the patient to tell others about the experience as a way of connecting and finding meaning
4 Assist the patient to develop new interpersonal relationships if needed, or to modify his existing relationships so as to obtain increased social support.

Grief and Loss: Identification in the Assessment/Initial Phase

In life, there are a myriad of experiences that involve grief and loss. IPT, which deals with real life and real people, should be open to all of these experiences. That means that if the patient conceptualizes or describes his experience as a Grief and Loss issue, then it is. It is not for the therapist to challenge or contend, it is the patient's experience that is important. The grief and loss experience of the patient is for the patient to define, not the therapist. The therapist's role is to understand and connect, to listen well, and to care deeply.

Practically speaking, the Grief and Loss issues in IPT can include, but are certainly not limited to, things like the death of a significant other, loss of physical health, divorce, or even loss of employment. Anticipating one's own death or that of a loved one, a severing of a relationship, or a crisis resulting in a loss of faith may be grief issues. It is always best for the therapist to place the patient's problems within the Problem Area that is the most meaningful for the patient.

Most frequently in IPT the identification of a Grief and Loss issue is readily apparent – it is the problem that has led the patient to seek therapy. On occasion, if the loss involves loss of health, anticipated loss, or loss of relationship, the therapist can gently point out a possible connection for the patient between life events and distress. In either event, the Grief and Loss issue should be identified in the Interpersonal Inventory and Formulation, and agreed upon as a focus of treatment.

In IPT grief need not be categorized as 'normal' or 'abnormal'– it is the task of the therapist to attempt to understand the patient's experience, not to pathologize or label it. To do otherwise leads to tremendous breaches in the therapeutic relationship, conveys to the patient that the therapist is not interested in listening but in diagnosing, and that the therapist, like others in the patient's social network, simply doesn't care. There is no need to categorize grief – listen well instead.

The Features of Grief and Loss

The experience of grief and loss shares much phenomenologically with depression, and their clinical differentiation is often challenging. While clinicians should not pathologize the experience of grief, constant vigilance should be maintained for the development of depression and other psychiatric difficulties in the context of grief. The closer the attachment and the more traumatic the circumstances surrounding the loss, the more vigilant the therapist should be.

While diagnosing depression in a bereaved individual is a complicated process, a few phenomenological features are useful clues to the presence of depression. These include:

- **Self-reproach**: In contrast to individuals with depression, individuals who are grieving are able to retain an intact sense of self and maintain their sense of self-esteem, and generally do not develop excessive guilt.
- **Suicidality**: While bereaved individuals may experience a sense of 'indifference to life' for a time after the loss, this seldom evolves into suicidal ideation or intent.
- **Psychomotor retardation or agitation**: Psychomotor agitation and retardation have been noted to be indicators of severe endogenous or 'melancholic' depression, and do not typically appear as physiological features of grief.
- **Psychotic symptoms**: Individuals with auditory or visual hallucinations should be evaluated for underlying psychotic processes.
- **Lack of reactivity**: Many bereaved individuals will describe a marked loss of interest in their usual activities, but the complete absence of reactivity should be regarded as clinically significant.

Box 16.1 lists additional features which are characteristic of both grief and loss and depression.

Box 16.1 The phenomenology of grief and loss

- Depressed mood or sadness
- Irritability
- Poor sleep
- Loss of appetite
- Loss of interest in usual activities
- Indecisiveness
- Anxiety symptoms such as panic attacks or obsessional thoughts

---

In IPT, there is no meaningful distinction between 'normal' and 'abnormal' grief. Grief is simply the experience of a patient following or anticipating a loss; there is nothing normal or abnormal about it. The primary goal of the IPT therapist is to understand the patient's experience with grief, not to pathologize it, and certainly not to dismiss it by describing it to the patient as 'nothing more than a normal reaction'. Patients request treatment for a variety of Grief and Loss issues; it should be assumed that patients who present for treatment with such issues will benefit from IPT, particularly if the grief or loss is identified as a significant issue from the outset of treatment. As it is not necessary for a patient to have a psychiatric diagnosis to benefit from treatment with IPT, self-identification of a Grief and Loss issue by the patient is sufficient grounds for evaluation for treatment.

Grief and Loss problems are conceptualized in IPT as resulting from two factors, both of which may be operative for the patient who seeks treatment surrounding a loss. The first factor is that the patient's social support system is not sufficient to sustain him through the loss experience. The second is that the patient may not be communicating his needs for support in a way that means others can respond effectively. Both of these factors are obviously strongly influenced by the patient's attachment style, as it influences the extent of the social support the patient has, as well as his capacity to utilize it.

In IPT, the therapist takes the temporary role of a support figure for the patient, and forms a relationship in which the patient can describe and work through his feelings about the loss. While this process might take place in social relationships, it often needs to occur first in the therapeutic relationship, particularly if the patient has difficulty utilizing his social support system. Similarly, those patients who have a limited social support network may also need to use the therapeutic relationship in this situation. Given this conceptualization in IPT, the terms 'complicated' or 'delayed' or 'prolonged' have no relevance. It is simply grief and loss. It is an individual experience. While grief and loss may have common themes, each experience is unique, and each requires careful and empathic exploration.

IPT places the different experiences of grief and loss in a context, a particular social environment: the patient's current social support system. For instance, grief that is experienced long after the physical loss or death is not conceptualized as 'delayed' but rather as an experience of grief and loss in a new social context. An obvious example of this is the experience that some women have following the birth of a child. After a live child is born, the woman has an entirely new experience of connection with her newborn – one she has never had before. As a result, she may experience earlier pregnancy losses such as miscarriages or abortions in a much different and deeper way than before. It is not that some complex repression or intrapsychic process has occurred; it is simply that the birth of her new baby and her experience of connection puts the previous loss in a perspective that was simply not possible before. And the loss is experienced in a new way.

Another example might be a man who has lost his father at a young age. He may have adapted to the loss, gone on to have many other productive and intimate relationships, and by his own estimation and that of friends and family, dealt with the loss well. Then an acute event occurs: graduation from college, or marriage, or perhaps even the birth of his first child – life events at which the absence of his father is acutely and painfully felt. As humans we yearn for our parents to be there – to be present and to share in our success; to have a father's hand on our shoulder as we celebrate our life events; to have a father tell us he is proud and loves us and that we have done well. No repression needed; the loss is simply experienced in new ways that are impossible to anticipate outside of the new context. It is not pathological or delayed or any other fancy psychological label; it is simply the individual's experience of loss.

Grief and Loss: Exploring in the Middle Phase

The basic tasks of working with grief in IPT are:

1 Clarifying the circumstances surrounding the loss
2 Helping the patient describe his experience of loss
3 Creating an environment of acceptance and connection with the therapist
4 Helping the patient tell the story of his experience to others to reduce isolation and facilitate connection.

Clarifying the Circumstances Surrounding the Loss

In the initial sessions, including the process of completing the Interpersonal Inventory, and more so during the middle sessions of IPT, the therapist must often rely heavily on clarification to help the patient better understand the circumstances of his loss. When the patient is in a markedly dysphoric or distressed state, the therapist should usually be less directive while encouraging more information and affect with empathic remarks. In contrast, if the patient's process affect is minimal, more directive questions about the circumstances surrounding the loss and his emotional reaction to it is quite helpful. Specific questions which may be helpful are listed in Box 16.2.

Box 16.2 Questions about grief and loss

- What has this loss been like for you?
- How were things with (the lost individual) around the time they died?
- What are your feelings about (the lost individual)?
- What are the most difficult things about (the lost individual) not being present anymore?
- What kind of support do you have now?
- What have you shared with others about your experiences with your loss?*

*The last question is particularly important as it focuses the patient on developing social support and extending his experience to others.

As the patient clarifies and describes his experiences, he has the opportunity to begin to share those experiences with the therapist, who serves in IPT as an empathic and understanding (but temporary) attachment. The therapist literally steps into the role of a support person for the patient: one who can empathize, understand, connect with, suffer alongside, and *be with* the patient. The extension of this process is the critical second stage of dealing with grief and loss in IPT, as the therapist should encourage the patient to begin to share the experience with others as well. The communication which occurs in therapy sets the stage for the communication which occurs later in the patient's social relationships. In essence, the therapist is literally helping the patient to reconstruct the experience in a way that it can be communicated meaningfully to other people.

Specific questions about the actual loss experience and the events surrounding the loss may be of great help in this process (Box 16.3). This is because the process of thinking about and describing concrete events and the circumstances surrounding them leads easily into the process of describing emotions and psychological reactions to the loss. Beginning with the facts usually leads the patient fairly rapidly into the emotions that accompany them.

Box 16.3 Questions about the loss experience

- How did you find out (the lost individual) had died?
- What was your reaction to this news?
- What was the funeral like?
- What was your mourning process like at the time?
- What kind of support did you get at the time?
- What would you have liked from others at the time?
- What kind of support are you getting now?
- What kind of support would you like now?

Helping the Patient Describe his Experience of Loss

The presence of painful and strongly felt emotions is for many patients the most distressing aspect of grief. Invariably, a patient's psychological coping mechanisms and attachment style will moderate how this manifests clinically. While the IPT therapist should not aim to overwhelm the patient, it is often helpful for the therapist to ask the patient to describe his experiences despite the temporary distress it may produce. In order for the patient to experience the affect associated with the loss within the session, he will need to feel secure within the therapeutic relationship.

The description of experience and connection with the empathic listener is conceptually important in IPT; it is not a matter of 'acceptance', 'resolution' or 'catharsis'. 'Acceptance' of the loss is not a goal because the term has no meaning across the experiences of different people. To some, acceptance might be experienced as a peace of mind, or seeing a greater purpose in a loss. To others, it may be a grudging acknowledgment that since the loss occurred, the best course is to cope with it and adapt as best as possible. To others, it may mean the realization of human frailty – a recognition that we cannot control our own destinies. Each individual is different; there is no target outcome or 'acceptance' that is optimal, and it is not for the therapist to impose one.

Likewise the concept of 'resolving' grief is not meaningful across experiences. The term implies that the grief will come to an end; that it will go away and not be experienced any more. Those of us who have lived real lives can attest to the fact that this is not the case. Simply asking someone to 'tell me about someone close to you that you have lost' will inevitably call back to mind difficult or painful losses. In IPT, these losses are seen as all the more beautiful because they can be experienced: they are testaments to the lost person. There is, to be sure, a qualitative difference between recalling a loss and feeling overwhelmed by it. But the goal in IPT is not to make the feelings or the experiences go away, nor to resolve the grief, but to connect with others as we share the human experience of loss, and to find meaning in the connections.

'Catharsis' implies that some intrapsychic processes have led the patient to repress or suppress the experience of loss, and that if they can simply discharge it, like water down a drain, the distress will diminish or go away. 'Catharsis' in this sense is an impossible goal. Instead, telling others about the loss is important. There is healing simply in *connecting with* and *telling to* someone else who cares. Telling others – first the therapist and then other people – is a way of gaining support and understanding of our experience, of decreasing our sense of isolation, and of finding meaningful connection in our shared experience of loss. It is forming community with fellow human beings in the deepest sense. It is attachment.

Because of this, the importance of developing a productive therapeutic alliance cannot be overstated. While recognition of grief and loss and therapeutic techniques are all helpful, the therapist must establish a caring and empathic relationship with the patient. There is great value in helping the patient to describe his experiences of grief to an empathic and understanding listener – this is the therapist's primary task when working with grief and loss. Once the patient begins to communicate his experience with loss in therapy, the therapist can help direct the patient to begin to share his experience with others outside of therapy as well.

The experience of grief commonly involves layers of feelings surrounding the loss. Assisting the patient to describe his experience in detail, to develop a 'three-dimensional' picture of the lost person, including a realistic assessment of the person's good and bad characteristics, is a helpful process in working with grief. On occasion, the patient will initially describe the lost person in idealized terms, and be unaware that this idealization (or devaluation) covers other feelings which may be difficult to accept. The discussion of and development of a balanced view of the lost individual greatly facilitates the mourning process. In essence, part of the grief work involves moving the patient to a securely attached way of experiencing, thinking about, and describing the lost individual as a 'whole person' with both positive and negative qualities.

This same process can be used for other losses as well, for example, the loss of a job, a divorce, or loss of physical functioning. In such instances it is also helpful for the patient to describe his experience of loss, and to move towards establishing new social relationships which will provide more support. Encouraging the patient to develop a more realistic and balanced view of his loss, then sharing it with others, will be of help.

Creating an Environment of Acceptance and Connection with the Therapist

Bowlby has described a 'secure base effect' in attachment relationships, in which the sense of emotional security in the relationship allows an individual to explore and take emotional risks that might otherwise be difficult.[1] This is absolutely crucial in IPT (and in all other kinds of therapy as well), and forms the basis for the therapeutic alliance. All of the interventions used in IPT rest upon this foundation.

The therapist should be sensitive to the profundity of the loss for the patient. Some patients may have a very deep sense of grief to losses others may consider minimal. As always in IPT, the therapist's job is to understand, not to diagnose, minimize, or prematurely reassure the patient. To minimize the importance of a loss, even with a well-meaning reassurance that 'things will get better' or 'thing will pass with time' serves only to cut off the conversation and to sever understanding. It is not helpful for the patient.

Moreover, the use of IPT should be open to anyone requesting help with a Grief and Loss issue. Whether depressed or not, patients requesting help with their grief experiences deserve help. It is what we do – it is what we are called to do. IPT is extremely well suited to working with grief and loss, to listening well, to providing support, and to caring for the people we work with. Those without 'diagnosable' depression are likely even better candidates for IPT and are likely to respond to brief treatment with it.

Helping the Patient Tell the Story of His Experience to Others to Reduce Isolation and Facilitate Connection

As the patient begins the process of understanding and integrating his grief experience, the distress of being isolated is often the most difficult experience of all. This is nearly always coupled with a sense that no one else can understand the depth of the loss, nor the depth of the patient's personal experience with it. The first step in IPT is for the therapist to literally step into this void and to provide support and understanding to the patient. If this is done well, the experience of connecting with the therapist and feeling better understood should lead the patient to want more of the same outside of therapy. The therapist can help the patient to initiate and develop new relationships (attachments) that help to reduce isolation, fulfilling many of his emotional, physical, attachment, and social needs.

No one can ever replace a loved one who is lost. There are no substitutes. Each person is unique; each relationship is unique. The therapist must take care never to state or even imply to the patient that the lost person can be replaced – to do so will destroy any sense of empathic resonance that has been established. Instead, it should be acknowledged that human relationships and social connections and attachment are important to everyone, and that the patient still has the need and the capability to maintain old relationships as well as to develop new ones – support and connection are to be found in them. Relationships give meaning and purpose to life, and the isolation that often occurs following a loss can leave the patient bereft of meaning as well as experiencing grief over the lost individual.

Grief work in IPT therefore involves helping the patient to begin to reconnect with others, and to form new relationships as well. This can be done in large part by encouraging the patient to begin to share his experience of loss with others. This accomplishes two things: it helps develop needed social support, and as the patient describes the experience to others, he will continue to understand it more fully and integrate it more fully into his own experience.

Grief and Loss: Additional Therapeutic Tactics

Dealing with Anticipatory Grief

Anticipatory grief and loss is not a diagnosis or category, but it may be used by some patients to describe their experience as they deal acutely with their own dying or the inevitable death of others they love. Patients whose spouses or parents are disabled with progressive dementing illnesses, or are dying of chronic or malignant diseases are examples of this kind of grief. The Grief and Loss Problem Area is extremely appropriate to use as a means of focusing treatment in IPT on experiences like these; helping patients to cope with anticipatory grief issues allows patients to describe and share their experiences with the anticipated loss as it is occurring. There may also be opportunities to discuss the upcoming loss with the person who is dying, giving patients the opportunity to attempt to address interpersonal conflicts with the involved person, rather than regretting not having done so.

When the anticipated death is caused by a process that allows the dying significant other to interact and communicate with the patient in a meaningful way, the patient can address the issues in the relationship that are conflictual both in therapy and with the significant other, working to put emotional affairs in order. Many patients will value the opportunity to explore this aspect of the loss, and this clinical situation is often one of the most fertile grounds for achieving change in IPT.

All of the techniques used for grief and loss can be used when dealing with anticipatory loss. For example, asking the patient to describe his reaction to the news of cancer, to a terminal diagnosis, or to a progressing dementia, can be very helpful. Asking what the patient expects to happen over the next few months or years, and even expectations about the funeral, are also useful. The utility of discussing these issues should be clear – dealing with them in an anticipatory fashion allows the patient to construct support before the fact, and to talk about what kind of support is needed and how it might be obtained ahead of time. This allows the patient and therapist to literally preempt potential problems that must be dealt with retrospectively in cases in which the death has already occurred.

Working with Dying Patients

The IPT therapist can use the anticipatory grief approach when working with patients who are anticipating their own deaths. The goals are to help the patients enlist social support during the end stages of their illness, and to communicate their experience to others. Further, creating a therapeutic relationship in which they can literally grieve their own anticipated loss is also extremely important. Several writers have described the pathway to accepting death,[2] perhaps the most well-known being Kubler-Ross,[3] who described a process of 'anger' giving way to 'denial' which proceeds to 'bargaining' and ultimately 'acceptance'. In IPT, though this theoretical perspective is helpful, it is critical not to impose a rigid structure or expectations for grieving upon the patient. To do so, particularly to convey or directly tell the patient that he has to go through particular 'stages' of grief, invalidates his personal and unique experience with grief. The therapist should serve instead as a listening ear for the patient, working towards encouraging and helping the patient to extend communication outward to his social support network.

The Patient Who has Difficulty Experiencing or Expressing Emotions

Some patients' affective experience may be so tightly defended psychologically that there appears to be little or no meaningful affect to work with. Those with fearful styles, though suffering immensely, may lack the vocabulary or ability to coherently describe their experience. In such cases, the therapist should slow the pace and work even harder to understand the patient. In situations like this, the temptation to reassure, normalize, or suggest that the patient is being defensive will only serve to cut off communication from a very sensitive and distressed patient – the exact opposite of the goal in IPT.

If the therapist believes that the patient is expressing distress as physical symptoms rather than affect, the therapist may choose to connect these symptoms to the loss experience. For instance, a patient with a more dismissive attachment style might present with somatic features such as pain or headache following the death of a parent. Such an individual will likely tolerate the therapist's attempts to link these physical symptoms with his loss experience if they are framed as part of the stress response that all people experience after a loss. A discussion about the patient's experience of stress would then lead naturally into the more affective components of the experience.

It is of paramount importance to pace the therapy appropriately with patients experiencing grief and loss. Rather than insist that the patient 'must resolve' his grief issues, the primary goal of the therapist should be to create an environment in which the patient can begin to share his experiences. This involves active listening, warmth, acceptance, and the conveyance of positive regard to the patient. The therapist should in essence create an attachment relationship with the patient to facilitate this process.

The therapist must not push the patient too quickly or beyond what he is able to tolerate. The goal of IPT is not to iatrogenically create anxiety about an issue to force the patient to confront it, and it is certainly not to precipitate more symptoms. The pacing should be determined by the patient's ability to tolerate the discussion rather than the therapist's agenda. Like other structural adaptations and pacing in IPT, this should be heavily influenced by the patient's attachment style and the therapist's accommodation to it.

There are several options for modifying IPT with patients who have difficulty in recognizing conflicted feelings about a loss. The first is to simply take more time. Rather than rush through therapy in a particular number of predetermined sessions, the therapist can slow down, spend more time exploring the details of the experiences around the loss, and simply *be with* the patient during times of silence. Simply *being with* is a way to listen well. Another option is to change the structure of the sessions so that they are more frequent but shorter, lessening the intensity to a level the patient can tolerate.

A medical analogy is helpful in clarifying this further. There are no elective medical procedures in which a physician can or should impose his agenda on the patient. Patients who are undergoing procedures such as lumbar punctures or endoscopy will often tell their doctor to 'slow down,' or remark, 'that hurts'. Physicians are obligated to slow down or even desist in such cases; it would be completely insensitive to press on despite the patient's distress. The patient–physician relationship demands that the patient give informed consent for the treatment; the therapeutic alliance demands that the physician be sensitive and caring, and not go faster than the patient can tolerate.

In the same way, when patients have difficulty in expressing or recognizing emotion, the therapist should not artlessly impose his agenda or interpretations upon the patient. The patient is in essence saying, 'slow down', and 'that hurts'. No psychotherapeutic treatment should inflict the therapist's agenda upon the patient. Pacing should be determined by the patient's needs in conjunction with clinical judgment.

The Patient Has Difficulty Connecting with Others in His Social Network

When offering the patient a supportive relationship that is in essence a 'secure attachment base', the therapist is – literally and with intent in IPT – temporarily meeting the patient's attachment needs for support and understanding. This is a completely appropriate response by the patient to a severe interpersonal stressor, and a completely appropriate stance on the part of the IPT therapist. Therapy always involves some degree of dependence on the therapist. Patients who do not have social support networks they can depend on during crises, or who are unable to effectively enlist the support that they do have, are behaving productively when they use therapy and the therapist to help resolve their crises.

The issue is not, therefore, dependency on the therapist, but rather dependency for a prolonged period. In IPT the therapist steps into the void to meet the patient's attachment needs for a brief period of time, gradually transitioning to a less intense relationship as the patient engages others in his social network for support and understanding. This should be done as quickly as the patient can tolerate, and will depend on his attachment style and social supports to a large degree. The key in IPT is that the therapist meets the patient's attachment needs for a short time.

Since IPT is conducted with a Maintenance Phase negotiated explicitly by the patient and therapist, there is much less pressure on the Conclusion of Acute Treatment. Were more dependent patients required to terminate with the therapist this might raise all kinds of transference issues and lead to return of symptoms or distress as termination looms. In contrast, the tapering of acute treatment followed by periodic maintenance allows a much more gradual and tolerable transition for the patient from the therapist to social supports outside of therapy.

Direct inquires about the patient's attempts at social connections, as well as assistance in finding appropriate venues for support, such as support groups or religious groups, are helpful in facilitating extra-therapy support and building attachments outside of the therapeutic relationship. The therapist can also give homework assignments to the patient to attend or become involved in such activities.

Case example 16.1: Rob

Rob was a 38-year-old man referred by his local doctor for a depressive illness with which he had struggled for the past 6 months. His local doctor had prescribed an antidepressant for him, although this had done little to alleviate the severity of his symptoms of depression. He described in the Interpersonal Inventory having a few male friends but otherwise little social support (Figure 16.1), and had not been engaged in any meaningful intimate relationships. Though living in his own apartment, he had a great deal of contact with his mother, who lived in the same city.

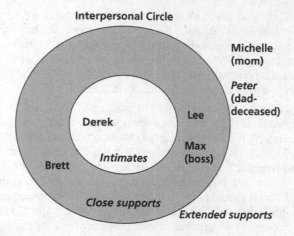

Figure 16.1 Interpersonal Circle – Rob

Rob described that he and his mother were constantly at odds, particularly since his father had died of colon cancer about a year earlier. Rob told the therapist that he had not been particularly close to his father, but felt 'sad that he had died'. He felt that there may have been some connection between his father's death and his depression, but had trouble describing in any detail how it was affecting him. The therapist was able to identify with Rob in the Interpersonal Formulation (Figure 16.2) that the onset of his mood symptoms did seem to correspond to his father's death, and that Rob's psychological distress was clearly impairing his ability to function.

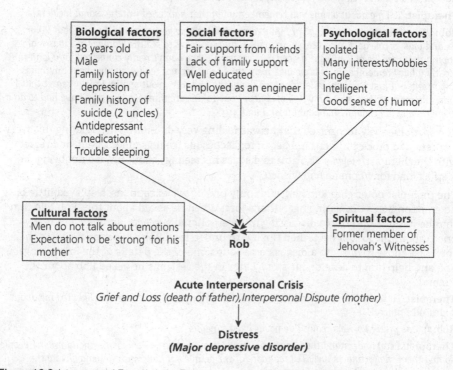

Figure 16.2 Interpersonal Formulation – Rob

Rather than considering his grief as 'normal' or 'abnormal', the therapist simply noted that Rob had identified issues related to the loss of his father, was having difficulty functioning since that time, and was seeking help. IPT was presented as a treatment likely to be beneficial in dealing with Rob's loss. The therapist and Rob agreed to about 12–14 sessions of IPT focusing primarily on Grief and Loss issues; Rob also wished to devote some time to resolve the Interpersonal Dispute with his mother.

As they discussed things in detail in the middle sessions of IPT, Rob told the therapist that he had not been close to his father as a teenager, and had difficulty recounting any specific interactions with his father during his childhood or teen years. He reported that he had contact with his father throughout his adult life, but spoke to him mostly about 'guy stuff' such as sports or home improvement projects. Rob stated he didn't feel losing his father was a particularly devastating blow, but noted that he had at times tried to 'convince himself' that it should have been. The therapist continued to explore Rob's relationship with his father with the goal of helping him to describe his experience more, and to bring coherence and understanding to his experience of the loss.

Therapist: *Rob, we've talked a lot about how things were with your father, including some of your regrets about the relationship. Perhaps we could talk more about the positives?*

Rob: *If there were any.*

Therapist: *I can't help but imagine that there were at least a few. You said as a boy you and he spent time together.*

Rob: *Yeah. We did a lot together.*

Therapist: *How did things change as you got older?*

Rob: *Well, we just didn't really 'connect' like we did when I was a kid.*

Therapist: *How did you connect back then?*

Rob: *Well, we didn't really. We just sort of talked about nothing.*

Therapist: *Tell me about a time you remember when that happened [Interpersonal Incident].*

Rob: *Well, there was one time when I invited my dad to a basketball game. I was about 20 or so, and was at college. My dad came up to visit, and we went to see the Hawkeyes. I was really hoping that we'd be able to have a good conversation … we hadn't really connected for a long time. Mostly what I remember is how we just spent time together, not really talking about anything important, but just being together to watch the game and talk about sports. I really regret that I didn't do more of that later – my dad was never one to initiate things, so I would have had to do it. I never really did though, and now I wish I had …*

Rob spontaneously recognized that he was feeling very different when relating this story (content and process affect), and began to discuss his feelings of loss, guilt, and regret with the therapist. He was also able to discuss his feelings about his dad not being the 'perfect' dad for whom he had wished.

The therapist noted that Rob had, with only one or two exceptions, displayed little or no emotion when discussing his father's loss. When he asked about this, Rob told him that he felt uncomfortable discussing more emotional subjects, and had 'not really cried' about the loss of his father. Hoping to understand Rob's experience better, the therapist chose to move to a discussion about some of the details of the loss to engage Rob and help him to develop his story. Later in the sessions he asked Rob about the funeral.

Therapist: *I'd really like to understand more about what your experience was like. Tell me about your Dad's funeral.*

Rob: *It was pretty horrible really. I've never liked funerals.*

Therapist: *I can understand that – funerals are almost always sad occasions, though many people do find them comforting as well. Tell me more of the details – what comes to mind? [Note the empathy with an invitation to extend the experience to comforting aspects as well. The therapist specifically asked Rob to tell him simply what came to mind rather than asking about a particular* *interaction or a difficult interaction – the pacing is given to Rob to share as he is able rather than forcing the issue.]*

Rob: *I guess what comes to mind was when they closed the curtain and the coffin disappeared.*

Therapist: *What was that like for you?*

Rob: *[Starting to cry] I thought that … that … I would never see him again.*

The therapist sat quietly with Rob while he wept and then began to compose himself. Rob told the therapist that he hadn't been able to cry about his father or the sadness he felt until that moment in therapy. The therapist then highlighted to Rob that it had only been recently that he had begun to describe his relationship with his father in more detail, and that the emotion had soon followed.

In later sessions, Rob and the therapist discussed the newly recognized impact of his father's loss. Rob recognized that he derived comfort from connecting with male friends, and he had begun to share his experiences with the loss of his father with a few of them. One friend in particular seemed to be able to connect well with Rob – this friend had also lost his father and had a similar experience with a father with whom he didn't feel connected. As Rob became more aware of his own reactions to his father's death, his relationship with his mother also improved. Rob's depressive symptoms improved, and in the concluding session he reported feeling 'sad rather than depressed'. This was an important qualitative difference for Rob, as he was able to identify and characterize his emotions, and he reported being able to experience them more fully. The 'sadness' felt appropriate to him, and he no longer had pervasive problems in functioning at work or socially. He told the therapist that the ability to explore his relationship with his father was critical to how he felt and that he was glad to have had the chance to 'put things right in his mind'. They agreed that maintenance sessions would be of help to 'check in', and made plans to meet again in 3 months.

Conclusion

In IPT, Grief and Loss is broadly conceptualized. It includes reactions to a death as well as anticipatory grief of another's or of one's own death. Loss of physical health, loss of relationships as a result of divorce, and a myriad of other types of loss can also be considered grief issues. As with the other Problem Areas, the primary point in IPT is to use the area to maintain the interpersonal focus of treatment rather than to make a 'correct' diagnosis. Listen to the patient and let him decide – it is, after all, his experience.

When working with a patient who is experiencing grief and loss, the therapist has two essential tasks. The first is to help the patient to begin to describe his experience, including emotional reactions in particular. This is done largely through the creation of a therapeutic relationship in which the patient feels secure in dealing with and sharing his experiences and feelings. The second task is to help the patient extend this process outside of therapy. The development of social support is crucial, and can be encouraged by having the patient begin to share his experience of loss with others.

References

1. Bowlby J. *Attachment. Attachment and Loss. Vol. 1.* 1969, New York: Basic Books.

2. Raphael B. *The Anatomy of Bereavement.* 1983, New York: Basic Books.

3. Kubler-Ross E. *On Death and Dying.* 1969, London: Macmillan.

Concluding IPT

17

Concluding Acute Treatment and Maintenance Treatment

Introduction

Acute Treatment with Interpersonal Psychotherapy (IPT) comes to a conclusion, not a termination. Rather than using the traditional psychoanalytic model in which 'termination' is a complete severing of the therapeutic relationship, the completion of Acute Treatment with IPT simply signifies the conclusion of a specific intensive phase of treatment. In IPT this does not signify the end of the therapeutic relationship – in fact, it is often agreed that the patient and therapist will have therapeutic contacts in the future, and provision is specifically made for these. Clinical experience has consistently demonstrated that a longitudinal therapeutic relationship is beneficial for most patients, and this is also clearly supported by empirical evidence. Not only are many of the major psychiatric disorders (such as depression and anxiety disorders) relapsing and remitting in nature, there is also clear evidence that provision of IPT as a maintenance treatment after recovery from depression is helpful in preventing relapse.[1,2] Because of the therapeutic benefit of maintenance treatment and the evidence supporting its utility, the therapist is obligated to discuss continuing Maintenance Treatment with all patients treated with IPT.[a]

Concluding Acute Treatment

Clinical experience and empirical evidence both make clear that IPT should be conceptualized as a two-phase treatment, in which a more intense Acute Treatment focuses on resolution of immediate symptoms and distress, and a subsequent Maintenance Phase follows with the intent of preventing relapse and maintaining productive interpersonal functioning. There are both theoretical and practical reasons for keeping Acute Treatment with IPT time-limited. The time limit theoretically may be effective in generating change, as it is often hypothesized that having an end point helps drive the patient to work more rapidly on improving her communication skills and on building a more effective social network. It should be noted, however, that despite the tempting intuitive conclusion that this is helpful with some patients, there is in fact no data supporting this claim.[3]

[a] Maintenance treatment should actually be discussed with all patients in all therapies.

239

With the exception of a few psychotherapies, there are no medical treatments which are terminated. It simply isn't done. Oncologists never tell their chemotherapy patients that they only get 16 sessions of chemotherapy and then they are terminated. Oncologists continue working with their patients acutely until they are well, then they provide follow-up care as needed. Surgeons don't tell their patients they only get 4 hours in the operating room and then surgery is terminated irrespective of the outcome. Surgeons continue working until the wound is closed. Once acute care is done, post-operative care is provided. Since there is no evidence that termination in IPT is of benefit, and since there are lots of data supporting Maintenance Treatment, IPT should not be terminated either.

There are reasons, however, to keep acute IPT time-limited and to make a distinction between Acute Treatment and Maintenance Treatment. The acute time limit influences both the patient and the therapist to focus on acute symptoms rather than on personality change or change in attachment style. In addition, to extend treatment beyond the 6–20-session limit that is typical of IPT is likely to lead to a shift in treatment as the therapeutic relationship becomes more prominent. As the relationship between patient and therapist assumes greater importance over time, transference moves to the fore and becomes the focus of treatment. In IPT, in contrast to more psychodynamic therapies, the goal is to avoid dealing directly with transference if possible, because it shifts the focus away from the patient's social relationships. While it is appropriate for the therapist to step in as a temporary attachment figure during a crisis, the point in IPT is to transition from support provided by the therapist to support provided by others as quickly as the patient can tolerate and manage it.

The development of transference as a focus of treatment is a function of three factors:

1 *The patient* – the more insecure the patient's attachment style, and the more maladaptive her communications, the more likely transference will become problematic and need to be addressed.
2 *Treatment intensity* – the more often therapy sessions are held (e.g. five times a week versus once weekly versus bimonthly) the more important transference becomes as a therapeutic issue.
3 *Treatment duration* – the longer intensive treatment continues, the more likely transference is to become a focus.

IPT is intentionally structured to minimize the likelihood that these factors will shift treatment from the patient's social relationships to a focus on the therapeutic relationship. This is why IPT is time-limited in Acute Treatment (treatment duration), why it is once weekly with tapering of frequency of sessions as conclusion nears (treatment intensity) and why treatment is not terminated (accommodating patients' insecure attachment styles).

Conducting Maintenance IPT

IPT can be conceptualized as a 'family practice' or 'general practitioner' model of care, in which short-term treatment for an acute problem or stressor is provided until it is resolved, and then maintenance or follow-up treatment is provided as needed. The relationship is ongoing: the patient is welcome to return should another acute problem arise, and is encouraged to return for periodic health maintenance. In IPT, once the acute crisis is resolved, the therapeutic relationship is *not terminated*; as does a general practitioner, the therapist makes herself available to the patient should another crisis occur, at which time another time-limited course of Acute Treatment can be undertaken. In the interim, the patient and therapist may elect, in the same fashion as the general practitioner, to schedule preventive sessions periodically.

In addition to providing quality clinical care, this model also meets the needs of a managed care practice. When there is a limit to the number of sessions that can be provided, whether because of financial limitations, insurance restrictions, institutional rules, or one of the many other irritating and arcane restrictions that may be in place, providing time-limited courses of therapy during crises is a viable way to maximize patient functioning.

This model of intermittent treatment is also extremely helpful in positioning the therapist as a stable attachment figure for the patient. Rather than completely terminating the therapeutic relationship, the therapist can simply make herself available for the patient should other crises occur in the future. Both theoretically and practically there is great benefit within an IPT framework in having the therapist serve as a stable attachment figure for the patient. Many of the patients who come to treatment have attachment styles which incline them to be overly sensitive to threats of abandonment, and forcing a complete 'termination' at the conclusion of Acute Treatment will iatrogenically move the therapy from symptom resolution and the patient's social relationships to a focus on the termination and the transference involved in this very real abandonment by the therapist. *There is no compelling clinical or theoretical reason to come to a complete termination with patients in IPT, and the data clearly support the benefit of Maintenance Treatment.*

Deciding When to Conclude Acute Treatment

In general, the best approach in IPT is to stick to the dosing range in the Treatment Agreement that was collaboratively established at the end of the Assessment/Initial Phase. The most important reason for this is to maintain therapeutic integrity. On the one hand, one of the most important qualities that the therapist brings to treatment is her integrity – the patient must believe that the therapist will follow through with what she agrees to do. Without this trust in the therapist, therapy will fail. On the other hand, the success of therapy is also dependent upon the patient's belief that the therapist is absolutely committed to helping her, and that her needs supersede nearly all other considerations, including a flexible agreement to conclude therapy after a particular number of sessions. Therapy is designed to benefit the patient, not the therapist; IPT should prioritize helping the patient instead of demanding rigid adherence to a manualized protocol, or rigidly demanding that only the exact number of sessions agreed upon can be used. If extending the therapy beyond the number of sessions initially agreed upon is clearly in the patient's best interest, then it should be extended.

The apparent conflict between maintaining the agreement and extending sessions when needed can be resolved quite simply by renegotiating a new Treatment Agreement with the patient when indicated. Clinical judgment and common sense should be used to make such decisions. The following case examples illustrate these practical issues.

Case example 17.1: Joe

Joe was a 38-year-old man who came to treatment for a mild depressive episode which he linked to the death of his father a year ago. Over the course of therapy, it became clear that despite a conflicted relationship with his father, Joe had maintained a mutually supportive marriage of 14 years, had developed a reasonable social support network, and had been productive at work. Joe and his therapist agreed at the end of the assessment to meet for about 12 sessions of IPT.

After making great progress in working through his grief, talking with his wife about his reactions to his father's death, and talking to a male friend who had also recently lost his father, Joe reported that his depression was essentially resolved and that he was doing well. At session 11, however, he requested that therapy be continued indefinitely, as he had 'really enjoyed talking to the therapist, and wanted to meet just in case something

241

else came up'. He began addressing the therapist by his first name, and also began to inquire about the therapist's personal life, such as whether the therapist enjoyed fishing and other outdoor activities Joe enjoyed. While much transference 'grist for the mill' was clearly developing, the therapist determined that Joe had benefited from the acute treatment and was functioning well. As Joe and the therapist had not agreed to long-term intensive treatment, nor did Joe appear to need it to maintain his level of functioning, the therapist determined that sticking to the initial agreement outweighed the potential benefits of continuing therapy. Moreover, the therapist also recognized that continuing therapy would involve a departure from IPT and a move to a more psychodynamic transference-based therapy.

The therapist responded to Joe's personal inquiries with pleasant self-disclosure, indicating that he did indeed enjoy fishing and camping. This comment was immediately followed by a statement from the therapist that such activities were clearly important to Joe, and that it would be of benefit to think about other friends with whom Joe could share these, particularly as they would be a great way to continue to build meaningful interpersonal relationships. Thus the therapist quickly shifted a potential transference encounter to a focus on continuing to develop interpersonal connections outside of therapy. The therapist also reiterated his opinion that it was best to stick to their therapeutic agreement, emphasizing that Joe had both done well in therapy and clearly had the ability to connect well with people.

At session 12, Joe indicated that he felt ready to conclude Acute Treatment. The therapist responded by reiterating that Joe could return in the future if needed – they had already discussed the fact that the death of Joe's mother, among other events, might be a point at which he could return should his symptoms recur.

Case example 17.2: Penelope

Penelope was a 27-year-old woman who entered IPT for the treatment of an acute and severe episode of postpartum depression. Because she was breastfeeding, she declined her physician's recommendation to use antidepressant medication, but did agree to start IPT.

During the course of therapy it became apparent that Penelope had a tendency to be somewhat passive in asking others for help. She tended to expect others to anticipate her needs, and when they did not, she tended to withdraw and isolate herself further. This was evident in her relationship with her husband: she described several instances in which she wanted him to help with household tasks and childcare but had not specifically asked him to do so. When he had not 'read her mind' and done these, she withdrew and described feeling more depressed. In addition, this style was manifest in therapy – early in treatment, she had been quite passive and somewhat difficult to engage as an active participant in solving her problems, often looking to the therapist to 'tell her what to do'.

Despite these tendencies, Penelope had done well in treatment. She had recognized that her communications with her husband were not effectively getting her needs met, and with encouragement, had begun to address her need for help with him directly. He had responded quite positively to her requests, and as she became more direct in her communication, she began to feel more supported and less depressed. With this success, she also changed her in-session behavior, and became more of an active participant in developing new ways to communicate more effectively. She also became involved in a postpartum support group, which she found to be of great help.

After 16 sessions of IPT, she indicated that she was doing well and was somewhat indifferent to continuing in treatment. Despite the transference implications of this statement, the therapist pointed out to her that her depression had been severe, and that both the research on postpartum depression and the therapist's own clinical experience suggested that relapse was a distinct possibility. This was a particular concern because she was not taking antidepressant medication. The therapist took the initiative to suggest monthly maintenance sessions over the next year, with the understanding that, should the depression recur, Acute Treatment would be reinstituted. Additional discussion focused on the possibility of returning to treatment even after the Maintenance Treatment was concluded, as Penelope was at risk for depression during subsequent postpartum periods, and she was planning on having more children.

Case example 17.3: Jane

Jane was a 35-year-old woman with what appeared to be a relatively straightforward episode of depression resulting from her divorce. She had been married for 5 years, and reported that she had felt that she had been cast adrift when her husband unexpectedly left. She had depended on him as her 'best friend' and had cut off several important relationships with female friends in order to be with him. She initially reported confusion about why he had left, and wanted to understand what had happened. An agreement to meet for about 12 sessions of IPT was established at the end of the assessment.

At session 3, Jane revealed that her ex-husband had been a heavy drinker; session 5 brought the revelation that he had been physically abusive to her. He had also been very adamant that she limit her contacts outside of the marriage, which had resulted in a constriction of her social network. In addition to exploring her ambivalent feelings about her ex-husband, therapy focused on re-establishing her social support network. She contacted several of her female friends and began socializing with them, including one woman who had also recently been through a difficult divorce. As her interpersonal support improved, her symptoms did as well, and she reported at session 10 that she felt she was functioning well and was no longer depressed.

During treatment, her fear that others would not meet her needs was manifest in therapy by a reluctance to disclose personal feelings to her therapist. This was evident in the delayed disclosure of the abusive relationship with her ex-husband, and in her concern that 'therapy might not be of help to someone like me', a statement she made early in treatment. At that time, the therapist chose to respond to her comment with reassurance that therapy was indeed quite likely to be of help, and that the therapist had previously had great success with other patients with problems similar to Jane's.

Near the end of session 11, when the conclusion of acute treatment was being discussed, Jane revealed to her therapist that she had been a victim of sexual abuse during her childhood. While the therapist appreciated that sticking to the original Treatment Agreement was important, she felt that it was far outweighed by the importance of this disclosure, and by the distress that Jane was experiencing in discussing it. Further, given Jane's difficulty in disclosing personal issues and the time invested in building a therapeutic alliance with her, the therapist judged it was best if she worked with Jane on the abuse issues rather than referring her to someone else. The therapist initiated a discussion with Jane about this, and they agreed to end IPT and move to open-ended work on understanding the impact of her abuse experience.

There are many other situations in which adding a session or two is of great benefit and clinically indicated. For instance, when working with women who have a pregnancy loss near the conclusion of therapy, when working with patients with new medical diagnoses which arise near the conclusion of therapy, or when working with patients with any variety of life events that happen near the conclusion of treatment who would benefit from several more sessions. Life events happen, and they are just as likely to happen near the conclusion of therapy as at any other point.

In sum, it is generally most beneficial to conclude Acute Treatment as agreed upon by the therapist and patient at the end of the Assessment/Initial Phase. The vast majority of well-selected patients will respond within this time frame and will be able to conclude Acute

Treatment without difficulty. There are both theoretical and practical reasons for concluding Acute Treatment as agreed; however, there are circumstances in which patients will clearly benefit from additional treatment, and in which more treatment is indicated. There will also be cases in which the patient has fully engaged in treatment with IPT, has not responded, and continues to need additional treatment, either from the therapist who provided IPT or from another clinician. In such cases, clinical judgment and common sense should be used to determine the best course of action.

Concluding Acute Treatment: Tactics

In addition to determining whether to conclude Acute Treatment, the therapist must also use clinical judgment to decide how to schedule sessions near the end of the Acute Phase. The clinician should be guided, as in other aspects of IPT, by both clinical experience and empirical data.

The empirical efficacy studies of Acute Treatment with IPT have all relied upon protocols which strictly dictate the use of weekly sessions of IPT, followed by an abrupt termination after a specified and inflexible number of sessions. In these studies, there is no latitude for therapists: sessions must be conducted weekly, and termination must occur – no treatment may be offered to patients at the end of the specified number of sessions, even if they remain symptomatic. These protocols have been used solely to maximize the internal validity of the research (i.e. its replicability), *not* because they reflect best clinical practice.

In contrast, clinical experience with IPT and other therapies strongly suggests that the best clinical practice is to extend the interval between Acute Treatment sessions once the patient is in recovery. Rather than continuing to meet weekly for the duration of treatment, the patient and therapist may choose to meet biweekly or even monthly towards the latter parts of Acute Treatment if the patient has recovered. Six to eight weekly sessions may be sufficient for more highly functioning patients to resolve their acute problems, but they often derive additional benefit from extending session intervals to biweekly or monthly once their functioning has improved. This gives them the opportunity to further practice communication skills, reinforce the changes that they have made, and develop more self-confidence while remaining in a supportive relationship – all of which facilitate better and more stable functioning.

It is also helpful to negotiate the number of *sessions* of therapy rather than a specified number of *weeks* of therapy. Therapy can be conducted weekly until the patient begins to improve; later sessions can be scheduled further apart after discussing the change with the patient. Most patients, if doing well, are quite happy to meet less frequently, and often initiate the discussion about doing so when they are feeling better.

In addition to providing more longitudinal care than acute weekly sessions can offer, coming to a gradual conclusion in Acute Treatment rather than an abrupt termination has other advantages. First, there is less need to focus on the sense of loss that the patient may experience at the conclusion of treatment, as the process is gradual rather than abrupt. Consequently, there is also little concern about the problematic transferential issues that would arise were a complete termination to occur. Second, the gradual conclusion more firmly fixes the therapist as a stable attachment figure while encouraging the patient to function independently. *The therapist should be available, but not necessary, for the patient.*

Finally, a gradual conclusion fosters the patient's hope for recovery and her faith in the treatment. Psychotherapy (at least some non-IPT forms) is the *only* form of treatment offered by healthcare providers in which an iatrogenically created abrupt termination to treatment is imposed. Instead of being terminated, patients expect that they will be provided with help as long as they are suffering – they do not expect that the dictates of a protocol will take precedence over their personal and individual needs. This is a reasonable and humane expectation, and one that is met in IPT.

While an abrupt termination can be theoretically justified as a means to increase the intensity of the transference reaction in long-term psychodynamic psychotherapy, there is no theoretical justification for artificially imposing an abrupt and potentially counter-therapeutic termination in time-limited non-transferential treatments such as IPT. The therapist should use her clinical judgment to determine if and when to schedule sessions at greater intervals as the patient recovers.

Goals for the Conclusion of Acute Treatment

A good conclusion to the intense therapy relationship which develops in IPT is of utmost importance, particularly as the focus of treatment is the patient's relationships and communication with her primary attachments, one of whom, at the conclusion of therapy, is the therapist. As a result of their attachment styles, many patients will be sensitive to the conclusion of the therapeutic relationship even if it is not terminated, and will experience feelings of loss or possibly even rejection. Thus handling the conclusion of therapy well is an essential task for the IPT therapist.

The primary goals of IPT are symptom relief, improvement in interpersonal functioning, and increased social support. A corollary of this is that the specific goals at the time of treatment conclusion are to foster the patient's independent functioning and to enhance her sense of competence (Box 17.1). The task is to help the patient appreciate that she has resources and skills to manage problems, and to squarely attribute therapeutic gain to the patient. As Acute Treatment ends, the therapist should make clear that the patient has improved, has made changes, and has the capability to function independently. The therapist is still available in the background should a future emergency arise, but the expectation is that the patient will not only function independently but do so quite capably.

Box 17.1 Goals of Conclusion of Acute Treatment

- To facilitate the patient's independent functioning
- To enhance the patient's sense of competence
- To reinforce new communication behavior
- To reinforce the use of social supports
- To contract for the provision of continuing Maintenance Treatment as needed

---

Metaphorically, IPT follows the old adage 'give a man a fish and he will eat for a day, teach a man to fish and he will eat for a lifetime'. Ideally, patients learn new communication skills, develop insight into how they communicate their needs, and establish more functional social support networks, all in the service of improving interpersonal functioning. These are all new or improved fishing skills. The metaphor can, however, be extended further in a way consistent with IPT. As with a fishing mentor or teacher, new situations arise in which the student or patient may again desire some expert help. When a patient is fishing for bass, a shark might appear on the line – if so, asking for additional advice is not only helpful but a darn good idea. When appropriate, patients should be encouraged to ask for additional therapy: recognizing when help is needed and asking for it in a gracious and effective manner is a goal in IPT.

At the Conclusion of Acute Treatment the therapist should take the stance that she is available to the patient should difficulties arise in the future. It is essential for the therapist to be experienced by the patient as a stable attachment figure even after Acute Treatment concludes – an attachment figure that should be called upon for help only when circumstances are dire, but one which is available nonetheless. The therapist is, temporarily at least, an important and appropriate part of the patient's social support network. If future crises arise, the ability to effectively call upon extended social support, including the therapist, should be reinforced.

Conclusion of Acute Treatment: Key Issues

The therapist should specifically discuss a number of issues with the patient prior to concluding Acute Treatment. These are:

- Maintenance Treatment
- Continued use of medication
- Discussion of potential future problems and signs of recurrence of distress.

The most important among these is a *discussion about Maintenance Treatment*. There are many alternatives for this, and a *specific and concrete agreement* should be established with the patient for whichever option is chosen. Options range from scheduling maintenance sessions at monthly intervals for patients at high risk to concluding Acute Treatment with an agreement that the patient will contact the therapist should problems recur for those at low risk.

Decisions about how to structure Maintenance Treatment should rely on clinical judgment. Often, they are also guided by logistical and other considerations. For instance, some patients will be receiving medication from a healthcare provider other than the therapist – in this case, there may be less concern about scheduling maintenance sessions as the physician can observe the patient for signs of relapse. Distance is another concern, as is cost; while the benefits of Acute Treatment may make the investment of time required to travel to appointments and the cost of Acute Treatment a wonderful investment for the patient, the cost-benefit equation may not support continued Maintenance Treatment at long distance or great financial cost.

Continued use of medication should also be discussed with the patient. Physicians conducting IPT can do this in the context of the therapy. Other mental healthcare providers should emphasize the need to continue medication even after the conclusion of IPT – patients should be firmly directed to continue medication until they have discussed stopping it with their physician.

The last item which should be discussed with the patient is the *recognition of early symptoms of recurrence*, which may signal another episode of illness or a return of interpersonal problems. Along with this, therapists should explicitly discuss future events which may lead to relapse or recurrence. Many of these will be obvious. A review of the onset of depression may reveal that sleep problems appeared before the full-blown episode occurred; if so, patients should be counseled to watch for such signs and to seek help should they return. In addition, there may be future life events or stressors during which patients are likely to have difficulties and would benefit from maintenance treatment. For example, a woman experiencing postpartum depression may have similar difficulties if she is planning subsequent pregnancies; a patient who has had difficulty grieving the loss of a parent may have similar problems at the death of her remaining parent; a student having difficulty making the transition to university life may have similar problems when beginning his first job. In IPT, therapists should anticipate these potential problems, discuss them with their patients, and plan for treatment in the future should they arise.

Conclusion of Acute Treatment: Techniques

Several specific techniques can be utilized to great effect during the Conclusion of Acute Treatment (Box 17.2). Primary among these is giving direct feedback to patients. In IPT, the therapist should review the progress made in therapy, giving as much positive feedback to patients as is genuinely possible. A review of the problems identified in the Interpersonal Inventory and progress in dealing with these, as well as a review of the associated symptomatic improvement, should be conducted. A specific summary of the positive changes that the patient has made in improving her communication and in developing a social support network should also be provided. Credit for change should be given to the patient – though the therapist has served as a 'coach', the patient has done the difficult work and has implemented the changes.

Box 17.2 Therapeutic techniques for concluding Acute IPT

- Positive reinforcement of the patient's gains
- Discussion of the patient's reactions to the Conclusion of Acute Treatment
- Therapist self-disclosure of reactions to the Conclusion of Acute Treatment
- Solicitation of feedback from the patient about the therapy

It is important to discuss the patient's reactions to the Conclusion of Acute Treatment. These are usually quite positive if sessions have been tapered as conclusion nears, and if the therapist makes clear that the patient can return in the future should the need arise. An iatrogenically created abrupt termination will lead to more difficulties at the termination of therapy. Even in cases in which the conclusion is handled well, however, the patient may have a significant sense of loss which should be directly discussed. The therapist may be one of the few people who have taken an active interest in the patient, or may be one of the few people who have treated her with unconditional positive regard. It is often the case that therapists underestimate the impact of concluding therapy: therapists have many patients, while a patient has only one therapist.

Discussion and acknowledgment of the patient's experience in the concluding phase is a key tactic when concluding IPT. The therapist should continue to listen well, and acknowledge that many people feel a sense of loss at the Conclusion of Acute Treatment, and that this reaction signifies both the effort that the patient has put into the work and the relationship that she has built with the therapist. The therapist should try to link these feelings with the sense of concern that some patients may experience as they fear that they will not be able to maintain their gains without the therapist's support. The therapist should also feel free to use judicious self-disclosure when discussing the end of therapy, and can relate her personal feelings about concluding treatment (assuming that they are positive). This serves three purposes:

1 It further acknowledges the patient's experience of loss
2 It models the direct communication of feelings
3 It reinforces the patient's ability to connect in a meaningful way with others.

For example, a therapist might state to her patient:

I have really enjoyed working with you, and will miss the interaction. I often find it difficult to conclude treatment with the people with whom I work, as I find myself feeling close to them and very invested in their success.

As IPT does not typically focus directly on the patient–therapist relationship, the discussions about concluding should not include questions about the patient's feelings about the therapist on a transference level, nor should they include questions which invite speculation by the patient about the therapist. Patients may ask personal questions of the therapist as the conclusion draws near – the therapist should respond openly and honestly with judicious self-disclosure, and may then redirect the patient to relationships outside of the treatment instead of querying the patient about their motives for asking, or interpreting any transference reactions.

Another helpful intervention when concluding is to ask for feedback from the patient regarding her experiences in therapy. One of the obvious benefits is that the therapist gets important information about what did and did not work well – invaluable information for a true scientist-practitioner, and wonderful information to add to one's store of clinical experience. Asking for feedback is also a great way of modeling, further encouraging the patient to do the same. It also emphasizes the collaborative nature of the therapeutic relationship, and reinforces the value of the patient's input to others.

A final consideration when concluding IPT is the management of post-therapy contacts. In traditional psychodynamic psychotherapy, such contacts are strictly prohibited. Research protocols also prohibit post-therapy contact of any kind. As the goals at the Conclusion of Acute Treatment with IPT are to facilitate independent functioning and reinforce the gains made by the patient, being receptive to the patient's request for post-therapy contact, or, in some cases, initiating a discussion about post-therapy contact, may be very helpful. For example, the therapist may determine that it would be helpful to have the patient call or email[b] the therapist a month or two after the conclusion to check in with the therapist. If there is concern about relapse with a patient who is unable to attend Maintenance Treatment, the therapist may even choose to call the patient a month or two after Acute Treatment has concluded. Requests by the patient to call or email (but please no texting) the therapist can generally be met positively as well. Clinical experience clearly indicates that for many patients, this kind of contact is very helpful.

Several principles need to be kept in mind, however. First, post-therapy contact of this kind should be mutually agreed upon. The therapist must keep up her end of the bargain – if she agrees to call the patient after a month, the therapist must follow through. Second, this type of post-therapy contact should be conceptualized by the therapist as a literal Maintenance Treatment, meaning that all of the therapeutic boundaries must be maintained as when face-to-face sessions were taking place. The same kind of therapeutic goals and techniques should also be in force. Therapists choosing to utilize this structure for concluding Acute Treatment and providing maintenance contact will also find that it generally diminishes the intensity of the conclusion as well, which is consistent with the non-transferential and supportive nature of IPT.

Conducting Maintenance Treatment

There are two primary differences between Acute and Maintenance IPT. The first is simply a quantitative matter – Maintenance IPT is less frequent and less intense. In some cases, the therapist may even choose to have maintenance sessions of shorter length – 20-minute or half-hour appointments may be sufficient for some patients who are doing well. The other difference is qualitative, as the goals of Acute Treatment are to resolve an interpersonal crisis, while Maintenance Treatment is designed to maintain functioning and prevent a return of symptoms (Box 17.3).

---

[b] Our 2003 book noted that the therapist may ask the patient to call or write to the therapist; sadly this very personal and meaningful way of communicating has been replaced by texting or email.

Box 17.3 Goals of Maintenance Treatment

- To review the original problem and the progress being made
- To consider new problems that can be dealt with preventively
- To continue to maximize the patient's interpersonal functioning
- To provide a continuing relationship for the resumption of Acute Treatment if needed

The first goal of Maintenance IPT is to review the patient's presenting problem and the progress that is being made. The therapist can make formal reference to the Interpersonal Inventory, or can simply update the status of the interpersonal problems the patient was struggling with prior to Acute Treatment. The purpose of this is both to imply to the patient that she should continue working on interpersonal communication, and to ensure that the problem has not resurfaced.

New problems which do not require acute intervention may also arise. The most common (and gratifying) is when patients bring new interpersonal problems to maintenance sessions after they have already started to resolve them. For instance, a patient who originally presented with a marital conflict may bring a conflict with an employer to a maintenance session. Ideally, the patient will have already started to apply some of the IPT problem solving techniques to the new problem, and will simply be informing the therapist about that work or asking for specific advice, as opposed to needing a burst of Acute Treatment. In other situations, the therapist may need to reinforce the patient's ability to cope with the new problem without needing to return to an Acute Treatment mode. More dependent patients, or those with preoccupied attachments, may feel less competent to deal with new problems, and their natural tendency is to flee back to treatment. The therapist should use her judgment to determine whether a resumption of Acute Treatment is needed.

The contract for Maintenance Treatment should be flexible, but all changes should be specifically discussed with the patient. For instance, a patient may come to a bimonthly maintenance session with a conflict in a new relationship. The therapist and patient may agree that since the patient is already familiar with IPT and has already put into practice some problem solving skills, three weekly sessions might be helpful. This is in contrast to a resumption of a 'full' course of 12–20 sessions of IPT, and also contrasts with the bimonthly sessions which had been established in the original Maintenance Agreement. The primary consideration is that changes in the agreement be specifically discussed and mutually agreed upon. Such changes should always be made if they are in the patient's best interest – it is the patient's needs rather than the agreement that is paramount. Clinical judgment should be used in making such decisions.

In situations in which the patient continues to function well, the therapist can help the patient to maintain this level of functioning with maintenance sessions. The therapist should be strongly encouraging and positively reinforcing, and should encourage the patient to be as independent as possible. This independence is important not only in the patient's social setting, but should be encouraged in session as well. For instance, rather than taking a more active stance while problem solving, the therapist should guide the patient to apply what has been learned in the Acute Treatment phase, and to generate her own solutions to new problems.

Finally, the provision of maintenance sessions gives the patient and therapist a platform from which they can resume Acute Treatment if needed. Continued contact, or the possibility of resuming contact if needed, makes the therapist a real attachment figure to whom the patient can return during a crisis. Continued contact also allows the therapist to monitor the patient's functioning, and for the therapist to suggest a return to more Acute Treatment if the patient appears headed for a recurrence of symptoms.

Maintenance Treatment: Tactics and Techniques

The basic techniques used in Maintenance IPT are no different from those used in Acute Treatment. The therapist's stance should be slightly less active, however, as the goal is to maximize the patient's independent functioning. Less activity in problem solving in particular is helpful, and encouragement that the patient 'knows how to solve the problem' is usually therapeutic as well.

Case example 17.4: Mary

Mary was a 27-year-old woman who presented for treatment following the death of her mother in an automobile accident. Her mother, who had been in good health, had been killed by a drunk driver about 3 months earlier. Mary described increasing problems with low mood, crying spells, feelings of guilt, and poor sleep. Though she continued to function at work, she felt that the quality of her work had deteriorated. The incident that compelled her to seek treatment was her anxiety about facing the driver of the other car for the first time at the upcoming trial.

Mary had no psychiatric history, and described an unremarkable childhood. She had been close to her mother, and had last seen her 2 days prior to the accident. She was able to relate a number of stories about her mother in great detail, and seemed to have a very balanced picture of her mother as a 'whole' person. Mary's father had been devastated by the death, and Mary described having for the first time to 'care for' her father. She described him as somewhat distant but strong – he was always there when others needed help. She had never seen him cry prior to her mother's funeral, and since then he had been unable to go back to work. He appeared to be severely depressed, and Mary had taken on the role of caring for him. She noted in the initial session that she felt that her concern for her father had made it difficult to think about her own reactions to her mother's death.

Mary had one brother who lived some distance away, and though they were not close, she felt they had connected when he had returned for the funeral. He had, however, returned home, leaving her to care for her father. Mary had been married for about 4 years, and described her husband as very supportive. Her husband attended an early session, and left the same impression with the therapist. Her social support was good – she was very involved in her church and had numerous friends at work and in her neighborhood.

As the Interpersonal Inventory (Figure 17.1) and Formulation (Figure 17.2) took shape, the therapist began to conceptualize the case as one in which a high-functioning, relatively securely attached individual was faced with an overwhelming interpersonal crisis. Mary's interpersonal relationships were good, her insight was quite good, and she seemed securely attached in her relationships.

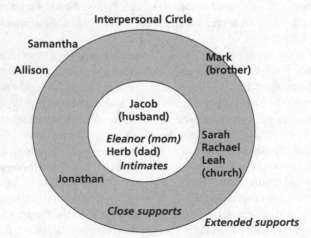

Figure 17.1 Interpersonal Circle – Mary

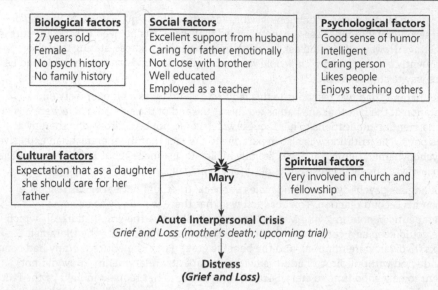

Figure 17.2 Interpersonal Formulation – Mary

Mary and her therapist agreed to meet for about 12 acute sessions of IPT with the goal of helping her to deal with the grief and the anxiety of the upcoming trial. Mary was able to make great progress – she was in touch with her emotions and could describe them in detail when recounting her experiences with the news of her mother's death and her funeral. With the therapist's encouragement, she talked in more detail about her feelings with her husband, then with several other close friends who were very supportive.

Mary also arranged for psychiatric treatment for her father after having used role playing in the session to work out more fully how she wanted to approach her father. He was willing to go to treatment, and appeared to be responding to antidepressant medication. She felt that she could be less physically involved in his care, and they began to talk about their experiences with her mother's death as well.

The most difficult situation was dealing with the driver who had killed her mother. After much discussion with the therapist and with others, Mary elected not to have any communication with him. She did attend the court proceedings (along with several friends she had asked to attend for support) but did not feel that it would accomplish anything to have further contact after he was sentenced. She spoke with her pastor about the anger she felt about the event, and her anger at God for allowing the accident to happen. Though she did not feel that she had 'resolved' the spiritual question, she seemed to be comfortable with the ambiguity the situation had caused, and continued with her religious activities.

Therapy was conducted once weekly until after the court hearing, and thereafter Mary requested that the therapy switch to once every 2 weeks. Since she was doing well and seemed to have very supportive relationships, the therapist agreed, and a new agreement was established to meet biweekly for the remaining five sessions. Towards the Conclusion of Acute Treatment, Maintenance Treatment was discussed in detail.

The Maintenance Agreement that was mutually established at the end of Acute Treatment was that Mary would return once monthly for 2 months, and then would return in the future if she felt that she needed to do so. Based on her solid attachments, social support, and lack of previous problems, the therapist was quite comfortable with this plan. The maintenance sessions were quite unremarkable, with the therapist simply reviewing Mary's general functioning, which continued to be quite good. At the end of the second maintenance session, both agreed that there was no need to schedule further meetings. However, Mary did ask for the therapist's email address, stating that she frequently corresponded with people via email and could envision that email would be a nice way to stay in touch.

The therapist had two reactions to this request. The first was a bit of anxiety and irritation at the fact that she had asked this at the end of the session. There were obvious transferential implications to her request which could not be addressed in therapy at this point. The irritation was also in part due to the fact that the therapist had extensive psychodynamic training, and was literally itching to ask more about Mary's request. The anxiety was largely because of the need for a rapid response.

Holding his psychodynamic tendencies in check, the therapist based his response upon his second reaction. This reaction was that there was likely to be some therapeutic benefit in giving Mary a 'transitional object' – the email address – which she could keep as a concrete way of continuing to feel attached to the therapist. The risks involved were minimal, and the benefits great. First, the entire therapy had been conducted without directly addressing the therapeutic relationship – now did not seem to be a good time to start. Second, responding to her request in light of the fact that there were no future contacts planned would increase the likelihood that Mary would contact the therapist if she needed help. Finally, denying her request would risk being perceived as rejecting right at the end of therapy, and would be completely inconsistent with the supportive therapeutic stance that the therapist had maintained throughout treatment.

The therapist did not hear from Mary until about a year later, when he received a short email with the news that she was doing well and that she and her husband were expecting their first child in several months. The therapist replied with a brief personal note that he was glad to have heard from her, congratulated her, and wished her well during the remainder of the pregnancy. A fleeting wish to ask Mary to write back after the delivery to update him about the birth and her new child was quashed on the grounds that an old supervisor wouldn't have approved, but the therapist did recognize that this would also have been consistent with Maintenance Treatment in IPT.

About five months later Mary called the therapist to set up an appointment. She had delivered a healthy baby boy, but had experienced a profound sense of sadness several weeks after the delivery. Though she did not appear to be depressed, she described that the birth had reactivated her feelings of loss regarding her mother. She stated that she had not expected the reaction, but after the birth had really wanted her mother, both to be there to see the baby as well as to provide physical help to her. A good friend of hers had recently also had a child, and Mary felt somewhat envious about the fact that this woman's mother had been there to help for about 2 weeks after the birth.

Mary and the therapist agreed to meet for four weekly sessions, during which they discussed Mary's reactions to the new circumstances. Once again, she was very articulate and was able to describe her emotional reactions, and shared these with other friends in detail. On a practical level, she invited her mother-in-law to stay for a week as she was making the transition back to work, which she felt was quite helpful even considering the fact that it was her mother-in-law. The therapist made a point of asking Mary to bring her child to one of the appointments, and spent quite a bit of time simply enjoying the experience with her. He had the impression that this was tremendously valued by Mary.

With the second Acute Treatment phase concluded and Mary recovered, Mary and the therapist agreed to continue the Maintenance Agreement as before.

Conclusion

Though there are many similarities, Acute Treatment and Maintenance Treatment are conceptualized in IPT as two distinct phases of therapy. The goals and intensity of each differ significantly: the goal of Acute Treatment is to resolve a current interpersonal crisis and improve social functioning, while the goal of Maintenance Treatment is to prevent recurrence of symptoms. While the techniques used in both are the same, Maintenance Therapy generally allows the therapist to be less active and to encourage the patient to apply the problem solving skills that she has learned. While discussion of Maintenance Treatment is literally mandatory for all patients, clinical judgment should guide the decisions that need to be made about the frequency and type of contact that will occur following Acute Treatment.

References

1. Frank E, *et al*. Three-year outcomes for maintenance therapies in recurrent depression. *Archives of General Psychiatry*, 1990, **47**(12): 1093–1099.
2. Frank E, *et al*. Randomized trial of weekly, twice-monthly, and monthly interpersonal psychotherapy as maintenance treatment for women with recurrent depression. *American Journal of Psychiatry*, 2007, **164**: 761–767.
3. Gelso CJ and Woodhouse SS. The termination of psychotherapy: what research tells us about the process of ending treatment, in Tryon GS (ed.) *Counseling Based on Process Research: Applying What We Know*. 2002, Boston: Allyn and Bacon.

Section 6

Additional Aspects of IPT

18

Psychodynamic Processes

Introduction

All human interactions have psychodynamic determinants. Whether it is a conversation with the milkman or an intensive psychotherapeutic exchange, psychodynamic processes influence all interpersonal interactions. The interactions that occur in Interpersonal Psychotherapy (IPT) are no exception to this rule, and in many ways the successful delivery of IPT hinges on the ability of the therapist to understand and manage them. This demands a great deal of skill as the time limit used in IPT requires that these processes be recognized and dealt with quickly.

Psychoanalysis and other psychodynamic approaches rest on two fundamental principles: psychic determinism and the proposition that unconscious mental processes are a primary influence on an individual's conscious thoughts and behaviors. According to psychoanalytic theory, people are largely unaware of the processes that drive their behavior, and it is these unconscious factors that lead to neurosis and psychopathology.[1] Freud emphasized the special therapeutic significance of these elements by stating that the term 'psychoanalysis' could be applied to every type of psychotherapy which recognizes the problems of transference and resistance, the basic importance of the unconscious, and the importance of early developmental history.[2] While recognized as important factors, in IPT these core principles are conceptualized somewhat differently, and are addressed in fundamentally different ways.

Transference

Transference in its most general sense refers to the repetition of early patterns of interpersonal relatedness with current partners.[3] The phenomenon is universal, and takes place in all relationships. Transference in its special application to the therapeutic process involves the patient transferring onto the therapist, as a specific interpersonal partner, his early experiences in interpersonal relationships. It is assumed in analysis to be an unconscious process outside of the awareness of the patient.

In psychodynamic psychotherapy, the transference of the experiences of early life relationships onto the therapist can be examined 'as if under a magnifying glass'.[3] The therapeutic task in psychodynamic psychotherapy is to create conditions in which the transference will be enhanced, so that it is more easily recognizable as such to the therapist.

A detailed examination of the therapeutic experience of the patient and his relationship with the therapist, particularly the transferential experience of the patient, is an essential element of psychodynamic psychotherapy. The therapist, as a neutral observer of the patient's reactions, is able to interpret, or give feedback, to the patient about his transferential reactions to the therapist, so that the patient can come to recognize the unconscious determinants of his distorted reactions to others.

A cardinal element of all psychotherapies (including IPT) is that the therapist should develop an understanding of the way he is perceived by the patient. A major task of the psychodynamic therapist is to help the patient discover how and why he experiences the therapist in a particular way.[4] In psychoanalytic therapy, this is hypothesized as the key to unlocking early experiences which have distorted the patient's subsequent relationships. All of the patient's responses to the therapist are colored by the transference and will therefore affect the outcome of treatment. If the patient's transference to the therapist is positive, the patient will experience the therapist as helpful and well-intended, and is likely to 'comply' with treatment interventions. On the other hand, if the patient's transference is negative or suspicious, all of the therapist's statements and interventions will be perceived in that light – the patient will not trust the therapist.

David Malan[5] has referred to a 'triangle of insight' in which the past and present experiences of relationships (in particular a parent figure) are linked through the experience of transference within psychotherapy. As the patient comes to an understanding of the way he reacts transferentially to the therapist, this understanding is generalized to other relationships in both the past and the present. It is the therapist's task to bring into the patient's conscious awareness these transferential patterns of behavior.

The concept of transference is quite similar to Sullivan's concept of parataxic distortion.[6] Sullivan believed that individuals form and maintain relationships with distortions or inaccuracies about the real qualities of the relationships, and that these distortions were the product of previous relationships. Like Freud, Sullivan also believed that these distortions were largely unconscious. Sullivan extended the concept of transference, however, by recognizing and emphasizing that transference, or parataxic distortion, does not occur in a vacuum – it is heavily influenced by the other individual in the relationship. In other words, the transference or distortion is affected by the 'real' qualities of the other individual – in the case of psychotherapy, by the therapist. Sullivan also recognized that both individuals in a relationship have parataxic distortions (including therapists) and that these reciprocal distortions also influence one another.

Bowlby's model of attachment takes this concept one step further.[7] Bowlby, in framing attachment behavior as a fundamental neurologically and physiologically based drive, largely dismissed the importance of the unconscious in relationships. Bowlby argued that rather than being held in the unconscious, the working model of interpersonal relationships that an individual develops is based on his real experiences, and reflects an accurate appraisal – accessible to the patient – of his prior relationships. The implications of Bowlby's model were profound from a theoretical standpoint, but did not lead to a dramatic shift in therapeutic technique. Using Bowlby's approach, the therapist still focuses on the therapeutic relationship as a means of understanding the patient's interpersonal distortions and characteristic pattern of engaging in relationships. This is because the patient's working model of relationships – his typical style of relating to others – is imposed upon the therapist, just like it is imposed on all other relationships. In contrast to psychoanalysis, however, the therapist helps the patient appreciate this pattern directly rather than interpreting the underlying unconscious elements of it.

IPT is based largely upon Bowlby's theories of attachment. While recognizing that there may be unconscious elements which influence an individual's interpersonal behavior, IPT focuses on those elements which are accessible to the patient. While a patient may initially have limited insight and not be aware of the patterns of behavior in which he engages, these interpersonal patterns are not presumed to be driven primarily by unconscious factors. Therefore, the therapist can help the patient to appreciate, and subsequently change, his behavior by examining patterns in the patient's relationships without the need to 'interpret' any unconscious motives which lie behind the patient's behavior. In simple terms, IPT is based on the premise that early life experiences have a profound impact on the patient's attachment style. A patient's real-life experiences lead him to his attachment style: in the case of abusive, critical, or absent relationships with parents, to an insecure attachment; in the case of warm and supportive relationships with parents, to a more secure attachment. This style is then pulled through adolescence and adulthood. Though heavily influenced by early experiences, all of the patient's relationships over time continue to influence it.

The attachment model – the working model of relationships – that the patient has developed is then imposed on current relationships, often inaccurately. In the case of insecure attachments, the working model makes it difficult for the patient to graciously ask for support and to give it to others. It takes a great deal of time and much lived experience to change a patient's fundamental attachment style, particularly give the time over which it has developed and solidified. Thus IPT, as a time-limited treatment, is not designed to change attachment style, but rather to help patients communicate more effectively given their underlying attachment style.

IPT also differs from psychodynamic approaches because it does not utilize the therapeutic relationship as the primary means of examining and understanding the transference, parataxic distortions, or maladaptive working models that the patient imposes upon relationships. Instead, IPT is concerned with the way the patient manifests these elements in his current interpersonal relationships. This is possible because all of the same factors (i.e. transference, parataxic distortions, and maladaptive working models) are operative in the patient's relationships outside of therapy. Focusing on the patient's current interpersonal relationships is desirable in IPT because it allows the patient and therapist to work on the most immediate problems the patient is experiencing, and allows the therapy to focus primarily on rapid symptom resolution rather than intrapsychic change.

Though IPT focuses on the patient's current social relationships, and though the treatment relationship is not a point of intervention in IPT, it cannot be emphasized enough that the therapeutic relationship is a veritable gold mine of information for the therapist. The therapist's experience of the patient provides information about the patient's attachment and communication style, informs the therapist about potential problems in therapy and how to flexibly structure treatment, about the patient's prognosis, and about specific problems that the patient is likely to be having with others outside of therapy. Though not directly addressed in therapy, it is crucial in IPT to have an appreciation of the transference and therapeutic relationship. This is best understood in IPT as being 'psychodynamically informed' as opposed to being 'psychodynamically focused'. Being psychodynamically informed is to acknowledge and consider psychodynamic processes such as transference without discussing them explicitly with the patient or considering them to be a focus of intervention. Being psychodynamically focused is not only to acknowledge the presence of transference and other factors within the therapeutic relationship, but also to discuss them explicitly as the primary mode of intervention within the treatment.

The difference between being psychodynamically informed and being psychodynamically focused in treatment can be illustrated metaphorically (Figure 18.1). In this analogy, the sharks represent problematic psychodynamic processes as they relate to the conduct of IPT or any other therapy. The psychodynamically informed swimmer on the surface of the water is aware of the sharks, and if they approach too closely will swim away or take appropriate measures to evade them. The goal of the therapist is to cross with the patient to the other side of the harbor while avoiding the sharks if at all possible. The scuba diver, on the other hand, is psychodynamically focused, and is not only prepared to swim with the sharks, but has the goal of seeking them out. To swim with sharks without being eaten takes many years of psychodynamic training and a working knowledge of the proper techniques to deal with them – sharks are very primitive and instinctual creatures with nasty aggressive streaks.

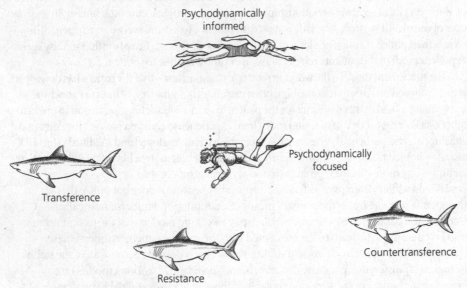

Figure 18.1 Psychodynamics and IPT.

Metaphorically, the goal of treatment is to cross a harbor full of sharks with the patient without being eaten. The goal in IPT is to get across the harbor by avoiding the sharks; the goal of psychoanalytic therapy is to root out and interpret the sharks. IPT is well suited to waters which have a few small sharks; a psychoanalytic approach is necessary in shark-infested waters as there is simply no way to avoid them all. Swimming in shark-infested waters is thus a useful metaphor for conceptualizing the difference between being psychodynamically informed and being psychodynamically focused: to be psychodynamically informed is to swim above the sharks and to be aware of their presence, taking evasive action when necessary; to be psychodynamically focused is to swim with the sharks and to be properly prepared to deal with sharks who bite!

Countertransference

In his writings about countertransference, Freud[8] conceptualized it as an unconscious interference with the therapist's ability to objectively understand his patients. Countertransference is the literal counterpart to transference – it involves the transferring of the therapist's experiences in early childhood relationships onto the therapist's relationship with the patient.[9] As with transference, the process is understood to be unconscious. As such, Freud regarded countertransference as at best a nuisance, and at times a barrier to the appropriate conduct of psychotherapy, because it prevented the therapist from objectively understanding the patient. Countertransference, if active, could lead the therapist to make inaccurate interpretations to the patient. The means to eliminate or minimize these countertransferential reactions was for the therapist to undergo analysis himself so that these processes could be brought into conscious awareness.

This conceptualization has been broadened by some authors so that it includes all of the reactions of the therapist to the patient, rather than just those that are believed to be unconscious and are derived from the therapist's early experiences.[10] Many authors have also argued that countertransference is as much a factor in therapy as transference, and that the broader countertransferential reactions of therapists should be examined by the therapists as part of the therapeutic process.[10,11]

Authors such as Ogden[12] conceptualize countertransference as psychodynamic phenomena in which the patient, through the process of projective identification, makes the therapist 'feel' his own intrapsychic experience. This process is the basis of some of the interventions used in object relations therapy. Similarly, self-psychology acknowledges countertransference as a pathway to empathy, a concept which is fundamental to some psychotherapies.[13] It is this process of empathic resonance – the product of the patient's projection of his experience onto the therapist – which forms the basis for the therapeutic relationship and subsequent change. In this model, the process is largely unconscious – the patient's projections upon the therapist are outside of the patient's awareness, and the therapist's task is to bring them into the patient's consciousness.

While recognizing the value of this broader conceptualization of countertransference, in IPT it is most useful to use a narrower concept. This is important so that a distinction can be made between those reactions which are 'native' to the therapist and those which are elicited by the patient. Those reactions to others which are intrinsic to the therapist or are 'classically' countertransferential do in fact interfere with the therapy, because they cause a distortion of the therapist's perception of the patient and his experience.

To put it in an attachment framework, the therapist's working model of relationships – just like the patient's – is influenced by his cumulative experiences. If this working model is not an accurate representation of the patient, it will color or distort the relationship between therapist and patient every bit as much as the relationship model imposed by the patient. If a therapist tends to have difficulty trusting others, tends to be overly self-reliant, or has a need to care for others, these tendencies or models will be played out in the therapy unless the therapist is aware of them and takes steps to counteract them. The obvious corollary to this is that IPT therapists need to have insight into their own attachment behavior and communication so that they can minimize the distortions in their interpersonal models and more accurately understand the experience of their patients. This clearly implies that personal psychotherapy should be encouraged for all therapists who wish to do IPT well.

As a complement to the more narrow view of countertransference, IPT also recognizes and strongly relies on the concept that the patient literally elicits reactions in the therapist during the course of therapy. This elicitation is not unique to the specific therapist; it is a reaction that nearly all therapists or people generally would have to the patient. This phenomena is described in Interpersonal Theory: the patient's direct and metacommunications in therapy pull for or elicit complementary responses from the therapist. For example, a patient who is hostile will likely elicit a hostile response from the therapist; a patient who is passive will tend to elicit a more dominant response from the therapist (at least initially); a patient who is dismissive will elicit a similar dismissive reaction from the therapist. These reactions are not considered to be countertransferential in IPT; they are natural responses that the patient elicits in the therapist. By extension, the patient is almost certain to be eliciting similar responses in others with whom they interact.

The key distinction in IPT is therefore to distinguish between those reactions that are generated because of the therapist's experiences independent of the patient which are unique to the therapist and his personal experiences, and those that are being elicited by the patient directly, to which nearly everyone would react. The former reactions, native to the therapist, are 'countertransferential' in IPT; the latter are responses elicited by the patient. The former are a barrier to a more accurate understanding of the patient and to developing a therapeutic relationship; the latter are an extremely important way to more fully understand the patient's attachment and communication style, and to begin to draw hypotheses about the interpersonal problems that the patient is having outside of therapy. Countertransference as it is narrowly conceptualized in IPT actually inhibits the development of empathy because it interferes with understanding, while appreciating the responses the patient is eliciting in the therapist (and by extension the responses they almost certainly elicit in others) is information used in developing a formulation of the patient's communication problems and for subsequent intervention.

This distinction between 'countertransference' and 'elicited response' is somewhat arbitrary and artificial, for the therapist (since he is a real human being with real experiences) always comes to therapy with a few attachment insecurities and slightly distorted relationship models which are influenced by his previous and current relationships. These interact with the patient's models and communications, which in turn influence the perception that both individuals have of each other. One can almost envision a spiraling maelstrom of elicited parataxically distorted relationship models whirling around the therapist's office with no possibility of determining whose distortion is whose. Rather than engaging in such therapeutic nihilism, however, it is best in IPT to simplify things to two fundamental principles: individuals (including therapists) can never fully understand one another; but as real people (and therapists) we do the best we can, and there is great beauty and value in the connections we form.

As a corollary to these concepts of countertransference and elicited responses, structured, focal, and time-limited treatments such as IPT offer an intervention that minimizes the impact of the negative responses that patients precipitate in the therapists with whom they work. Patients who are difficult to relate to or work with may benefit from a time-limited intervention in part because the time limit minimizes therapist 'burn out' by the patient. An angry borderline patient is much easier to tolerate for 15 sessions as opposed to 4 years. Of course, these more difficult patients may ultimately require long-term treatment with heroic therapists. However, the structured nature of IPT often allows the therapist to offer a patient who might otherwise be labeled as 'difficult' or 'unlikable' the opportunity for a collaborative interaction and perhaps his first experience of a warm and caring relationship.

Resistance

In 1892, Freud's description of 'Elizabeth von R' introduced the concept of resistance to psychotherapists.[8] As a construct in psychotherapy, resistance is perhaps best considered as the patient's attempts to maintain his intrapsychic status quo. As applied to the analytic situation, resistance can be broadly construed as any action or attitude of the patient that impedes the course of the therapy.[14] From a psychoanalytic standpoint, resistance is pervasive in all therapies as it is theorized that all patients have an unconscious desire to avoid change and to avoid the recognition of painful, shameful, or embarrassing affect, memories, or fantasies. Fromm-Reichmann[3] defines resistance as:

the reactivation, outside of the patient's awareness, of the motivating powers which were responsible for the patient's original pathogenic dissociative and repressive processes.

In her view, it is an unconscious process which protects individuals from overwhelming or unacceptable anxiety, and is a mechanism of literal 'self-preservation'. Psychological defenses outside of the patient's awareness are responsible for the resistance. In therapy, resistance is manifest in many ways, but all are characterized by avoidance in one form or another of issues which cause the patient to feel anxious.

A primary goal of psychoanalytically oriented psychotherapy is to uncover the genesis of a patient's anxiety – i.e. the unacceptable underlying impulses which the patient is unable to successfully defend against – and it is therefore focused on revealing and understanding the nature of the patient's resistances. In contrast to other therapies that evade or ignore resistance, psychoanalytically oriented therapies seek to uncover the 'cause, purpose, mode, and history' of resistances.[11] Freud[4] stated that the working through of resistances:

is a part of the work which effects the greatest changes in a patient and which distinguishes analytic treatment from any other kind of treatment.

In IPT, it is the conscious elements of resistance that are therapeutically important. In simple terms, 'resistance' in IPT means nothing more than a patient's natural inclination to avoid change. There is no need in IPT to pathologize it; all humans are resistant to change to some degree, and it is a natural and normal reaction. Those patients with less secure attachment styles will be less likely to adapt well to change, and have likely had bad experiences with change previously. Their reactions are therefore understood as a natural reaction, and as an extension of their attachment style. There is no need in IPT to invoke a more complex model, and viewing the patient as actively attempting to undermine or resist therapy is not only not necessary, but is detrimental to the therapeutic relationship.

As an example, what might in psychodynamic psychotherapy be labeled 'resistance' is often apparent in situations in which treatment is compulsory – patients who are legally required to be in treatment but who do not want to be may intentionally withhold information, refuse to answer questions, or be generally uncooperative with treatment, and be fully aware that they are doing so. In IPT, the therapeutic perspective is that this is a normal and expected reaction given the patient's experience to date. Why should he be any more trusting of the therapists than other authority figures, many of whom have been unreliable or untrustworthy. The dismissing or fearful attachment style has developed because the patient has been in many relationships in which he could not trust others, or if he did, that trust was abused. What would be unusual would be if the patient suddenly entered therapy securely attached and fully trusting. Other examples might be a patient involved in marital therapy who intentionally withholds information about a current affair, an adolescent patient who refuses to speak in a family therapy session, or a patient who intentionally misses an appointment because he is angry at the therapist. Again, these are understood in IPT as flowing from a maladaptive attachment style that the patient has come by honestly. The dissembling, refusal to cooperate, or acting out is communication based on a maladaptive and insecure attachment style.

'Resistance' in IPT can also be understood as a natural reaction to change that is common to all individuals, even the most securely attached. This reaction is particularly common among psychotherapy patients, as the fear of the unknown, and the fear of change, is often what drives patients to seek treatment. It can even be conceptualized as an acute crisis – a Role Transition. This difficulty in changing behavior is conceptualized in IPT as something that the patient is aware of and has come by honestly – in other words, the patient's real-life experiences have led to an understandable fear of particular kinds of change. This is influenced in large part by the patient's attachment experiences and his attachment style. For instance, if the patient has had real experiences of rejection by others, it is completely understandable that he would have difficulty in forming new relationships, and would feel that doing so would be very threatening. A patient who has had experiences with others in which he has been abused would have a natural and understandable fear of being in a position in which he has to trust others. As with Bowlby's concept of attachment behavior, this is based upon real-life experiences, and does not require unconscious processes.

In IPT, the therapeutic response which this conscious fear of change calls forth is very different from that which is indicated in psychodynamic psychotherapy. Rather than intervening by interpreting the patient's unconscious resistance, the IPT therapist can respond to the patient's difficulties with empathy. Given the patient's experiences, it is little wonder that he finds a particular kind of change difficult. The IPT therapist's job is to understand the difficulty, to empathize with the patient, and to help problem solve and provide positive reinforcement for attempts at change. As a stable attachment figure who provides the patient with unconditional positive regard, the therapist can empathically facilitate change on a conscious level.

In sum, people change for one of two reasons. Either their suffering has become intolerable, or they are able to recognize that they will benefit from the change. The latter requires a fair amount of insight and a high capacity for delayed gratification – changes such as subjecting oneself to graduate school to facilitate a long-term goal would fall into this category. Nearly all psychotherapy patients, however, change because they are in intolerable circumstances – they come to treatment because they are suffering, not because they are seeking greater insight or self-actualization and are eager to undergo a lengthy and expensive process. Even in Iowa, the complaint that, 'I'm suffering because I'm having an awful dispute with my spouse' is heard far more frequently in the therapist's office than the statement, 'I'm here for therapy because I want to be self-actualized!'

In medicine, decisions are made with reference to a 'risk–benefit' assessment. In this process, the desired clinical outcome, e.g. abolition of a bacterial infection with antibiotics, is pursued using a treatment at a predetermined dose or level based on the empirical literature and clinical experience. Just as some patients may be sensitive to the average recommended doses of antibiotics, some patients may also be sensitive to therapeutic interventions which are designed to foster interpersonal change. As the dose of antibiotics may need to be decreased for some patients, so the pacing of therapy may need to be modified for patients for whom change is difficult. This type of 'resistance' or sensitivity to change calls not for interpretation but for empathy, and for positive reinforcement of the change that the patient is able to attempt.

Conclusion

IPT is subject to the same psychodynamic processes that affect all psychotherapies and all clinical interactions. In IPT these are generally not specifically addressed as part of the treatment unless they appear to threaten the patient's ability to engage in treatment. All of the processes, however, are important as sources of information for the therapist, and understanding them is integral to IPT.

References

1. Brenner C. *An Elementary Textbook of Psychoanalysis*. 1973, New York: Anchor Press.
2. Freud S. The history of the psychoanalytic movement, in Freud S (ed.) *The Basic Writings of Sigmund Freud*. 1938, New York: Random House.
3. Fromm-Reichmann F. *Principles of Intensive Psychotherapy*. 1960, Chicago: University of Chicago Press.
4. Freud S. Remembering, repeating, and working through, in Strachey J (ed.) *Standard Edition of the Complete Psychological Works of Sigmund Freud*. 1962, London: Hogarth Press.
5. Malan DH. *A Study of Brief Psychotherapy*. 1975, New York: Plenum.
6. Sullivan HS. *The Interpersonal Theory of Psychiatry*. 1953, New York: Norton.
7. Bowlby J. *Attachment. Attachment and Loss. Vol. 1*. 1969, New York: Basic Books.
8. Freud S. *The Complete Psychological Works*. 1946, London: Hogarth Press.
9. Freud S. The future prospects of psycho-analytic therapy, in Strachey J (ed.) *Standard Edition of the Complete Psychological Works of Sigmund Freud*. 1962, London: Hogarth Press.
10. Abend S. Countertransference and psychoanalytic technique. *Psychoanalytic Quarterly*, 1989, **58**: 374–395.
11. Greenson R. *The Technique and Practice of Psychoanalysis*. 1967, New York: International Universities Press.
12. Ogden TH. The concept of internal object relations. *International Journal of Psychoanalysis*, 1983, **64**: 227–235.
13. Kohut H. *The Analysis of the Self*. 1971, New York: International Universities Press.
14. Strean HS. *Essentials of Psychoanalysis*. 1994, New York: Brunner Mazel.

19

Applications of Interpersonal Psychotherapy

Introduction

Interpersonal Psychotherapy (IPT) has been easily adapted to different populations because of its universally applicable interpersonal orientation. The three IPT Problem Areas are relevant to many different diagnostic categories, relationship problems, and distress generally. Because of its flexibility and range, *once the basic IPT is model is mastered, clinicians should be able to easily apply it to a variety of populations and disorders.* It is advisable, however, to develop expertise in the particular area in which IPT is being used: e.g. to have experience with adolescents if applying IPT to adolescents, perinatal women if applying to postpartum depression, or geriatric patients if applying IPT to older patients.

IPT for Depression

IPT for Adolescent Depression

IPT has been adapted for use with adolescents.[1-3] IPT is efficacious in treating adolescent depression, and a number of randomized controlled clinical trials have demonstrated its efficacy.[4-6] Key modifications of IPT for adolescents address developmental aspects, including the emerging autonomy of the adolescent and the development of more intimate and affiliative relationships. The need to integrate the patient's unique family ecology into the treatment is also emphasized.

IPT for adolescents typically utilizes a 12–16-session model; within this there is scope to integrate the patient's parent(s) into the therapeutic process during both the Initial/Assessment and Middle Phases. IPT has been validated for children aged 9 and above when a parent or caregiver is included throughout treatment.[7] All of the adolescent modifications utilize more psychoeducation and interventions such as communication and problem solving in addition to regular mood monitoring.

IPT in Late-life Depression

Reynolds and colleagues have adapted IPT for geriatric patients.[8] Their modifications place particular emphasis upon Grief and Loss and Role Transitions. This includes complex themes such as retirement, aging, and distress when one partner becomes ill or shows signs of dementia. IPT is usually provided in shorter sessions and is flexible with problems such as hearing impairment or decreased mobility.

There is a great deal of research supporting IPT for older adults,[8-10] including the Maintenance Therapies for Late Life Depression study, a randomized, double-blind, placebo-controlled trial comparing nortriptyline, IPT (alone or in combination) and treatment as usual.[11] The IPT-nortriptyline combination was superior to the other conditions; patients in the 60–70-year-old category fared better than patients 70 years and older.

IPT for the Cognitively Impaired Elderly

Many depressed geriatric patients show evidence of cognitive decline such as memory loss or impaired executive dysfunction. The latter deficit is a common precipitant of Role Disputes between patients and caregiving family members. These can occur because caregivers often misattribute features of executive dysfunction as willful opposition. Miller and colleagues adapted IPT for the cognitively impaired elderly by engaging both caregivers and identified patients throughout therapy.[12,13] This approach uses flexible individual or joint meetings as the clinical situation dictates. A great emphasis is placed on providing the caregiver with extensive education about depression, dementing illnesses, cognitive impairment and its potential effect upon interpersonal functioning. IPT with the cognitively impaired works towards a 'steady state', after which the frequency of visits can be lengthened. As cognitive impairment worsens, therapy is restructured to address the emerging challenges for the patient and his family.

IPT for Perinatal Women

A number of studies have used IPT for perinatal women and their partners. These include IPT for pregnant women[14-17] and for the postpartum.[18,19] Perinatal modifications include the integration of partners,[20] the addition of ethnographic interviewing as a means of enhancing engagement in treatment,[16,21] and groups for postpartum depression.[22,23] General modifications include a focus on psychoeducation about child development and perinatal sexual functioning, and recognition of perinatal losses that might impact the current depression. IPT is being used in clinical settings for infertility and pregnancy loss.

IPT for Dysthymic Disorders

IPT has also been adapted for patients with dysthymic disorder.[24] In the original description of this work nearly two decades ago, the chronicity of the symptoms of dysthymia were believed to make it inappropriate to use an acute interpersonal focus for IPT; thus a now abandoned Problem Area labeled 'iatrogenic Role Transition' was created. Rather than being developed collaboratively, this Problem Area was imposed on the patient by the therapist, and was conceptualized as a Role Transition from a depressed to less depressed state. This imposition allowed the therapist to avoid using the now discarded interpersonal deficits or sensitivities Problem Area, which was recognized even in early work with IPT to be a far less productive area on which to focus. The equivocal evidence of efficacy using the iatrogenic Role Transition Problem Area suggests that it was no better than the interpersonal deficits area it was intended to replace.

Initial research did not support the efficacy for IPT for dysthymic disorder.[25] In a randomized controlled trial comparing IPT, sertraline, and a brief supportive psychotherapy control, sertraline alone or combined with IPT were equally efficacious, and both were superior to IPT alone, which was in turn superior to brief supportive psychotherapy. In a later trial, IPT was compared with brief supportive psychotherapy for dysthymic patients with comorbid alcohol abuse. IPT was superior in treatment of mood symptoms and had a modest impact on alcohol use.[26]

Since the original description of IPT for dysthymia, the Problem Area of interpersonal deficits/sensitivities has been eliminated; instead, it is understood in IPT that long-standing fearful attachment is a far better way to conceptualize this pattern of interpersonal behavior. There is now much greater emphasis on developing an acute problem focus in collaboration with the patient rather than focusing on a chronic problem – there is nearly always some acute crisis that leads a patient to finally seek out therapy even in the context of chronic illness. That acute crisis – a Grief and Loss issue, an Interpersonal Dispute, or a Role Transition – should be the focus of IPT.

Rather than imposing an 'iatrogenic' Problem Area on patients with chronic depression or dysthymia, therapists should listen well and help the patient determine what acute problem led them to seek therapy at that particular moment. Though dysthymia is chronic, there are nearly always specific events which influence patients to seek help – an understanding consistent with the theoretical underpinnings of IPT. Iatrogenically imposing anything on the patient runs completely counter to the spirit of IPT, therefore the therapist's task with dysthymic patients is to collaboratively identify the acute stressor and focus on that acute Problem Area, recognizing that treatment may be lengthier because of the patient's paucity of interpersonal support and attachment insecurities. Concluding Acute Treatment, rather than terminating it, and the transition into Maintenance Treatment with IPT also play a critical role with these patients.

IPT for Bipolar Disorder

While the mainstay of management of bipolar disorder is medication, psychological therapies can assist bipolar patients to make appropriate modifications of lifestyle habits to better manage their illnesses. Disturbances in circadian rhythms, such as altered sleep habits, destabilize bipolar disorder.[27] Using this as the basis for modification, Frank *et al.* have integrated social rhythm therapy with IPT to create Interpersonal and Social Rhythm Therapy (IPSRT) for bipolar disorder.[28]

Rather than a modification, IPSRT is best considered a combination therapy. It is a comprehensive psychosocial management approach to bipolar disorder, combining IPT with psychoeducation and behavioral interventions to stabilize daily routines. The IPT component of IPSRT assists patients to adapt to and cope with the multiple psychosocial and relationship problems associated with bipolar disorder. There is a special emphasis in the IPT component of IPSRT on the Problem Area of Grief and Loss to address the impact of the illness on the healthy self. A randomized controlled trial of IPSRT demonstrated onset of fewer affective episodes during a 2-year follow-up period, although the effect was greater for depressive episodes.[28] The large-scale Systematic Treatment Enhancement Program for Bipolar Disorder (STEP-BD) compared cognitive behavioral therapy (CBT), IPSRT and Family Focused Therapy in subjects with bipolar disorder who were on specific standardized medication regimens. At 12-month follow-up, all three groups demonstrated similar recovery rates and all were superior to the control arm (a brief psychoeducation intervention).[29]

IPT for Non-affective Disorders

IPT for Eating Disorders

IPT was first utilized in a large clinical trial for bulimia nervosa by Fairburn and co-workers.[30,31] While CBT was superior to IPT at the end of Acute Treatment, IPT was found to be equally beneficial at long-term follow-up,[32] a finding since replicated.[33] The IPT condition used in this trial was extensively modified to remove any behavioral components, leading many to conclude that a version of IPT that integrated the behavioral interventions commonly used with eating disorders might have greater efficacy. This comprehensive approach has since been described and appears to have great promise.[34] Group IPT for eating disorders has been described by Wilfley *et al.*[35] Apart from demonstrating the benefits of IPT for this population, this work provided a valuable template for the application of IPT in groups.[36–38]

The efficacy of IPT for anorexia nervosa is less convincing. To date one randomized controlled trial showed that IPT and CBT were inferior to treatment as usual.[39] One critique of this finding is the assertion that anorexia nervosa requires a comprehensive management approach incorporating skilled medical, family, and individual psychological management. Therefore an integrated approach to treatment is likely to be superior over stand-alone interventions.

In our detailed discussion of the adaptations of IPT for post-traumatic stress disorder (PTSD) below, it seems clear that there should be a paradigm shift in psychotherapy development and research for many psychiatric disorders. Rather than using IPT, CBT, or any other therapy as a 'stand-alone' treatment, integrated or sequential approaches which utilize behavioral, interpersonal, dynamic, and mindfulness techniques and tactics should be developed and tested. These integrated approaches are far more likely to be of benefit with all patients, particularly those with eating disorders, PTSD, anxiety disorders, substance abuse disorders, and personality disorders. Good surgeons use a variety of instruments with each case as the need dictates, good psychotherapists should do the same.

IPT for Social Phobia

Lipsitz and colleagues adapted IPT for social phobia.[40] Despite long-standing impairment, nearly all patients with social phobia, like those with dysthymia, have an acute crisis that leads them to seek treatment. It may be a relationship dispute or transition which might seem trivial to some, but for these patients it carries great importance given their paucity of social contacts. As with dysthymic patients, it is the task of the IPT therapist to listen well and to help the patient identify the acute crisis, recognizing that therapy with these patients, most of whom have fearful attachment styles, will require a longer course of Acute Treatment. Concluding Acute Treatment rather than terminating it, and the transition into Maintenance Treatment are critical. A small-scale open trial indicated some potential efficacy of IPT for social phobia,[40] although a larger-scale randomized controlled trial found that IPT was superior to placebo but inferior to CBT.[41]

IPT for Borderline Personality Disorder

IPT has been utilized with patients with borderline personality disorder (BPD).[42–44] Modifications include providing treatment in two phases. In the first acute phase, the patient receives 18 IPT sessions over 16 weeks. Goals are to establish a therapeutic alliance, limit self-destructive behaviors, explain the IPT model, and provide initial symptomatic relief. If the patient tolerates this first phase, a continuation phase of 16 sessions in as many weeks follows. Goals of the continuation phase treatment include developing more adaptive interpersonal skills, and maintaining a strong therapeutic alliance as termination approaches. Patients with BPD thus can receive up to 34 IPT sessions over 8 months.

A trial including 35 patients with BDP and major depression compared fluoxetine plus CBT to fluoxetine and IPT over 32 weeks.[44] Apart from some minor differences in quality of life and interpersonal functioning, there was no difference in outcome between the treatment groups. A second study including 55 patients with BPD and major depressive disorder compared fluoxetine and clinical management to fluoxetine plus IPT over 32 weeks. In this study, remission rates did not differ significantly between subgroups. Combined therapy was more effective in reducing anxiety and improving self-reported social functioning. Treating borderline patients with IPT that is terminated does not appear to be more efficacious than good clinical care. It is intuitively obvious that borderline patients are likely to react negatively to a forced termination and that their long-standing problems are more likely to require longer treatment.

The adaptation of IPT for BPD highlights some of the conceptual problems in the earlier work with IPT. The theoretical basis for IPT emphasizes the need to focus on acute interpersonal stressors, understanding that underlying attachment and personality issues complicate treatment, but are not a focus of IPT because the duration of the time-limited treatment is too short for substantial change in attachment to occur.

In the original adaptation of IPT for BPD, an additional Problem Area called 'self-image' was added.[42] In contrast to the acute problem foci for which IPT has demonstrated efficacy, this 'self-image' problem area was a long-standing problem; moreover, it was intrapsychically oriented rather than interpersonally focused. As such, the self-image problem area, like the discarded interpersonal sensitivities/deficits area, is not theoretically or practically consistent with IPT. An approach in which borderline personality disorder and attachment insecurity were conceptualized as complications of treatment which focused on an acute interpersonal problem – a Role Transition, Interpersonal Dispute, or Grief and Loss issue – would be consistent with IPT and would be expected to have an impact on mood and interpersonal functioning, though it would also be expected to have much less impact on the patient's underlying attachment style and personality.

Another conceptual and practical problem with all of the adaptations of IPT for patients with BPD was that the therapy was terminated. This presents enormous problems generally and with IPT specifically. Generally speaking, terminating treatment under any circumstances with patients with BPD causes iatrogenic distress. As noted throughout this guide, termination of therapy shifts the focus from interpersonal crises outside of therapy to a crisis within the therapeutic relationship. To terminate treatment with a borderline patient precipitates a real abandonment crisis. The therapist is literally abandoning the patient – there is no way to sugar-coat this fact. To terminate after a longer period of treatment (34 weeks in some cases) only intensifies the significance of the abandonment. Fuel is added to the fire with borderline patients when the therapy is continued weekly and then abruptly terminated. Discussion of termination does not mitigate their experience of termination as a real abandonment, *because it is an abandonment*. There is no theoretical or practical reason to terminate treatment, and every reason with insecurely attached patients to make a smooth transition from the Conclusion of Acute Treatment to Maintenance Treatment.

IPT for Post-traumatic Stress Disorder

IPT has been applied to the treatment of post-traumatic stress disorder (PTSD) by a number of clinicians.[45–50] The ways in which adaptations to IPT have been made are well illustrated with PTSD. We describe these with PTSD as an example of the processes that can be used to modify IPT for other affective and non-affective disorders.

Introduction to PTSD

The psychological and physiological effects of traumatic stress are neither uniform nor inevitable. Complex biological, psychological, and social factors (both before and after the trauma) determine its ultimate impact. The types of psychological traumatic stress are also variable.

There is a growing body of evidence for the treatment for PTSD. Antidepressants, particularly the serotonin reuptake inhibitors (SSRIs), help to reduce the core symptoms of PTSD and are recognized as mainstream treatment.[51] Van Etten and Taylor[52] analyzed 61 treatment trials for PTSD, including pharmacotherapy and psychotherapies such as Exposure Therapy and Dynamic Psychotherapy. Overall, there was greater efficacy for Exposure Therapy than for any other treatment. Other reviews of psychotherapeutic approaches[53] have shown significant improvements in PTSD symptoms both post-treatment and at follow up.[54,55] Recent reviews support a combination of treatments including psychoeducation, cognitive and behavioral techniques, and substantive interventions for comorbid mood, substance use, and anxiety disorders.[53,56,57]

Despite the evidence supporting psychotherapy, academicians have argued that 'there is no gold standard treatment program for PTSD, nor has any particular treatment approach received universal acceptance among clinicians'.[58] Moreover, there appears to be a general consensus that individual treatment modalities are not effective in addressing the full range of clinical problems, such as the interpersonal difficulties frequently observed in traumatized individuals.[58,59] While these observations strongly suggest that the interpersonal focus of IPT is likely to address the interpersonal stressors faced by individuals with PTSD, they also suggest that IPT is likely to be more effective as part of an integrated treatment that combines interpersonal, behavioral, cognitive, and exposure-based approaches.

IPT for PTSD – conceptual issues

A number of authors have described phases of psychological response to traumatic events. According to Horowitz,[60] trauma survivors progress through phases of 'outcry', 'denial', 'intrusion', 'working through', and 'completion'. Herman[61] has conceptualized treatment interventions for PTSD in several phases which parallel the psyche's processing of trauma. She advocates for the creation of an environment of safety which facilitates a period of 'remembrance and mourning' and ultimately a process of 'reconnection'. The latter emphasizes the need for an interpersonal focus to trauma. Van der Kolk and others also advocate a phased treatment program for PTSD.[62] Their approach includes phases of stabilization, reconstruction of trauma-disrupted cognitive schemas, reconnection, and enhanced interpersonal efficacy.

Based on this work, a conceptual approach to the traumatized patient emphasizing a hierarchy of needs akin to the theory of Maslow has been developed[63] (Figure 19.1). Each dimension implies a therapeutic intervention. Immediate needs such as safety and a stable ecology are the first priority. After traumatic stress, particularly related to manmade disasters, these two needs are the primary focus of intervention within traumatized communities.

Following this, the traumatized patient seeks some sort of physiological homeostasis and relief from psychological distress. Beyond this are questions of an existential nature such as the meaning of traumatic events, notions of retributive and restorative justice, and a resolution or sense of closure over an event. Many of the latter have significant interpersonal components.

Adapting IPT for PTSD

In light of this phased approach to PTSD and in recognition of the interpersonal aspects of trauma, IPT has been adapted for PTSD by a number of investigators.[45–49] All three of the IPT Problem Areas are salient for this population.

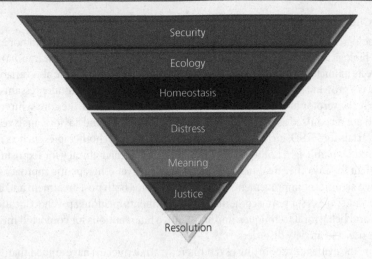

Figure 19.1 Post-traumatic stress disorder (PTSD) hierarchy

Interpersonal Disputes may exacerbate the course of PTSD or arise as a consequence of it, particularly the hyperarousal and avoidant symptoms (Table 19.1). PTSD has a detrimental effect on self-awareness, intimacy, sexuality, and interpersonal communication, all of which are key elements for the maintenance of healthy interpersonal relationships and the avoidance of conflict.[64] It can also impact Role Transitions or 'family life stages' including courtship, marriage, childbirth and childrearing, and retirement.[65] These various developmental tasks and their associated changes in family and marital functioning are frequently disrupted by avoidance or PTSD symptom intensification. The core issues underlying these crises derive from an inability to develop trust, a sense of guilt, and feelings of detachment or estrangement from others, all of which are associated with PTSD.

Table 19.1 Interpersonal Disputes arising from post-traumatic stress disorder (PTSD)

Symptom cluster	Examples of Interpersonal Disputes
Intrusive symptoms	Problems around trauma-specific phobias Unable to share bed due to nightmares
Avoidant symptoms	Avoiding important social engagement Poor communication style Inhibited problem solving style
Hyperarousal symptoms	Irritability Aggressive outbursts or episodic dyscontrol Hostile interactions

One of the most difficult tasks facing the trauma survivor is the adjustment to a new internal psychological state in the aftermath of trauma. Janoff-Bulman[66] described it as a process of adjusting to the 'shattered assumptions' of the world that the trauma survivor experiences. Prior to a traumatic event, the world is predictable and safe, and the individual has confidence in his capacity to participate in it. In the wake of trauma, these assumptions are 'shattered' and the individual faces an internal and external world that is unpredictable and fragmented. This abstract existential concept can be addressed as a Role Transition which focuses on a pre-trauma and a post-trauma role. In the case of recently developed PTSD, the adjustment to a potentially chronic illness process and its treatment may challenge a patient's self-concept in his 'old (pre-trauma) role' as well as necessitate a modification of his expectations of self and future in the 'new (post-trauma) role', particularly when poor control of symptoms means that return to work or to a previous level of social functioning may be unrealistic.

This conceptualization of the reaction to trauma is consistent with the attachment model undergirding IPT. The pre-trauma attachment (more secure) is shifted to a post-trauma attachment style (more insecure) because the working model of others has shifted. The trauma negatively impacts the internal model of trusting others and asking for help, and is a tragic illustration that current or recent events can impact attachment.

Grief and Loss is also a frequently used Problem Area when treating PTSD. Bereavement, particularly if it is sudden or unexpected, is associated with PTSD in between 9–36 percent of cases.[67] Bereavement resulting from a loss due to a traumatic event may constitute an acute crisis that may precipitate or exacerbate symptoms of PTSD. When PTSD symptoms have been complicated by 'survivor guilt', the IPT techniques used with Grief and Loss help patients identify with the concrete aspects of the loss, such as clarifying ways their attachment needs may be met by others in their remaining social support networks. This approach de-emphasizes in-depth discussion of the existential meaning of an individual's survival and loss, and instead focuses on helping the patient identify ways that his current attachment needs can be met.

It is well established that survivors of trauma, particularly combat veterans, experience long-term problems in interpersonal relationships. PTSD adversely impacts individuals' attachment styles; pre-traumatic attachment may be altered by the traumatic experience, leading to difficulties in current attachment and interpersonal functioning.[64] While the old Problem Area of interpersonal sensitivity/deficits was once used as a way to define this vulnerability, current work with IPT places it squarely in the realm of fearful or dismissive attachment. As noted, trauma impacts attachment, greatly diminishing the patient's perceived sense of safety and security, and his ability to trust others and ask for help when distressed. This fearful or dismissive style exacerbates the acute problems that drive the patient to seek treatment. Thus the long-term disruption to interpersonal functioning arising from trauma is conceptualized as the result of a maladaptive attachment style; treatment is focused on acute crises in the context of this attachment style.

A trauma-based maladaptive attachment style is relevant to nearly all patients with PTSD, and is directly discussed with all patients as sequelae of the trauma, framed in terms of difficulties trusting others and making oneself vulnerable. Therapeutic interventions emphasize the impact of PTSD symptoms upon interpersonal functioning and attempt to define these processes as being as much a part of the disorder as flashbacks or nightmares.

Group IPT for PTSD

While individual therapy is the most common approach to PTSD, group psychotherapy is a valuable adjunct. Group psychotherapy is well suited to addressing the impact of PTSD on an individual's relationship with others, as the modality provides the opportunity for social support, social reintegration, and interpersonal learning.[68,69] The challenge for the therapist working with groups is to create a 'healing matrix', where patients can risk exposure and restore a sense of self-worth, feeling safe, and feeling connected to others.[70] In IPT terms, the group must be secure and have a high degree of inclusion.

Case example 19.1: James

James was a 56-year-old man who had recently retired from his liquor store business after obtaining a war service pension. He had served in the Australian Navy in the Vietnam War, and had volunteered to be a gunner in a US Army helicopter regiment. James's combat exposure had been heavy; his regiment had likely been responsible for the deaths of dozens of Vietnamese combatants and civilians, as their role had largely been offensive operations. James felt he was responsible for much of the carnage as he had operated one of his helicopter's M60 machine guns. Despite this, James's most distressing recollections were of incidents where there was a threat to himself or his comrades. His father had fought in the Second World War as an infantryman in the Pacific and had suffered with severe anxiety throughout most of his adult life before dying of complications of alcoholism in his forties. James had volunteered for combat 'to do my duty like my father did'.

After his military service he became a prison officer. He remained in that role for 20 years, running a high-security prison block and dealing with the worst offenders. He was involved in a number of violent incidents and suicides. James had taken early retirement 5 years prior to seeking treatment and had bought a liquor store. The business had struggled because of James's worsening irritability and avoidant behavior. This had led to escalating levels of alcohol consumption.

James had already completed a CBT program for PTSD. He had obtained some symptomatic benefit from it, and was an active group participant. However, James had required seven admissions to hospital in the 6 months following completion of the CBT program. These had invariably been associated with conflicts with his wife or step-daughter, all in the context of alcohol abuse. He had taken antidepressant medication, but it had only been of modest benefit.

James lived with his wife, although his step-daughter frequently visited for long periods. His wife had been treated for depression and his step-daughter had suffered from eating disorder symptoms, episodes of deliberate self-harm and mood swings. His first marriage had ended in estrangement and there had been domestic violence involved. He had one son from that marriage, from whom he was completely estranged. He had been the step-father of his step-daughter from age 8. Her sister had died in adolescence from a brain tumor, which had heralded her eating disorder symptoms and her mother's chronic depression (Figure 19.2).

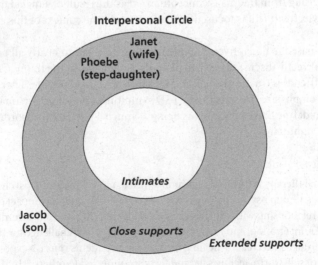

Figure 19.2 Interpersonal Circle – James

James was referred for group IPT based upon his previous experience in the CBT group, but also because of the perceived role of the family conflict in his symptom exacerbations. During the pre-group individual session he had presented as guarded, prickly, and controlling. He frequently peppered his narrative with expletives, but had become tearful and distressed when discussing his wife's and step-daughter's 'problems'. As one therapist had noted:

> **James presents as having no redeeming features until he talks about his wife and step-daughter, and then his façade just crumbles and he is like a scared little kid.**

James was diagnosed with PTSD, although much of his functional impairment seemed associated with comorbid narcissistic personality traits, depressive symptoms, and the effects of alcohol abuse. He was abstinent from alcohol at the start of treatment. During the Interpersonal Formulation in the individual intake session (Figure 19.3), James noted that the acute problem which had led him to therapy was an Interpersonal Dispute involving his step-daughter.

James was on time for the first group session and chose a seat with his back against a corner of the room. As other group members arrived he became visibly more vigilant and agitated. When asked to introduce himself to the group he quickly snapped, 'I have a problem with my kid and I'm no bloody good in dealing with people.'

During the middle sessions of the group, James would occasionally respond to questions and began to disclose more about his step-daughter. He said

> **I could never be close to her because of all the kid molesters I had to deal with in the jails, and when her sister died, I just had nothing to say. I have seen death all around ... hell I even caused a lot of death, so I had nothing to say.**

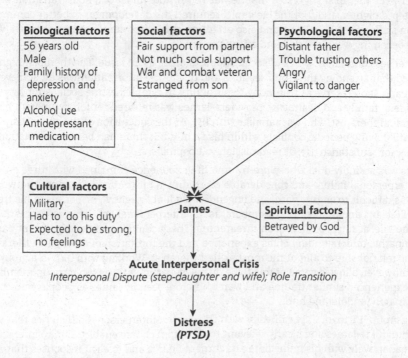

Figure 19.3 Interpersonal Formulation – James

Another group member confronted him, asking, 'Mate, did you think you were a father to her back then?' to which James replied angrily, 'About as much as mine was to me.'

The group therapist tried to elicit the specific details of interactions between James and his step-daughter. This was difficult because of James's reluctance to participate in the group process. When invited to role play an interaction with his step-daughter, he responded, 'I told you, I'm not doing any of that garbage. If you insist on it, I'm leaving right now.' Rather than abandon the point entirely, the second group therapist asked James if he could remember what he actually said to his step-daughter, so as to recount an Interpersonal Incident. When he described this, it was apparent that his communication was both vague and inflammatory. The therapist invited group members to offer suggestions for other styles of communication that may have been better. It was suggested by another member that James might want to set up a conversation with his step-daughter to practice less confrontational communication. The therapist called attention to James's affect during the interaction within the group and highlighted that his distress seemed to indicate he cared for his step-daughter.

In the following session, James reported that he had a conversation with his step-daughter and that they had been able to talk about events, and even about her sister's death. Three days later, though, they had another argument. In clarifying the argument, it became apparent that James had lost control when his irritability and 'short fuse' escalated. As he described and attempted to justify it: 'It's just like when they show all that Afghanistan war stuff on TV, I just go off.' Another group member asked, 'Buddy, how do you deal with the Afghanistan stuff?' to which James replied, 'I do the breathing and distraction stuff earlier rather than later, so I can avoid a blowup.' One of the therapists suggested that perhaps a similar behavioral strategy could be applied to interactions with his step-daughter.

In subsequent discussions, James's disclosed his shame and sadness at 'being such a bad father'. The therapist suggested that he was now in the midst of a Role Transition with his step-daughter, and that the 'new role' required the development of better communication skills, problem solving, and also attention to his emotional responses to her, which were becoming warmer and more affectionate.

In later sessions, James's lack of social supports arose as an issue. The therapist highlighted that attending the group sessions and disclosing information was an achievement and should serve as testimony to his ability to establish some social supports outside of family and healthcare providers. James was referred for follow-up with his individual therapist, who was familiar with IPT. At the conclusion of the group, James was still having periodic conflicts within his family, but there had been no escalation in aggression, substance use, or readmission to hospital.

James was an individual whose pre-trauma life experience combined with three decades of interpersonal failure and considerable morbidity in his immediate support network. He was difficult to engage with, and engendered a lot of negative responses in his treating clinicians and in the group members, as his interpersonal style was confrontational and hostile, at times bordering on threatening. These could have been significant barriers to empathic understanding of his experience and the formation of a workable therapeutic relationship to all but the most skilled therapist. Working with him in a group setting, however, allowed some of this to be diffused, particularly as other group members had experienced similar trauma and were therefore seen by James as people who could legitimately understand him.

Using group IPT to intervene directly with the current interpersonal difficulties that were meaningful to James and clearly relevant to symptom course enabled him to interact more adaptively with his immediate attachment figures and to elicit responses that helped him gratify his attachment needs. He had clearly sought interpersonal interactions, either with his family members or professional caregivers. His pattern of interaction prior to IPT for PTSD had been to elicit unfavorable and unwanted responses from them, which created a downward spiral of symptom intensification, substance abuse, and worsening interpersonal interactions. Being a focal intervention, IPT for PTSD enabled the therapists to quarantine problematic transference and countertransference problems and provide him with a series of gratifying interpersonal interactions within the group therapy setting, which could be generalized to relationships outside of therapy.

It is not clear whether James would have tolerated the same interventions in individual therapy or whether an individual therapist would have become 'bogged down' in problematic countertransference. The cohesive group, focused upon Interpersonal Problem Areas, maintained a working state and generated a momentum for change that may not have been created in an individual therapeutic frame. As Wilfley et al.[36] highlight, the group format in IPT provides an 'interpersonal laboratory' with numerous opportunities for interpersonal interactions that may be therapeutic. James likely benefited from empathic and practical responses from group members working collaboratively on a focal area. Such interactions, explicitly highlighted by the group therapist, seemed to provide stimulus for further change and a restitutive emotional experience.

Evidence supporting IPT for PTSD

Several studies have evaluated the efficacy and effectiveness of IPT in PTSD; the majority of these have used a group format. Krupnick et al.[49] found group-based IPT for PTSD effective in reducing symptoms of PTSD, depression, and some aspects of interpersonal functioning in a sample of 48 low-income, predominantly minority women who had sustained interpersonal trauma. Bleiberg and Markowitz[47] provided IPT to 14 subjects with PTSD in an open trial, and found that 12 of them no longer met the diagnostic criteria for PTSD.

Robertson and colleagues[45,46] used group IPT for 13 patients with chronic PTSD. Quantitative outcomes indicated no change in the severity of PTSD symptoms, but substantial gains in social functioning, generalized well-being, and mood symptoms did occur. Their qualitative analysis of participant exit interviews highlighted themes of interpersonal connection and enhanced interpersonal efficacy emerging in the course of therapy with IPT.

Ray and Webster[48] applied group IPT to nine military veterans using the approach developed by Robertson et al. At 2- and 4-month follow-up, there were improvements in PTSD and depressive symptoms with some qualitative data suggesting the participants experienced improvements in anger management and interpersonal functioning. Meffert and co-workers[50] conducted a trial of IPT with 22 Sudanese refugees in Cairo, and found reductions in PTSD and depressive symptoms in addition to anger and interpersonal violence.

Conclusion

IPT has been adapted to a wide variety of psychiatric disorders, including a spectrum of affective disorders, eating disorders, and some anxiety disorders. In all of these adaptations, IPT is distinguished because of its primary interpersonal focus and use of the IPT Problem Areas. The application of IPT to PTSD is an example of the way that the interpersonal aspects of a disorder or distress are identified and IPT is modified to address them. The application of IPT with PTSD also illustrates its potential use in a sequential or integrated psychotherapeutic approach.

There are many disorders to which IPT can be applied. Without doubt, IPT should be of benefit in improving mood and interpersonal functioning in a wide range of problems and distress. Our hope is that new investigators will continue the development and investigation of IPT for an even greater variety of problems.

References

1. Mufson L. *Interpersonal Psychotherapy for Depressed Adolescents*, 2nd edn. 2004, New York: Guilford Press.

2. Mufson L, Moreau D and Weissman MM. The modification of interpersonal psychotherapy with depressed adolescents (IPT-A): phase I and phase II studies. *Journal of the American Academy of Child and Adolescent Psychiatry*, 1994, **33**: 695–705.

3. Rosselo J and Bernal G. The efficacy of cognitive-behavioral and interpersonal treatments for depression in Puerto Rican adolescents. *Journal of Consulting and Clinical Psychology*, 1999, **55**: 379–384.

4. Mufson L, *et al*. A randomized effectiveness trial of interpersonal psychotherapy for depressed adolescents. *Archives of General Psychiatry*, 2004, **61**: 577–584.

5. Rosselo J, Bernal G and Rivera-Medina C. Individual and group CBT and IPT for Puerto Rican adolescents with depressive symptoms. *Cultural Diversity and Ethnic Minority Psychology*, 2008, **14**: 234–235.

6. Tang TC, *et al*. Randomized study of school-based intensive interpersonal psychotherapy for depressed adolescents with suicidal risk and parasuicide behaviors. *Psychiatry and Clinical Neurosciences*, 2009, **63**: 4.

7. Dietz LJ, *et al*. Family-based interpersonal psychotherapy for depressed preadolescents: An open-treatment trial. *Early Intervention in Psychiatry*, 2008, **2**: 154–161.

8. Reynolds CF, *et al*. Treating depression to remission in older adults: a controlled evaluation of combined escitalopram with interpersonal psychotherapy versus escitalopram with depression care management. *International Journal of Geriatric Psychiatry*, 2010, **25**: 1134–1141.

9. Heisel MJ, *et al*. Adapting interpersonal psychotherapy for older adults at risk for suicide: preliminary findings. *Professional Psychology: Research and Practice*, 2009, **40**: 156–164.

10. Miller MD. Using interpersonal therapy (IPT) with older adults today and tomorrow: a review of the literature and new developments. *Current Psychiatry Reports*, 2008, **10**: 16–22.

11. Reynolds CF, *et al*. Treatment of bereavement-related major depressive episodes in later life: a controlled study of acute and continuation treatment with nortriptyline and interpersonal psychotherapy. *American Journal of Psychiatry*, 1999, **156**: 202–208.

12. Miler M and Reynolds CF. Expanding the usefulness of interpersonal psychotherapy (IPT) for depressed elders with comorbid cognitive impairment. *International Journal of Geriatric Psychiatry*, 2007, **22**: 101–105.

13. Miller MD. *Clinician's Guide to Interpersonal Psychotherapy in Late Life: Helping Cognitively Impaired or Depressed Elders and their Caregivers*. 2009, New York: Oxford Press.

14. Spinelli MG and Endicott J. Controlled clinical trial of interpersonal psychotherapy versus parenting education program for depressed pregnant women. *American Journal of Psychiatry*, 2003, **160**: 555–562.

15. Spinelli MG and Weissman MM. The clinical application of interpersonal psychotherapy for depression during pregnancy. *Primary Psychiatry*, 1997, **4**: 50–57.

16. Grote NK, *et al*. A randomized controlled trial of culturally relevant, brief interpersonal psychotherapy for perinatal depression. *Psychiatric Services*, 2009, **60**: 313–321.

17. Bledsoe SE, *et al*. Feasibility of treating depression in pregnant, low-income adolescents using culturally relevant, brief interpersonal psychotherapy. *Journal of Women's Health*, 2010, **19**: 1781.

18. O'Hara MW, *et al*. Efficacy of interpersonal psychotherapy for postpartum depression. *Archives of General Psychiatry*, 2000, **57**: 1039–1045.

19. Stuart S and O'Hara MW. The use of interpersonal psychotherapy for perinatal mood and anxiety disorders, in Steiner M and Riecher-Rössler A (eds) *Perinatal Depression: From Bench to Bedside*. 2005, Basel: Karger, pp. 150–166.

20. Carter W, Grigoriadis S and Ross LE. Relationship distress and depression in postpartum women: literature review and introduction of a conjoint interpersonal psychotherapy intervention. *Archives of Women's Mental Health*, 2010, **13**: 279–284.

21. Grote NK, Swartz HA and Zuckoff A. Enhancing interpersonal psychotherapy for mothers and expectant mothers on low incomes: adaptations and additions. *Journal of Contemporary Psychotherapy*, 2008, **38**: 23–33.

22. Reay R, *et al*. Group interpersonal psychotherapy for postnatal depression: a pilot study. *Archives of Women's Mental Health*, 2006, **9**: 31–39.

23. Mulcahy R, *et al*. A randomised control trial for the effectiveness of group interpersonal psychotherapy for postnatal depression. *Archives of Women's Mental Health*, 2010, **13**: 125–139.

24. Markowitz J. *Interpersonal Psychotherapy for Dysthymic Disorder*. 1998, Washington DC: American Psychiatric Press.

25. Mason BJ, Markowitz JC and Klerman GL. Interpersonal psychotherapy for dysthymic disorder, in Klerman GL and Weissman MM (eds) *New Applications of Interpersonal Psychotherapy*. 1993, Washington DC: American Psychiatric Press, pp. 225–264.

26. Markowitz J, *et al*. Pilot study of interpersonal psychotherapy versus supportive psychotherapy for dysthymic patients with secondary alcohol abuse of dependence. *Journal of Nervous and Mental Disorders*, 2008, **196**: 468–474.

27. Ehlers C, Frank E and Kupfer DJ. Social zeitgebers and biological rhythms. *Archives of General Psychiatry*, 1988, **45**: 948–952.

28. Frank E. *Treating Bipolar Disorder: A Clinician's Guide to Interpersonal and Social Rhythm Therapy*. 2005, New York: Guilford Press.

29. Miklowitz D, *et al*. Psychosocial treatments for bipolar depression: a 1-year randomized trial from the systematic treatment enhancement program. *Archives of General Psychiatry*, 2007, **64**: 419–427.

30. Fairburn CG, *et al*. A prospective study of outcome in bulimia nervosa and the long-term effects of three psychological treatments. *Archives of General Psychiatry*, 1995, **52**: 304–312.

31. Fairburn CG, Jones R and Peveler RC. Three psychological treatments for bulimia nervosa: a comparative trial. *Archives of General Psychiatry*, 1991, **48**: 463–469.

32. Fairburn CG, Jones R and Peveler RC. Psychotherapy and bulimia nervosa: the longer-term effects of interpersonal psychotherapy, behavioural psychotherapy, and cognitive behaviour therapy. *Archives of General Psychiatry*, 1993, **50**: 419–428.

33. Agras WS, *et al*. A multicenter comparison of cognitive-behavioral therapy and interpersonal psychotherapy for bulimia nervosa. *Archives of General Psychiatry*, 2000, **57**: 459–466.

34. Arcelus J, *et al*. A case series evaluation of a modified version of interpersonal psychotherapy (IPT) for the treatment of bulimic eating disorders: a pilot study. *European Eating Disorders Review*, 2009, **17**: 260–268.

35. Wilfley DE, *et al*. Adapting interpersonal psychotherapy to a group format (IPT-G) for binge eating disorder: toward a model for adapting empirically supported treatments. *Psychotherapy Research*, 1998, **8**: 379–391.

36. Wilfley DE, *et al*. *Interpersonal Psychotherapy for Group*. 2000, New York: Basic Books.

37. Rieger E, *et al*. An eating disorder-specific model of interpersonal psychotherapy (IPT-ED): causal pathways and treatment implications. *Clinical Psychology Review*, 2010, **30**: 400–410.

38. Wilfley DE, *et al*. A randomized comparison of group cognitive-behavioral therapy and group interpersonal psychotherapy for the treatment of overweight individuals with binge-eating disorder. *Archives of General Psychiatry*, 2002, **59**: 713–721.

39. McIntosh V, Jordan J and Carter F. Three psychotherapies for anorexia nervosa: a randomized controlled trial. *American Journal of Psychiatry*, 2005, **162**: 741–747.

40. Lipsitz JD, *et al*. Open trial of interpersonal psychotherapy for the treatment of social phobia. *American Journal of Psychiatry*, 1999, **156**: 1814–1816.

41. Stangier U, *et al*. Cognitive therapy versus interpersonal psychotherapy in social anxiety disorder: a randomized controlled trial. *Archives of General Psychiatry*, 2011, **68**: 692–700.

42. Angus L and Gillies L. Counseling the borderline client: an interpersonal approach. *Canadian Journal of Counselling*, 1994, **28**: 69–83.

43. Markowitz J, Skodol A and Bleiberg K. Interpersonal psychotherapy for borderline personality disorder: possible mechanisms of change. *Journal of Clinical Psychology*, 2006, **62**: 431–444.

44. Bellino S, Zizza M and Rinaldi C. Combined therapy of major depression with concomitant borderline personality disorder: comparison of interpersonal psychotherapy and cognitive psychotherapy. *Canadian Journal of Psychiatry*, 2007, **52**: 718–725.

45. Robertson MD, Humphreys L and Ray R. Psychological treatments for post traumatic stress disorder: recommendations for the clinician. *Journal of Psychiatric Practice*, 2004, **10**: 106–118.

46. Robertson MD, *et al*. Group interpersonal psychotherapy for post traumatic stress disorder: clinical and theoretical aspects. *International Journal of Group Psychotherapy*, 2004, **54**: 145–175.

47. Bleiberg K and Markowitz J. A pilot study of interpersonal psychotherapy for posttraumatic stress disorder. *American Journal of Psychiatry*, 2005, **162**: 181–183.

48. Ray R and Webster R. Group interpersonal psychotherapy for veterans with posttraumatic stress disorder: a pilot study. *International Journal of Group Psychotherapy*, 2010, **60**: 131–140.

49. Krupnick J, *et al.* Group interpersonal psychotherapy for low-income women with posttraumatic stress disorder. *Psychotherapy Research*, 2008, **18**: 497–507.

50. Meffert SM, *et al.* A pliot randomized controlled trial of interpersonal psychotherapy for Sudanese refugees in Cairo, Egypt. *Psychological Trauma: Theory, Research, Practice, and Policy*, 2011, **5**: 1–10.

51. Stein D, Ipser J and Seedat SCR. Pharmacotherapy for post traumatic stress disorder (PTSD). *Cochrane Database of Systematic Reviews*, 2006, 1.

52. Van Etten M and Taylor S. Comparative efficacy of treatments for posttraumatic stress disorder: a meta-analysis. *Clinical Psychology and Psychotherapy*, 1998, **5**: 144–154.

53. Solomon S and Johnson D. Psychosocial treatment of posttraumatic stress disorder: a practice-friendly review of outcome research. *Journal of Clinical Psychology*, 2002, **58**: 947–959.

54. Bradley R, Greene J and Russ EA. A multidimensional meta-analysis of psychotherapy for PTSD. *American Journal of Psychiatry*, 2005, **162**: 214–227.

55. Foa EB, Keane TM and Friedman MJ. *Effective Treatments for PTSD. Practice Guidelines from the International Society for Traumatic Stress Studies*, 2nd edn. 2008, New York: Guilford Press.

56. Basco M, *et al.* Cognitive-behavioral therapy for anxiety disorders: why and how it works. *Bulletin of the Menninger Clinic*, 2000, **64**: 52–70.

57. Andrews G and Hunt C. Treatments that work in anxiety disorders. *Medical Journal of Australia*, 1998, **168**: 628–634.

58. McFarlane A and Yehuda R. Clinical treatment of posttraumatic stress disorder: conceptual challenges raised by recent research. *Australian and New Zealand Journal of Psychiatry*, 2000, **34**: 940–953.

59. Shalev A, Bonne O and Eth S. Treatment of posttraumatic stress disorder: a review. *Psychosomatic Medicine*, 1996, **58**: 165–182.

60. Horowitz M. *Stress Response Syndromes*. 1976, New York: Aronson.

61. Herman J. *Trauma and Recovery*. 1992, New York: Basic Books.

62. van der Kolk B, McFarlane A and van der Hart O. A general approach to treatment of posttraumatic stress disorder, in van der Kolk B, McFarlane A and Weisath L (eds) *Traumatic Stress*. 1989, New York: Guildford Press.

63. Maslow A. A theory of human motivation. *Psychological Review*, 1943, **50**: 370–396.

64. McFarlane A and Bookless C. The effect of PTSD on interpersonal relationships: issues for emergency service workers. *Sexual and Relationship Therapy*, 2001, **16**: 261–267.

65. Scaturo D and Hayman P. The impact of combat trauma across the family life cycle: clinical considerations. *Journal of Traumatic Stress*, 1992, **5**: 273–288.

66. Janoff-Bulman R. *Shattered Assumptions: Towards a New Psychology of Trauma*. 1992, New York: Free Press.

67. Zisook S and Shuchter S. PTSD following bereavement. *Annals of Clinical Psychiatry*, 1998, **10**: 157–163.

68. Allen S and Bloom S. Group and family treatment of post-traumatic stress disorder. *Psychiatric Clinics of North America*, 1994, **17**: 425–437.

69. Kollar P, Marmar C and Kanas N. Psychodynamic group treatment of posttraumatic stress disorder in Vietnam veterans. *International Journal of Group Psychotherapy*, 1992, **42**: 225–246.

70. Klein R and Schermer V. Introduction and overview: creating a healing matrix, in Klein R and Schermer V (eds) *Group Psychotherapy for Psychological Trauma*. 2000, New York: Guilford Press.

20

Research in Interpersonal Psychotherapy

The highly significant research in Interpersonal Psychotherapy (IPT) includes the initial studies in the 1970s by Klerman and Weissman,[1-3] the National Institute of Mental Health Treatment of Depression Collaborative Research Program (NIMH TDCRP),[4-6] the maintenance studies of Frank *et al.*,[7-9] the international studies of IPT,[10-12] and the recent meta-analyses of IPT.[13,14] A complete list of references can be found at the IPT Institute at www.iptinstitute.com.

There is much that is *not known* about IPT. There are many elements which have yet to be empirically demonstrated. The use of weekly sessions, for instance, follows clinical tradition – there are no data supporting weekly over biweekly, monthly, or even twice-weekly sessions. The use of hour-long appointments, as opposed to half-hour, 15-minute, or 2-hour sessions, is not empirically derived – there are no data regarding the optimal duration of sessions of any psychotherapy.

While efficacy studies are based on the entire 'treatment package' of IPT, there are no data regarding which parts of the package are essential. Many of the techniques and tactics used in IPT (and other psychotherapies) are based primarily on clinical experience and historical precedence. Deconstruction studies have not been conducted in IPT. The impact of assigning homework (or not), of constructing a Biopsychosocial/Cultural/Spiritual Formulation (or not), or of conducting an Interpersonal Inventory (or not), has not been studied.

The impact of strict adherence to IPT has not been studied. Clinical experience suggests that allowing therapists to use their clinical judgment leads to better outcome; empirical evidence supports this as well.[15-17,18] The requirement that therapists strictly adhere to a manual prevents them from combining therapeutic approaches. For instance, a therapist may believe that adding a behavioral activation technique to IPT will help a particular patient. A discussion about cognitions may be of great benefit to some IPT patients. However, only a therapist who is 'allowed' to do so rather than 'required' to follow a rigid protocol will be able to use this kind of combined approach. There is little doubt that patients do in fact benefit from a variety of techniques, and that a 'mix and match approach' is often taken in therapy. While widespread in practice, this has not been tested empirically.

In addition, there are no data regarding the impact of adherence to IPT as opposed to the delivery of quality IPT. Adherence is not difficult to assess – a simple yes/no checklist can be used. But adherence and quality are not the same. Conducting an Interpersonal Inventory adherently, for example, is not the same as doing it well. Virtuoso IPT requires that the therapist makes adaptations to individual patients. Adherence is a fine goal, but we should aspire to conduct high-quality IPT.

There are two responses to the lack of data about the specific elements of IPT. The first is to insist that since the data are derived from a specific IPT protocol or manual, all of the elements of that specific IPT protocol must be delivered precisely as defined or it won't be efficacious. There are no data supporting this. It might be a reasonable position to take if all of the IPT protocols were consistent, but there is great variability. Some have used more than 20 sessions, others six. Some have used five Problem Areas, some three. Some provide Maintenance Treatment, some do not. Some include homework, and some do not permit it.

The better response is to base the clinical practice of IPT on a combination of the empirical evidence, clinical experience, and clinical judgment. Adding a measure of common sense is also wise. To suggest that empirical data alone should dictate treatment is both naïve and unrealistic – there are simply too many aspects of IPT that have not been empirically studied. Further, to insist that the practice of IPT be based solely on empirical data ignores the vast wealth of information that has accumulated from clinical experience with IPT. While the empirical literature supporting the efficacy of IPT should strongly influence treatment, clinical experience and clinical judgment are equally important factors in determining how IPT is delivered. Evidence-based practice should rest in part on practice-based evidence.

References

1. Klerman GL, *et al*. Treatment of depression by drugs and psychotherapy. *American Journal of Psychiatry*, 1974, **131**: 186–191.

2. Weissman MM. The psychological treatment of depression. Evidence for the efficacy of psychotherapy alone, in comparison with, and in combination with pharmacotherapy. *Archives of General Psychiatry*, 1979, **36**: 1261–1269.

3. Weissman MM, *et al*. The efficacy of drugs and psychotherapy in the treatment of acute depressive episodes. *American Journal of Psychiatry*, 1979, **136**(4B): 555–558.

4. Elkin I, *et al*. NIMH Treatment of Depression Collaborative Treatment Program: background and research plan. *Archives of General Psychiatry*, 1985, **42**: 305–316.

5. Elkin I, *et al*. Conceptual and methodological issues in comparative studies of psychotherapy and pharmacotherapy, I. Active ingredients and mechanisms of change. *American Journal of Psychiatry*, 1988, **145**: 909–917.

6. Elkin I, *et al*. Conceptual and methodological issues in comparative studies of psychotherapy and pharmacotherapy, II. Nature and timing of treatment effects. *American Journal of Psychiatry*, 1988, **145**(9): 1070–1076.

7. Frank E, *et al*. Three-year outcomes for maintenance therapies in recurrent depression. *Archives of General Psychiatry*, 1990, **47**(12): 1093–1099.

8. Frank E and Spanier C. Interpersonal psychotherapy for depression: overview, clinical efficacy, and future directions. *Clinical Psychology: Science and Practice*, 1995, **2**: 349–369.

9. Frank E, *et al*. Randomized trial of weekly, twice-monthly, and monthly interpersonal psychotherapy as maintenance treatment for women with recurrent depression. *American Journal of Psychiatry*, 2007, **164**: 761–767.

10. Bolton P, *et al*. Group interpersonal psychotherapy for depression in rural Uganda: a randomized controlled trial. *Journal of the American Medical Association*, 2003, **289**(23): 3117–3124.

11. Bass J, *et al*. Group interpersonal psychotherapy for depression in rural Uganda: 6-month outcomes: randomised controlled trial. *British Journal of Psychiatry*, 2006, **188**(6): 567–573.

12. Verdeli H, *et al*. Group interpersonal psychotherapy for depressed youth in IDP camps in Northern Uganda: adaptation and training. *Child and Adolescent Psychiatric Clinics of North America*, 2008, **17**: 605–624.

13. Cuijpers P, *et al*. Psychotherapy for depression in adults: a meta-analysis of comparative outcome studies. *Journal of Consulting and Clinical Psychology*, 2008, **76**(6): 909–922.

14. Cuijpers P, *et al*. Interpersonal psychotherapy for depression: a meta-analysis. *American Journal of Psychiatry*, 2011, **168**(6): 581–592.

15. Barber J, Crits-Christoph P and Luborsky L. Effects of therapist adherence and competence on patient outcome in brief dynamic therapy. *Journal of Consulting and Clinical Psychology*, 1996, **64**: 619–622.

16. Barber J, *et al*. The role of the alliance and techniques in predicting outcome of supportive-expressive dynamic therapy for cocaine dependence. *Psychoanalytic Psychology*, 2008, **25**: 461–482.

17. Barber J, *et al*. The role of therapist adherence, therapist competence, and the alliance in predicting outcome of individual drug counseling: results from the NIDA collaborative cocaine treatment study. *Psychotherapy Research*, 2006, **16**: 229–240.

18. Castonguay L, *et al*. Predicting the effect of cognitive therapy for depression: a study of unique and common factors. *Journal of Consulting and Clinical Psychology*, 1996, **64**: 497–504.

Integrated Case Example

This chapter is a synthesis of all of the components discussed throughout this book. The case illustrates the flexible structure of Interpersonal Psychotherapy (IPT), the Interpersonal Inventory, Interpersonal Formulation, Problem Areas and techniques.

Case Example 21.1: Allan

Part I: Clinical Assessment

Background

Allan was a 42-year-old married father of two teenage daughters. He worked as a proof reader, a job he had held for 10 years. He had initially presented to his family physician complaining of insomnia and abdominal pain. His family physician had diagnosed a major depressive disorder and had instituted treatment with a serotonin selective reuptake inhibitor (SSRI) antidepressant. After 3 weeks, Allan had not had much benefit from medication, and a referral was made to a therapist.

Assessment/Initial sessions

Allan arrived half an hour early for his appointment. After he arrived, the therapist's secretary told him that the therapist was running 5–10 minutes behind schedule. This appeared to irritate Allan, though he did not directly communicate his annoyance.

Once the session began, Allan described having difficulty sleeping over the previous 3–6 months. He reported feeling irritable and frustrated, and had complaints of non-specific abdominal pain and headaches. In her referral letter, Allan's family physician reported that Allan had been experiencing depressed mood for most of the day with a tendency for his mood to lift through the afternoon. She noted both initial and terminal insomnia characterized by early morning wakening. Allan confirmed this, and further described having a decreased level of interest in his usual activities, and a reduced capacity to enjoy things. Allan also reported that he had been experiencing difficulty with concentration which had affected his job performance. He matter-of-factly divulged that he had intermittent suicidal thoughts, and had contemplated overdosing on his medication and alcohol, though he did not have any specific intent at the moment. The therapist inquired specifically about psychotic symptoms, which were not present, and then further clarified Allan's suicidal ideation. Though Allan reported that he had thoughts at times that he might be better off dead, he had no intent to do anything. Further, he stated that he would never commit suicide because it would be devastating for his family.

In addition to the antidepressant medication, Allan's family doctor had prescribed a benzodiazepine for sleep. Allan had doubled the dose on his own. He denied consuming alcohol or other illicit substances, and denied that he had been obtaining prescriptions for sedatives elsewhere.

Past psychiatric history

Allan denied previous consultation with any mental healthcare professionals. On closer inquiry, however, he described several prolonged periods of dysphoria, as well as two occasions in his early adolescence and young adulthood where he had significant depression that lasted for months. He had not, however, sought any form of psychiatric treatment or counseling.

Past medical history

Allan reported being in good health. His only medications were the antidepressant and the benzodiazepine.

Family psychiatric history

Allan was an only child. His mother had been hospitalized throughout his childhood with episodes of severe depression. He believed that the onset was after Allan's birth. He had been raised by a variety of caregivers throughout his childhood, and described that his father became detached from him and his mother. Allan did not recall feeling particularly affectionate or close to any of his caregivers, nor was he able to recall any meaningful relationships with school teachers or peers. Speaking in the neutral voice he used nearly all of the time, Allan reported that his mother had recently suffered another episode of severe depression and had been hospitalized again:

> She tends to spend a long time in the hospital. I'm not sure she ever really gets better. I've never known her to be 'normal'.

Allan was unaware of any other family members who had experienced psychological problems.

Social and developmental history

Allan was carried to term in an uncomplicated pregnancy and delivery. There was no evidence that his mother had been depressed antenatally. He was not aware of any delay in reaching his developmental milestones. Allan described few meaningful attachments as a child, and recalled that he was generally anxious and avoidant in his behavior. He reported that he was isolated at school with few friends, and was described by his teachers as a 'shy but pleasant child'. There was no evidence of separation anxiety or somatizing symptoms as a child. Allan completed 5 years of secondary education before leaving to join the civil service, where he worked in a low-level administrative capacity for the next 10 years. Throughout his employment in the civil service he had few social contacts, but he did get involved in solitary physical activities such as going to the gym for exercise and running.

Allan met his wife Pam at a church function during his early twenties. She had been on a vacation from abroad, and after meeting they formed a relationship which he described as 'initially close, more of a friendship than lovers'. Pam migrated to live with Allan and they were married after 2 years. Eliza was born after 12 months; Anna 3 years later. Allan described being happy as a father, particularly with Eliza, to whom he felt close. He recalled spending a lot of time with Eliza when she was younger, and he particularly enjoyed going on long runs with her. He had been less close to Anna, but still felt that their relationship was good. He had grown closer to Eliza as his relationship with Pam had deteriorated over the years.

Eliza had begun to spend increasing amounts of time away from the family and seemed to Allan to have been avoiding contact with him, particularly over the previous 6 months. Allan stated that approximately 2 months before he had become aware of a relationship Eliza was developing with an older woman, which he believed was sexual. He had no strong feelings about the relationship itself, but was aware that as she was spending much less time at home, he had felt more isolated. Allan summed up his social relationships by stating rather blandly: 'I feel completely alone – there's nobody for me'.

Premorbid personality

Allan described a long-standing difficulty with intimate relationships. He reported that he found strong emotional states such as anger and sadness intolerable. He described a pattern of exploding in torrents of rage, only to become deeply ashamed at losing control. This difficult cycle of rage and shame was greatly distressing to him. The therapist noted, however, that when Allan described what he called 'rage' in detail, it was quite limited. In fact, the therapist observed that what Allan labeled 'rage' would have been called nothing more than simple anger by most people. It appeared that Allan was most concerned about losing control of his emotions, and felt that any display of anger was a 'rage'.

The therapist came to the view that Allan had a tendency to rely on obsessional and perfectionistic coping strategies, such as working longer hours, trying to atone for his perceived failings by repetitively attending to tasks, and by overemphasizing order and goal achievement. There seemed to be a tendency for him to view the world in an 'all or nothing' way, focusing primarily upon the negative aspects of life. The therapist felt there was evidence that this was a stable pattern of personality functioning that had probably been present since childhood.

Cultural and spiritual factors

Allan described his work environment as a 'culture of silence'. It was expected that people were productive; particularly among the men the expectation was to talk about the Hawkeyes or the Roosters games and not much else. No one revealed much personal information, and Allan felt that to do so would be perceived as a weakness by others. Allan described himself as spiritual, but he did not attend church regularly. He described going with Pam on occasion at holidays, but disliking the crowds of people and what he perceived to be the superficial relationships there.

Mental state examination

Allan was a fit-looking, middle-aged man who was casually attired in jeans and a collared shirt. He wore a neatly trimmed beard with glasses, and had short cropped hair. The therapist had great difficulty establishing rapport with Allan, and found him to have little or no warmth. He had difficulty maintaining eye contact. Allan's affect was flat and he described his mood as 'quite depressed'. While there was no disorder of thought, there appeared to be significant self-reproach and hopelessness in his thought content, though it was not delusional in intensity. There were no perceptual disturbances evident. Allan had fair insight into the severity of his problems – he acknowledged that some of his vegetative symptoms were excessive and might be indicative of an illness, but he was very hopeless, and felt that there was nothing he could do that would be of help, aside from taking medication.

Diagnostic formulation

The therapist made the following *Diagnostic and Statistical Manual of Mental Disorders* (DSM)-IV diagnoses (Table 21.1):

Table 21.1 GAF, Global Assessment of Functioning

Axis I	Major depressive disorder
	Dysthymic disorder
Axis II	Obsessive-compulsive personality traits
Axis III	None
Axis IV	Family and marital disputes
	Illness of mother
	Social isolation
Axis V	GAF = 55

Interpersonal Inventory

The psychiatric assessment, in large part based on the therapist's perception that it would be helpful to prioritize the therapeutic alliance rather than rush or impose a rigid agenda, was done over the first two sessions. In session 3, the therapist invited Allan to work with him to construct an Interpersonal Inventory. He realized that it was especially critical to give Allan a sense of collaboration. He gave Allan brief instructions on how to write in the names of people in his Interpersonal Circle, handed the paper to Allan, and sat back in his chair.

Allan quickly wrote in Pam, Eliza, and Anna. Interestingly, he placed Eliza much closer to the center of the circle than he did Pam. Pausing a bit, he then asked the therapist who else should be added. The therapist responded:

> Whoever is in your social support network, especially if they have relevance to the problems you are having right now.

Allan pushed for more clarification, as if there were a right answer that the therapist was withholding. Despite that, the therapist warmly encouraged Allan that it was his circle to complete, that there were no right or wrong answers, and that he simply wanted to have a visual sense of Allan's social network so that he could understand Allan and his distress better.

Allan then wrote in his mother on the very outer edge of the paper. On the other side, he wrote in his father in parentheses indicating he had died. The only other name he added was a colleague at work, John, whom he placed in the outer circle. Before handing the paper back to the therapist, he took one last look at it, and then drew a circle around Eliza and an arrow pointing towards the outside of the circle. When asked to describe it, he said it represented her leaving for another relationship (Figure 21.1).

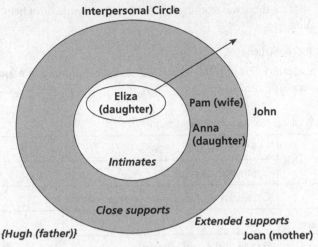

Figure 21.1 Interpersonal Circle – Allan

When the therapist asked more about his relationship with his wife, Allan replied:

> Pam doesn't have much time for me anymore. She seems to have fallen out of love and I don't think she wants to be with me. I don't think I'm a particularly pleasant person to be with at the moment. Things just seem to be falling apart.

On further inquiry, it became apparent that Allan and Pam had been arguing a great deal, and that their relationship had become 'cold and stale'. When the therapist inquired further about Allan's relationship with his daughters, Allan reported that he had a 'falling out' with his older daughter Eliza, and that Anna had become increasingly difficult at home, annoying both Allan and his wife.

When asking about Allan's interests and activities outside of work, the therapist found that there was very little evidence of any social support. Allan had little or no contact with anybody outside of his immediate family, and he seemed quite socially isolated and unsupported.

Attachment style

The Interpersonal Inventory provided a great deal of information about Allan's attachment style. It seemed clear that Allan's social isolation was a significant factor in the genesis of his mood symptoms and distress. Allan described his typical style of interacting as a tendency to do things alone or to avoid people; the therapist concurred but also held the more sophisticated view that Allan had a combination of fearful and dismissive attachment styles. To evaluate this further, the therapist gathered some additional information:

Therapist: *Allan, in addition to the family conflicts we've discussed, I wanted to talk more about the general sense of isolation you are feeling.*

Allan: *Yes – it is a problem.*

Therapist: *You told me earlier that you tended to rely on Pam to 'break the ice with people'.*

Allan: *That's right.*

Therapist: *What makes it difficult, do you think?*

Allan: *Well, I've never really tried, I guess.*

Therapist: *Tell me more about that.*

Allan: *I've never had much luck in relationships. Not since I was a kid, and certainly not as an adult.*

Therapist: *Perhaps we could look at a few examples of relationships in which you felt this has been a problem, and see if there is a pattern.*

Allan: *You mean like dragging over old ground?*

Therapist: *Well, even though we are working on your current relationships, I think we can learn about your current problems by paying some attention to what has happened in the more recent past.*

Following this exchange Allan and the therapist discussed a few examples of instances in which Allan had tried and failed to initiate interpersonal contact. It appeared that the common theme throughout all of these relationship failures had been Allan's tendency to place high expectations upon those around him, only to find that they did not follow up with further contact. Allan described that if a particular social contact had not followed through with a request or not met an expectation, then Allan would express disapproval. Typically, Allan would not initiate further contact and ultimately the relationship would dissolve. The therapist also asked Allan to tell a story as another way to assess his attachment style:

Therapist: *It would be helpful for me to understand things even better if you could tell me a story or two about your interactions with other people. What comes to mind?*

Allan: *[pausing for a bit] Nothing really. What do you mean by a story?*

Therapist: *What I'm looking for is an example. I've found that many times I can understand people even better from the interactions they describe in stories. Perhaps there is one with Pam that would be a good example.*

Allan: *[pausing again] I still can't really think of anything. I mean, we've had our share of fights, and a few good times, but I can't think of any specific stories.*

Therapist: *Perhaps a holiday or family event might be an example.*

Allan: *[pausing yet again] Well, I guess this last Valentine's Day would be a good example. We both bought each other some cards, more out of obligation really. Then on the way home from work I felt a bit guilty, so I stopped off to get her some flowers. It was late in the day, so most of the nice ones were picked over. I ended up with daisies ... she didn't get me anything at all, and then we were mostly silent over dinner. I think for both of us it was disappointing, but more like it was just the same. Nothing different, both of us at a distance. It's kind of depressing just thinking about it again.*

Interpersonal Formulation

Just as he had done with the inventory, the therapist realized that the therapeutic alliance could be further strengthened by engaging Allan in collaboratively developing the formulation. After drawing the boxes, he again handed the paper and pencil over to Allan so that he could write in the relevant elements. Together they developed a tentative formulation (Figure 21.2), which included Allan's family history and his limited social contacts as major factors in his current distress. The psychological elements in particular were handled very carefully by the therapist; his conceptualization was that Allan had an attachment style with both dismissive and fearful elements, and that he also had substantial avoidant and obsessive personality traits. For purposes of the formulation, however, they used the words Allan had used to describe himself: 'likes more individual activities, not very affectionate, and doesn't really like social activities.'

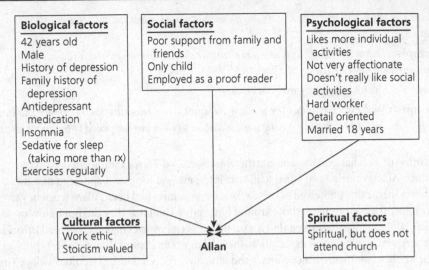

Biological factors
42 years old
Male
History of depression
Family history of
  depression
Antidepressant
  medication
Insomnia
Sedative for sleep
  (taking more than rx)
Exercises regularly

Social factors
Poor support from family and
  friends
Only child
Employed as a proof reader

Psychological factors
Likes more individual
  activities
Not very affectionate
Doesn't really like social
  activities
Hard worker
Detail oriented
Married 18 years

Cultural factors
Work ethic
Stoicism valued

Allan

Spiritual factors
Spiritual, but does not
attend church

Figure 21.2 Initial Interpersonal Formulation – Allan

Therapeutic considerations

The therapist considered a number of treatment approaches to Allan's problems. He was mindful of the fearful and dismissive styles of attachment as evidenced by the account of Allan's early environment, his current interpersonal functioning, and his interactions during the first session. Another consideration was the presence of significant personality traits, as evidenced by Allan's description of his long-term pattern of social relationships. The therapist considered the following possible therapeutic interventions:

- **Cognitive behavioral therapy** – CBT had merit for a number of reasons. The first was its focal and structured nature. While not engaging problematic aspects of attachment and psychodynamics, CBT would still be likely to help Allan address the dysfunctional nature of his cognitions and underlying schemas, particularly the obsessional aspects of his thoughts and behavior.
- **Psychodynamic psychotherapy** – It was clear to the therapist that Allan had a life-long history of 'empathic failures' by caregivers. Allan's account of his childhood, particularly his relationship with his chronically ill mother and distant father, his history of multiple caregivers, and his description of few if any nurturing relationships as a child, suggested that a long-term therapeutic relationship which was focused on the childhood antecedents to his problems and provided him with an experience of empathic understanding would be beneficial.
- **Family therapy** – Allan's account of his family functioning highlighted significant problems in his relationships with his wife and daughters. There was certainly evidence that the family system was not functioning well, and treatment of the system would impact the family's long-term functioning and its effect upon Allan's depressive illness.
- **Interpersonal Psychotherapy** – While there were clear biological and psychological reasons for Allan to have developed depression, perhaps the most compelling aspect of his presentation was the current relationship difficulties he was experiencing in his marriage and with his daughters in the context of his social isolation. These acute crises, which led Allan to seek treatment, could be understood as the trigger for depression which interacted with Allan's biopsychosocial, cultural, and spiritual vulnerabilities. A treatment which was interpersonally focused would offer Allan a good chance of symptom relief, and IPT would be completely compatible with medication. Moreover, IPT was intuitively appealing

because it was directed towards Allan's presenting complaints and his attributions for the development of his depression.

The therapist was also guided by the empirical literature. First, efficacy studies were clear that IPT would be an evidence-supported treatment for Allan's depression,[1] as well as for his dysthymia.[2] Second, there was evidence from the National Institute of Mental Health Treatment of Depression Collaborative Research Program (NIMH TDCRP) that IPT might be better suited to patients with more obsessive traits, as opposed to treatment with CBT.[3] There was also empirical evidence that combined treatment with both medication and IPT would be of additional benefit to Allan.[4]

The potential for a problematic therapeutic relationship, given Allan's history of relationship failures, suggested to the therapist that his approach with IPT would need to be modified to accommodate Allan's fearful attachment style. First, the therapist recognized that he needed to spend more time to develop a therapeutic alliance with Allan, and would need to take special care to listen well. Empathy would have to be used judiciously and carefully: enough to build the alliance, but not too much, as there was a risk that Allan would see it as excessive and reject it. Second, the pacing of IPT would need to be modified, as Allan would likely need more time to develop a sense of trust in the therapist and to be able to disclose his feelings more freely. This meant spending time simply getting to know Allan rather than rushing to an agenda or specific therapeutic tasks. Finally, the therapist recognized that he would need to work very carefully to convey to Allan that he was interested in truly understanding him, and that he needed to be flexible so that Allan did not perceive that the therapist was imposing an agenda upon him.

At this point in the Interpersonal Formulation, after considering the various treatment options, the therapist summarized:

Allan, my sense is that the distress you're experiencing really comes from a sense of isolation and a feeling that no one understands you well. As you described it, the tipping point – the crisis you are faced with – is a big change in your relationship with Eliza. Though things have not been going well for some time with your wife, it sounds to me that things were tolerable until the last several months. I think I can begin to understand how that has been difficult for you as you've sensed the change in your relationship with Eliza.

There seem to be a number of factors that have interacted to produce this episode of depression at this point in your life – you did a good job of listing them on the formulation we just finished. I'm particularly struck by the genetic factors: the history of your mother's severe depression suggests that you've almost certainly inherited a vulnerability to depression.

I think that there are a number of psychological vulnerabilities that have also led you to become depressed. While you're clearly a hard working and detail-oriented man – indeed this has helped you achieve much in your work – I suspect these traits have also been an 'Achilles heel' for you in dealing with this crisis. While it has worked well for you in the past to deal with problems by working harder, things recently have come to a point where this strategy doesn't seem to be working any more.

Most compelling for me, however, is the context in which you've become depressed. You've described to me how your marriage with Pam has deteriorated to the point where you feel it's failing. You've also told me that your relationship with Eliza has also changed, and this seems to have been a great loss for you as well.

Culturally you described a sense at work – your relationship with John, for instance – in which people simply don't talk about personal issues or let other people know that they are struggling. I can understand why that would be a difficult place to get much support. And you mentioned that, though you have a sense of spirituality, there isn't really a religious group or organization that you feel a part of. [Taking the paper and drawing lines from the various boxes] All of these factors seem to have come together right now as you're in the midst of a big change in your relationship with Eliza, and it seems to be complicated by the chronic problems with Pam. It seems like the change with Eliza has tipped the scale, and now you're depressed and distressed. What do you think about that as a start to describing why you're having trouble right now?

Allan responded by saying, 'I don't like to admit it, but I have to agree that the biological part must be playing a role. I had always thought that I could control that; that it wouldn't get the best of me. But you're right, as I look at the paper we put together, it seems pretty clear that's what's going on. I'm just disappointed that I can't manage it on my own.'

With a hopeful smile, the therapist continued:

Based on our assessment then, I think that a diagnosis of major depression is warranted. You've done a good job of describing the distress you are experiencing far beyond symptoms – especially the isolation, and I'd like to learn much more about that. All of it: the depression, distress, sense of isolation, seems directly connected to the changes in your relationships with Eliza and the problems with Pam.

Given the biological elements, medication clearly has an important place in your treatment, and I strongly recommend continuing it. In addition, I believe that we can address many of your relationship issues using psychotherapy. Psychotherapy, like medication, has many varieties. For example, some treatments might examine your thinking patterns, or perhaps the way in which your family is interacting. With the relationship elements playing such a strong role, however, I think that Interpersonal Psychotherapy, or IPT, will be the most helpful for you.

IPT is a treatment that looks primarily at your current relationships. It's been shown in numerous scientific studies to be helpful in the acute treatment of depression, and this seems to be because it helps individuals deal with their unique interpersonal problems. I believe that we can make the best use of it by focusing on your interpersonal relationships and helping you to make changes in them. What are your thoughts about this?

Allan responded to the therapist that he thought that perhaps there was some hope in working with his relationships. While he was a bit skeptical about the value of talking with someone about his problems, he agreed to start IPT.

The therapist was careful to frame his summary of the Interpersonal Formulation in the language that he and Allan had used to develop it. Since it was collaborative, there was literally no danger that it would miss the target – Allan had contributed a great deal to it. The alliance and engagement in treatment was enhanced by using Allan's language: the therapist consistently talked about his thoughts rather than his feelings, and asked Allan to respond in the same way by asking about his thoughts about the summary as opposed to asking about his feelings. The therapist also highlighted Allan's strengths rather than framing the formulation as a summary of his weaknesses, which Allan would likely take as criticism. Finally, the therapist also framed the formulation as a hypothesis they had developed together, rather than as a definitive interpretation, and carefully invited Allan's feedback about it.

Developing foci for treatment

With a solid formulation in hand, the next task was to clarify with Allan the specific interpersonal problems on which to focus treatment.

Pam and Allan had met while she was visiting from New Zealand on a working holiday. Overlooking the fact that she was a Kiwi, Allan had enjoyed spending time with Pam in the early years, particularly since 'she was better at social contact'. Allan described that Pam had been solely responsible for organizing the couple's social life, and that he would 'go along for the ride' so long as Pam 'was prepared to break the ice'. While Allan did not feel he was excessively socially anxious, he felt more comfortable in this passive role.

Allan reported that recently Pam had become increasingly 'fed up with my behavior'. He reported that Pam consistently 'would not do what I requested, particularly around the house', and that he would often argue with her. Allan reported that their conversations frequently became arguments, and that things were now at the point where nothing could really be discussed. Allan told the therapist that Pam was now spending more time with her friends and was increasing the number of hours she was at work. Over the last several years, Allan had been working afternoon shifts and Pam working during the day. The only contact they now had was for a few moments in the evening, after Allan had arrived home from work, when he would usually find Pam already asleep. On weekends Pam continued to make arrangements 'with the girls', from which Allan was obviously excluded. Allan reported that their sexual relationship had all but ceased, and that there was now little affection between the couple.

The therapist asked for some specific Interpersonal Incidents in which the couple came into conflict and Allan reported the following interaction.

Therapist: *Tell me about the last time you and Pam argued.*

Allan: *Well... just the other night we had a bit of a fight.*

Therapist (sitting back in an invitation to Allan to tell a story): *Tell me more about what happened.*

Allan (neutrally and curtly): *I arrived home from work, the trash had not been put out, and there were dirty dishes in the sink.*

Therapist: *What happened then?*

Allan (with mild indignance): *I reminded her that I had specifically told her to take out the trash and clean up the dishes.*

Therapist: *Tell me more: how did you ask her to do that?*

Allan: *What words exactly?*

Therapist: *Yes – I'd really like to understand better how the communication went.*

Allan (feigning politeness): *I said, 'Pam, I have asked you before to put the garbage out. The house is becoming a mess. You know that just drives me crazy.'*

Therapist: *And how did Pam respond?*

Allan: *She didn't say anything.*

Therapist: *What was the emotional message you conveyed? Were you upset, angry, neutral?*

Allan (with no emotion or affect): *Well, mostly I was angry. My voice got pretty loud, and then I felt guilty afterwards because I lost my temper. I need to do a better job of controlling my emotions.*

It was not rocket science for the therapist to infer from this and several other Interpersonal Incidents that there was very poor communication between Allan and Pam and there was a need to specifically focus upon this within the treatment.

Allan and Eliza had enjoyed a close relationship until approximately 9 months before, when she decided to leave school in the fifth year of high school to go to work. This had disappointed Allan, as he had wanted Eliza to complete her final exam at school and go to college. Allan reported that his relationship with Eliza was, in most ways, closer than that with Pam. He fondly recalled jogging and swimming with Eliza, and having a friendly competition to 'improve our personal bests'.

The therapist noted that as Allan was discussing the loss of his relationship with Eliza, his affect became more bland and restricted, despite the clearly significant loss he was describing. When the therapist asked about Allan's views of Eliza's relationship with an older woman, he responded that he had always imagined that Eliza would be at home, and that they would continue to have the close relationship they had developed over the years. Intellectually, he said, he realized that she was growing up and would eventually move on, but emotionally he had chosen to deal with it by ignoring it. It was, according to Allan, 'too difficult to think about'.

The following dialogue ensued.

Therapist: *Allan, I can see that you have many reactions and feelings about the changes with Eliza, and it sounds like you've tried to deal with them by pushing them to the side. What I'd like to do is understand better what is happening in your relationship with Eliza right now, and how it affects you and your depression. We've talked some about the three Problem Areas in IPT – how would you characterize the problems you and Eliza are having now?*

Allan: *I certainly feel a loss, so I guess grief might fit. Can you tell me more about Role Transitions again?*

Therapist: *Well, Role Transition looks at changes in relationships and how they affect each person differently. Many people who have developed psychological symptoms in the context of a Role Transition have had a Loss experience, and they often feel great sadness or anxiety about it. While I can see that grief certainly reflects how you are feeling at the moment, Role Transition might also fit. I think that either Grief or Role Transition would work, but I also think that it needs to be your decision.*

Allan: *Well, I guess that I have to still be her dad, so perhaps looking at this as a Role Transition would probably work best.*

Therapist: *Let's add that to the formulation then – do you want to write it in?*

Allan: *Sure.*

Allan and the therapist concluded by mutually agreeing to add the following foci to the Interpersonal Formulation (Figure 21.3):

- An Interpersonal Dispute with Pam
- A Role Transition with Eliza.

The therapeutic agreement

At this point, Allan and the therapist had met for three sessions. They had completed a thorough psychiatric evaluation, an Interpersonal Inventory, and an Interpersonal Formulation. Allan, despite his less secure attachment style and limited social support, appeared to be a reasonably good candidate for IPT, and had agreed to it.

It was only at this point that they developed a formal Treatment Agreement to meet for about 12 additional 50-minute sessions of IPT over the next several months. They agreed

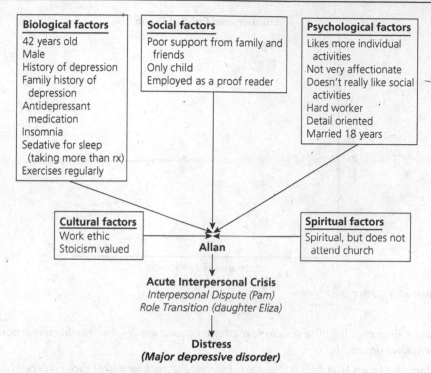

Biological factors

42 years old
Male
History of depression
Family history of
  depression
Antidepressant
  medication
Insomnia
Sedative for sleep
  (taking more than rx)
Exercises regularly

Social factors

Poor support from family and
  friends
Only child
Employed as a proof reader

Psychological factors

Likes more individual
  activities
Not very affectionate
Doesn't really like social
  activities
Hard worker
Detail oriented
Married 18 years

Cultural factors

Work ethic
Stoicism valued

Allan

Spiritual factors

Spiritual, but does not
  attend church

Acute Interpersonal Crisis
Interpersonal Dispute (Pam)
Role Transition (daughter Eliza)

Distress
(Major depressive disorder)

Figure 21.3 Interpersonal Formulation – Allan

to continue meeting weekly, with an explicit discussion of the possibility of meeting less frequently as Allan improved. Allan agreed to be prompt and to give at least 24 hours' notice should he need to change appointments.

Part II: Middle Sessions

Interpersonal Dispute: Session 4

The middle sessions were focused on the dispute and transition issues. Allan elected to start with the dispute with Pam, and the therapist began by using clarification to get more information. The therapist had long ago learned from his supervisor the clinical pearl 'when in doubt, clarify'. In order to get more information, the therapist began by asking Allan to help him visualize and better understand the dispute by working on a Conflict Graph. Taking a piece of paper, the therapist drew two lines and began the interaction (Figure 21.4).

Therapist: *Allan, it would be helpful to me if you could help me to visualize the conflict between you and Pam. If you'd be willing to do it, I'd like you to plot your view of where the conflict is. The x-axis simply represents the importance of the relationship between the two of you, and the y-axis the severity of the conflict. I'm looking for a single point at the intersection of severity and importance as you see it.*

Allan: *I can do that, but how come there are no numbers? I'm thinking that the severity is pretty high – about an 8 or so.*

Therapist: *I've found that numbers, though they might seem to be helpful, actually hinder my understanding of the problem. It's kind of like rating pain: numbers don't carry much meaning, because what is an 8 for you might be a 10 for me, or a 2 might be a 5 for another person. I've*

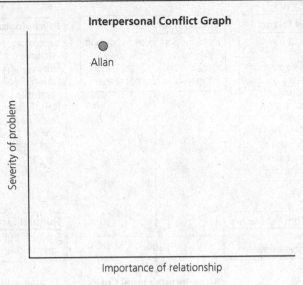

Figure 21.4 Conflict Graph – Allan

found it much more helpful to describe your experience using words – that way the other person can really understand better.

Allan: *OK, I guess I can do that. [Pausing to examine the graph for a bit] I guess I'd put it here: pretty serious problem, but I'm not sure how invested I am in the relationship.*

Therapist: *Tell me more about that.*

Allan: *I was thoroughly committed, but now it just seems mundane – distant. I don't want to leave, and I don't have any energy for another relationship or anything, but it just isn't important anymore. Our relationship feels like a relationship at my work – we both have things to get done, we can talk about schedules, and going to the store, or fixing the toilet, or taking care of the car, but it's nothing more than that. I find myself bored a lot at home ... alone too I guess.*

The therapist proceeded to ask Allan more about the relationship, using the graph as a way to facilitate his verbal description of the relationship. After about 15 minutes, the therapist then shifted.

Therapist: *We've got a pretty good start on understanding where you are in the relationship – where do you think Pam would mark your relationship on the graph?*

Allan: *I don't know – I hadn't really thought of her perspective ...*

Therapist: *It might be interesting to find out what she thinks ...*

Allan: *Maybe so ... [pausing nearly 30 seconds to think] I guess she'd put it somewhere about here – pretty important, but I think she's more invested in the relationship at the moment than I am ... I really don't know ...*

Therapist: *It would be interesting to find out what she thinks ... I wonder what she would say ... [Figure 21.5].*

Session 5

In session 5, the therapist developed several more Interpersonal Incidents to further elaborate other examples of disagreements between Allan and Pam. The therapist was able to highlight two factors which were related to the dispute. The first was that the way Allan was

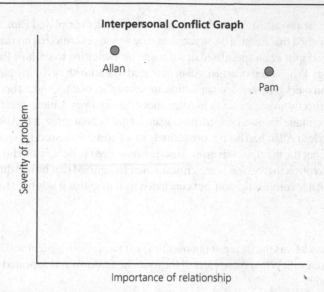

Interpersonal Conflict Graph

Figure 21.5 Conflict Graph – Allan and Pam

communicating his needs to Pam was not conveying his message adequately. Second, the therapist felt that Allan's expectations of Pam were not realistic.

Allan's generalization was that 'Pam never listens to me', and he described feeling angry, disappointed, and frustrated. The therapist was able to introduce the possibility that Pam may have also felt angry and frustrated by Allan's requests, possibly because of the way the two of them were communicating. Allan acknowledged that this might be the case, but was still of the view that his expectations of Pam were not unreasonable, although he admitted that he might need to look at alternative ways of discussing them with her.

The session began with the therapist focusing on the interpersonal issues discussed the week previously:

> Allan, last week we discussed your dispute with Pam in some detail. Can you tell me what has happened with her during the week?

Allan responded that there had been two or three further arguments along similar lines to those already reported. The therapist asked Allan to provide more examples of some specific communications. Allan gave numerous verbatim examples of his statements such as 'you never do what I ask, you don't show me any respect' and 'Pam, I've told you a thousand times to take the trash out on Monday nights'. Several specific incidents were discussed, each of which was in essence a repetition of the initial incident that Allan reported.

The therapist suggested to Allan that there might be some alternative ways of approaching the subject with Pam, and that by utilizing role playing, there might be some opportunities to work on modifying the problematic communication. The rest of the session was spent with the therapist and Allan role playing and discussing an instance in which he was unhappy with some aspects of Pam's home care. The therapist and Allan started the role play with the therapist playing Allan. In this reverse role play, the therapist attempted to model non-confrontative ways of communicating with Pam, including statements such as, 'Pam, how about we talk over a cup of coffee about getting on top of this housework?' or 'Pam, what ways do you see that we can make this house run more smoothly?'. Allan saw potential merit in this approach, but continued to externalize the problem, though he did acknowledge that his communication style could be improved.

The therapist also asked Allan what he was experiencing as he played Pam. After a brief pause, he described that he felt a bit attacked, as if he would get criticized no matter what he said. The therapist again speculated that it might be interesting to see how Pam would describe things. When they switched, Allan managed to start with two fairly pleasant comments, but quickly reverted to communicating in an accusatory and rather irritable way. Rather than directly giving feedback to Allan about this communication style, the therapist asked him to critique his own performance, again adapting his approach to Allan's dismissive and fearful style. If Allan had been more securely attached a more direct approach might have been feasible, but the therapist was aware that he would need to be very careful not to give Allan the perception that he was being critical. Allan recognized that he had quickly moved into more irritable communication, but concluded by noting that it was hard to change old habits.

Session 6

Session 6 began late, as the therapist ran over time with a previous patient and needed to take an urgent phone call. When Allan entered the room he sat down and appeared quite angry. He then stated:

> I can't believe you are this disorganized! You finished 4 minutes early at the end of the last session and today you are running 15 minutes late. I bet you still charge me the same fee!

The therapist was quite taken aback by this exchange. He was initially at a loss as to how to respond, and then finally stated:

> Allan I am sorry that you feel that I don't value your time. I do my best to stick to my schedule, but sometimes my day gets out of control with phone calls and other emergencies. Despite that, I can certainly understand why you're angry with me, and appreciate the fact that you let me know how you feel.

As the therapist was responding, Allan became visibly upset and tearful. This was startling for the therapist, as this was the first time Allan had shown any real affect. After Allan had regained his composure, the therapist attempted to link this affect with what Allan was experiencing at the time by examining his process affect. Allan responded:

> I can't believe that just happened. Everybody I ever deal with lets me down, and the relationship goes nowhere. You're the only person who has been able to make any sense to me and now this is going to go bad as well.

The therapist tried to validate Allan's concerns by reflecting his understanding of what Allan had said, and then responded:

> Allan, I hear your concerns and your frustration. I wonder if what just happened here tells us something about what's happening in your other relationships, particularly with Pam. I haven't been aware of your concerns about time pressure, although I know you have expectations about this. I'm wondering if this is the same pattern that leads to problems with Pam. If we can trace how this emerged with Pam, I think we can better understand your conflict with her.

The therapist considered a number of options in using the therapeutic relationship. One possibility would have been to examine the ways Allan had communicated his expectations to the therapist. He was mindful of how distressed Allan had become, and felt that it was better not to deal with this directly, particularly given Allan's insecure attachment style. The therapist therefore moved to an exploration of the similarities in Allan's relationship with

Pam. Allan, presumably motivated by his new affective experience, was able to finally link his expectations with the dispute with Pam. The session ended, on time with the therapist stating:

> Allan, I think this has been one of the most productive sessions we have had so far. I appreciate how difficult it was for you to give me feedback about being late, but I think that taking that risk really helped me to understand you much better. I also appreciate the reminder to keep my schedule in order.

Session 7

Session 7 began on time with Allan apologizing for his previous behavior. The therapist acknowledged the apology, and again reinforced the fact that Allan's comments had been helpful in understanding him better. For Allan, the experience of addressing his frustration and resolving it with the therapist seemed to have reassured him that it was possible with Pam. He reported to the therapist that he had discussed his expectations with Pam, following his role playing rehearsal. Allan stated that he felt that the problem had improved, and that he would like to concentrate on the problems with Eliza.

They briefly reviewed both the Interpersonal Inventory and Formulation. The therapist then directed the discussion to an exploration of the transition:

Therapist: *It seems like you feel that you've lost something significant with Eliza's growing up – is that accurate?*

Allan: *It's hard to describe really. She continues to change, and I guess I do as well, but we just aren't close like we used to be.*

Therapist: *Change leaves a lot of us vulnerable at times.*

The therapist and Allan then discussed the particular difficulties he faced in dealing with Eliza's relationship with the 'older woman'. Rather than being concerned about her sexuality, Allan was concerned that Eliza was going to be exploited by this older woman and 'get hurt'. The therapist stated that he had talked with many patients about the difficulty parents have dealing with the changes that occur as their children become adults, and that this was a frequent source of distress. The therapist felt that his relationship with Allan had progressed to a point where he could judiciously disclose some of his own life experiences, though just a little bit.

Therapist: *I think I can begin to understand your difficulty. I can remember when my kids were growing up, it was always hard to strike a balance between giving them their freedom, their own choices and knowing when to come in to bail them out. You never stop worrying though, do you?*

Allan: *You've got that right. I seem to be constantly worried about Eliza, though I can't seem to bring myself to tell her why.*

The therapist then suggested a homework task for Allan: he could have a conversation with Eliza about her relationship, but rather than focus on his concerns, he could ask her how her relationship with the older woman had evolved, and where she saw things going, in a friendly and interested way rather than as a concerned parent.

Session 8

Session 8 began with Allan reporting that the homework assignment, which he completed the evening following the previous session, was very successful. He had finally talked with Eliza about her relationship, and had also invited her partner over to visit as well. He stated:

> I guess my relationship is going to be this way. I still miss my little girl but she isn't a little girl anymore. I guess I'm going to have to deal with her as a young woman.

The therapist asked Allan how this impacted his relationship with Emma, his younger daughter, to which Allan replied:

> She's been responding to a lot of what is going on around her. I think as things have settled down with Pam and Eliza and me that she's felt calmer and things have sorted themselves out.

With his distress diminished and progress in the Problem Areas, the therapist elected to move to general social support. During the Interpersonal Inventory the therapist had noted a consistent pattern in which Allan's expectations of others were often unrealistic and poorly communicated, leading to disappointments in his social relationships. Allan appeared to be developing some understanding of this; however, the therapist was concerned that introducing this as a problem might be perceived as criticism and undermine Allan's improving self-esteem. Rather than giving direct feedback to Allan about his social skills, the therapist chose to focus on Allan's general social support.

Therapist: *As we discussed some time earlier, good social support is often a way to protect against depression and psychological distress. Now that things are going better, what are some ways you could get some additional support outside of your family?*

The therapist used the technique of Problem Solving to help Allan generate potential ways to increase his social support. Allan listed three possibilities:

- Approaching a colleague for a drink after work
- Joining a hiking club
- Attending a church function.

Allan agreed to a homework assignment to consider which option looked best for him and to make some preliminary inquiries.

Session 9

In session 9, Allan told the therapist that he had made some inquiries about hiking clubs and had some contact details. He said that he had chosen to approach a colleague at work with whom he felt some connection. The rest of the session was devoted to Allan rehearsing potential communication strategies through role playing. A homework task was set for Allan to approach the colleague and invite him out for a beer after work.

They also discussed the Conclusion of Acute Therapy at length. The topic was actually first broached by Allan, who felt that he was doing better, and that biweekly sessions would fit his schedule better at this point. The therapist concurred, and they agreed to meet biweekly for two sessions, then once a month later, and then move to Maintenance Treatment. Allan stated that he was comfortable in spacing out the meetings, as he also felt that he was doing well. He added, however, that he was not prepared to stop therapy at this point, and liked knowing that he would still be able to see the therapist even though it would be a while before the next appointment.

Session 10

Two weeks later session 10 began with Allan reporting that he had invited a colleague out, and had an enjoyable drink after work. He said that this colleague had then invited Allan and Pam to his place for a barbecue the following weekend. The therapist noted a considerable improvement in Allan's mood, although Allan reported some ongoing difficulties with his sleep. Allan agreed that he was improving, noting that he felt less stressed about his relationships and that his marriage was improving.

The therapist then returned to the previous discussion and asked about the possibility of joining a hiking club. The rest of the session was then devoted to Allan practicing his communication meeting the members of the group who had been planning a hike in the bush outside of the city that weekend.

Session 11

At session 11, Allan reported that he was continuing to do well. He had continued with social contacts at work, and though they were limited, he felt that they were of benefit. Allan expressed some surprise that he was able to initiate some of these, and felt pleased that he had begun to develop some confidence in his social skills. His relationship with Pam had also continued to improve, as had his relationship with Eliza. After a review of progress to date, the following dialog ensued.

Therapist: *Allan, we're nearing the end of our Acute sessions. I have found this a good point to tie things together in order to set the scene for Maintenance Treatment. There is a quote from Winston Churchill I always like to use here: 'this is not the beginning of the end, this is the end of the beginning ...'*

Allan: *You didn't do the accent that well, but I think I know what you mean.*

Therapist: *Allan, what are your thoughts about moving to maintenance and meeting less frequently?*

Allan: *Oh, I think that I'll do fine – I'm not really concerned. After all, we'll still be meeting, and I can contact you if I really need to, so it isn't as if I'll never see you again.*

Therapist: *I'm glad that we will have the chance to meet periodically too – I like to keep track of the people I've worked with to make sure that they're doing well. I've worked with a lot of patients, though, who still felt that finishing up the weekly meetings was hard.*

Allan: *I suppose that it will be a bit hard for me – I do enjoy talking to you now – at least after we got over the time when you were late. It seems a lot easier though, since we've already been meeting less frequently – every other week and then last month I mean. I'll probably will miss this though – it's been a good way to talk through some problems. And I never really thought that talking about things was all that helpful before.*

Therapist: *I want to let you know that I'll also miss meeting with you regularly. I've really enjoyed working with you, and it's been great to see you make so much progress. I'm looking forward to seeing how much more progress you make when we meet next month.*

At this point, the therapist considered continuing this line of questioning about Allan's reactions to the impending conclusion. However, based on Allan's responses, the therapist felt that pressing the issue further would not be productive, particularly given Allan's attachment style. Further, to continue to press Allan for more reactions would move the therapy into a discussion of the therapeutic relationship, which would be a move strongly against the precedence set in the treatment. The therapist could see no particular point in doing this, especially since Allan was doing well. Moreover, the therapist had intentionally structured the therapy so that the conclusion would be less abrupt – both the spacing of the later sessions and the specific contract for provision of maintenance treatment in the future were designed to lessen the impact of the conclusion.

The therapist therefore decided to return to the original Interpersonal Inventory and Formulation and highlighted the progress that Allan had made in each of the Problem Areas. The therapist reminded Allan that the Interpersonal Dispute had originally been quite severe, but had improved as he had examined his communication and his expectations of Pam.

Allan reported that he and Pam had enjoyed a significant change in their relationship, and that Pam had even asked to accompany Allan on one of his bushwalks.

They then looked at the Role Transition with Eliza and noted that though Allan had experienced a loss of the relationship with his young daughter, he had acquired a new relationship with his adult daughter. The therapist praised Allan for his ability to adapt to the circumstances and also his courage in inviting his daughter's partner to the family home for a meal. Allan reported that he felt quite happy with his progress in this area and was more confident that Eliza would be able to come and 'talk to me father to daughter, but as a woman rather than my little girl'.

The therapist also praised Allan for his ability to initiate new social contacts. The therapist noted that Allan's improving ability to socialize had led in part to his recovery. The therapist gave Allan one final homework task for their concluding session, which was to develop a list of problems which might arise in the future.

Session 12

The last Acute Treatment sessions occurred one month later, and began with Allan admitting he was feeling a little sad about the conclusion. The therapist replied by stating that while the change was difficult, they would continue clinical contact for Maintenance Treatment. Since the clinical contact was continuing, the therapist encouraged Allan to contact him should acute problems emerge.

Allan then reported a number of potential future problems following the homework task. One of those included the recurrence of his problematic communication with Pam. The therapist and Allan then discussed how he might apply his new skills in this regard. When discussing potential problems with Eliza, Allan felt that there could be further complications in her relationship with her partner, but that continuing to treat her as an adult was the best way to help her to deal with this.

Allan and the therapist then went on to discuss the issue of Allan's general social supports. Allan was aware that his tendency to isolate himself could re-emerge, and stated that he would try to pay attention to how he communicated his needs and expectations with his friends and acquaintances. Near the end of the session, they formally agreed, as they had discussed before, to meet again in 3 months and to do so for at least the next year as a Maintenance Treatment. Both put the date of the next appointment in their calendars, and the therapist reiterated that Allan should contact him should future problems arise.

The therapist then concluded:

Allan, when we first met I was very concerned about how much distress you were experiencing, and to be perfectly honest I was very worried about you and your safety. I was also concerned that psychological treatment may have been a problem because of your initial reluctance to talk to someone about your problems and your relationships in particular. Despite my concerns, you've done extremely well – I've been impressed not only with the way you've dealt with Pam and Eliza, but with the way you've been able to discuss things with me. This has been a very rewarding experience for me, particularly as you've worked so hard and have made so much progress.

Allan blushed and smiled. He stood, shook the therapist's hand and moved to the door, exactly 50 minutes after he had entered. 'See you in 3 months,' he said, as he left the office.

References

1. Cuijpers P, *et al.* Psychotherapy for depression in adults: a meta-analysis of comparative outcome studies. *Journal of Consulting and Clinical Psychology*, 2008, **76**(6): 909–922.

2. Browne G, *et al.* Sertraline and interpersonal psychotherapy, alone and combined, in the treatment of patients with dysthymic disorder in primary care: a 2 year comparison of effectiveness and cost. *Journal of Affective Disorders*, 2002, **68**: 317–330.

3. Barber JP and Muenz LR. The role of avoidance and obsessiveness in matching patients to cognitive and interpersonal psychotherapy: empirical findings from the treatment for depression collaborative research program. *Journal of Consulting and Clinical Psychology*, 1996, **64**: 951–958.

4. Thase ME, *et al.* Treatment of major depression with psychotherapy or psychotherapy-pharmacotherapy combinations. *Archives of General Psychiatry*, 1997, **54**(11): 1009–1015.

IPT Institute and Certified Training in Interpersonal Psychotherapy

The IPT Institute is an international organization devoted to the certification of IPT clinicians, supervisors, and trainers. The IPT Institute also sponsors training in IPT around the world. More information about the IPT Institute and training opportunities can be found on the web at www.IPTInstitute.com.

The Mission of the IPT Institute is to:

- Establish IPT training standards
- Ensure that IPT is delivered with a high level of adherence and at high quality
- Develop a cadre of highly trained and certified IPT clinicians, supervisors, and trainers
- Conduct research regarding IPT training and adherence.

The IPT Institute was founded in 2009 to develop and promote clear standards for IPT training and certification. The IPT Institute was also developed to coordinate efforts with the International Society of Interpersonal Psychotherapy (ISIPT). Certification is not required to practice IPT, but is available for interested clinicians. Listings of certified clinicians and supervisors can be found on the IPT Institute website.

IPT Certification Requirements

Level A: Introductory Course in IPT

- Participation in an IPT Institute accredited training course lasting 2 days or more.

Level B: Clinical Training in IPT

Prerequisites

- Completion of a Level A IPT course.
- Familiarity with the IPT manuals.
- Professional clinical training in mental health treatment.

IPT supervision

- Supervision by a certified IPT Institute supervisor for two complete IPT cases.
- Supervision must be provided in individual or group formats.
- Supervision must be based on audio or videotaped recordings of sessions.
- Supervision must be a minimum of 1 hour of supervision per 2 hours of therapy.
- IPT treatment must meet clinical training standards for adherence and quality.
- Submission of a satisfactory IPT portfolio including:
    - Case reports of two completed IPT cases
    - Supporting documents for the two cases including the IPT Formulation and Interpersonal Circle
    - Adherence and Quality Ratings (supervisor submitted).

Level C: Clinical Certification in IPT

Prerequisites

- Completion of clinical training (level B) in IPT.
- Nomination by a certified IPT Institute supervisor.

IPT supervision

- Supervision by a certified IPT Institute supervisor for two additional complete IPT cases.
- Supervision must be provided in individual or group formats.
- Supervision must be based on audio or videotaped recordings of sessions.
- Supervision must be a minimum of 1 hour of supervision per 2 hours of therapy.
- IPT treatment must meet clinical certification standards for adherence and quality.
- Submission of a satisfactory IPT portfolio including:
  - Case reports of two completed level C IPT cases
  - Supporting documents for the two cases including the IPT Formulation and Interpersonal Circle
  - Adherence and quality ratings (supervisor submitted).

Level D: IPT Supervisor Certification

Prerequisites

- Completion of IPT clinical certification (level C).
- Nomination by a certified IPT Institute supervisor.
- Evidence of continuing practice of IPT.

Training

- Completion of certified IPT supervisor training course.
- Must meet ongoing level D standards for IPT supervision.

Independent evaluation of supervision

- An IPT supervision portfolio must be submitted for independent evaluation.
- Supervision portfolios must include portfolio materials from an IPT supervisee and documented evaluations of supervision.
- IPT supervision must meet standards for adherence and quality as judged by an independent IPT Institute supervisor.

Level E: IPT Trainer Certification

Prerequisites

- Completion of IPT clinical certification (level C).
- Nomination by a certified IPT Institute trainer.
- Evidence of continuing practice of IPT.

Training and supervision

- Completion of an IPT Institute certified IPT trainer workshop.
- Satisfactory co-facilitation of an accredited introductory course in IPT.
- Must meet ongoing level E standards for IPT training.

Independent evaluation of supervision

- An IPT training portfolio must be submitted for independent evaluation.
- Training portfolios must include videotape of an IPT training course and documented course evaluations from participants.
- IPT training must meet the institute standards for adherence and quality as judged by an independent IPT Institute trainer.

Clinicians interested in training opportunities in IPT or supervision in IPT can contact the IPT Institute through the IPT Institute website at www.IPTInstitute.com or can contact Dr Scott Stuart directly at scott-stuart@uiowa.edu.

Interpersonal Inventory Form

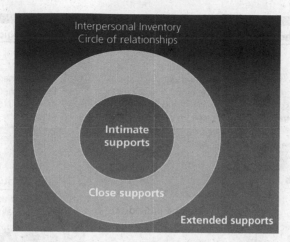

The Interpersonal Inventory form

Interpersonal Formulation Form

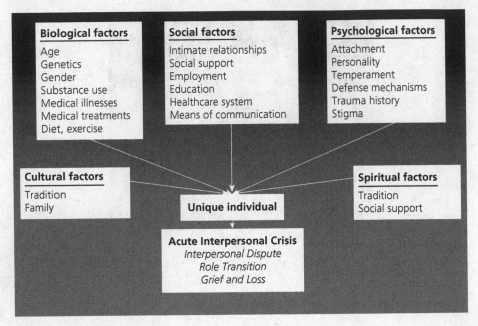

The Interpersonal Formulation form

Appendix D

International Society of Interpersonal Psychotherapy (ISIPT)

The ISIPT is an academic organization of clinicians, researchers, and other individuals interested in clinical work, teaching, and research in IPT.

The mission of the ISIPT is to:

- Disseminate IPT internationally
- Promote training in IPT
- Promote research in IPT
- Provide a forum to further develop IPT.

The ISIPT was founded in 2000 by Michael Robertson and Scott Stuart. The first ISIPT meeting was held at the American Psychiatric Association meeting in Chicago in May 2000, and was attended by clinicians from the USA, Canada, Great Britain, Iceland, Scandinavia, Australia, New Zealand, Germany, and Luxembourg. Since that time the organization has grown to include members from six continents and over 40 countries. The ISIPT has convened four International ISIPT meetings including 2005 in Pittsburgh, 2007 in Toronto, 2009 in New York, and 2011 in Amsterdam. The fifth international meeting will be held in Iowa City, Iowa, USA, in June 2013.

More information about the ISIPT can be found at the ISIPT website at www.interpersonalpsychotherapy.org.

Index

Printed in the United States
by Baker & Taylor Publisher Services

Printed in the United States
by Baker & Taylor Publisher Services